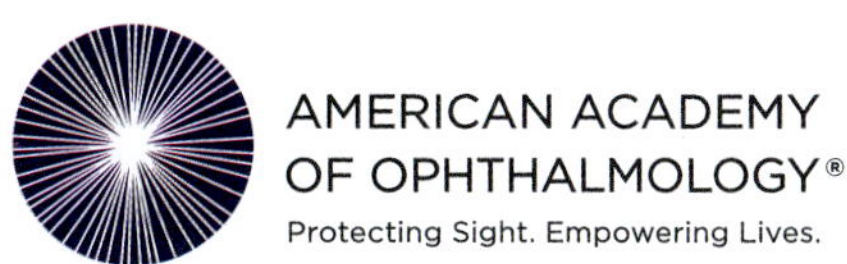

9 | Uveitis and Ocular Inflammation

Last major revision 2019–2020

2021–2022

BCSC

Basic and Clinical Science Course™

EB

Published after collaborative review with the European Board of Ophthalmology subcommittee

The American Academy of Ophthalmology is accredited by the Accreditation Council for Continuing Medical Education (ACCME) to provide continuing medical education for physicians.

The American Academy of Ophthalmology designates this enduring material for a maximum of 10 *AMA PRA Category 1 Credits*™. Physicians should claim only the credit commensurate with the extent of their participation in the activity.

CME expiration date: June 1, 2022. *AMA PRA Category 1 Credits*™ may be claimed only once between June 1, 2019, and the expiration date.

BCSC® volumes are designed to increase the physician's ophthalmic knowledge through study and review. Users of this activity are encouraged to read the text and then answer the study questions provided at the back of the book.

To claim *AMA PRA Category 1 Credits*™ upon completion of this activity, learners must demonstrate appropriate knowledge and participation in the activity by taking the posttest for Section 9 and achieving a score of 80% or higher. For further details, please see the instructions for requesting CME credit at the back of the book.

The Academy provides this material for educational purposes only. It is not intended to represent the only or best method or procedure in every case, nor to replace a physician's own judgment or give specific advice for case management. Including all indications, contraindications, side effects, and alternative agents for each drug or treatment is beyond the scope of this material. All information and recommendations should be verified, prior to use, with current information included in the manufacturers' package inserts or other independent sources, and considered in light of the patient's condition and history. Reference to certain drugs, instruments, and other products in this course is made for illustrative purposes only and is not intended to constitute an endorsement of such. Some material may include information on applications that are not considered community standard, that reflect indications not included in approved FDA labeling, or that are approved for use only in restricted research settings. **The FDA has stated that it is the responsibility of the physician to determine the FDA status of each drug or device he or she wishes to use, and to use them with appropriate, informed patient consent in compliance with applicable law.** The Academy specifically disclaims any and all liability for injury or other damages of any kind, from negligence or otherwise, for any and all claims that may arise from the use of any recommendations or other information contained herein.

All trademarks, trade names, logos, brand names, and service marks of the American Academy of Ophthalmology (AAO), whether registered or unregistered, are the property of AAO and are protected by US and international trademark laws. These trademarks include, but are not limited to, AAO; AAOE; AMERICAN ACADEMY OF OPHTHALMOLOGY; BASIC AND CLINICAL SCIENCE COURSE; BCSC; EYENET; EYEWIKI; FOCAL POINTS; FOCUS DESIGN (logo on cover); IRIS; IRIS REGISTRY; ISRS; OKAP; ONE NETWORK; OPHTHALMOLOGY; OPHTHALMOLOGY GLAUCOMA; OPHTHALMOLOGY RETINA; OPHTHALMOLOGY SCIENCE; OPHTHALMOLOGY WORLD NEWS; PREFERRED PRACTICE PATTERN; PROTECTING SIGHT. EMPOWERING LIVES.; THE OPHTHALMIC NEWS AND EDUCATION NETWORK.

Cover image: From BCSC Section 8, *External Disease and Cornea*. Fluorescein brightly stains the base of the herpes simplex virus epithelial dendritic lesions in a cornea after LASIK. *(Courtesy of Arie L. Marcovich, MD, PhD.)*

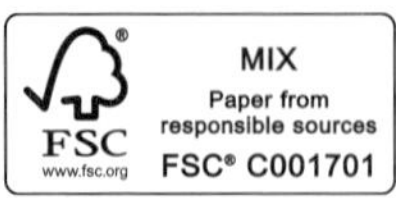

Copyright © 2021 American Academy of Ophthalmology. All rights reserved. No part of this publication may be reproduced without written permission.

Printed in China.

Basic and Clinical Science Course

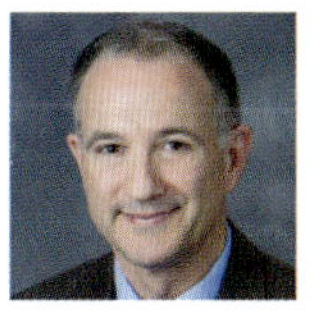

Christopher J. Rapuano, MD, Philadelphia, Pennsylvania
Senior Secretary for Clinical Education

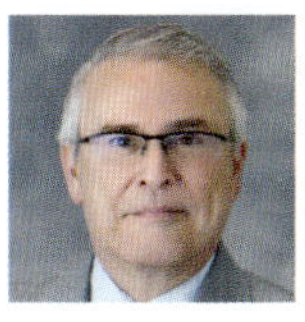

J. Timothy Stout, MD, PhD, MBA, Houston, Texas
Secretary for Lifelong Learning and Assessment

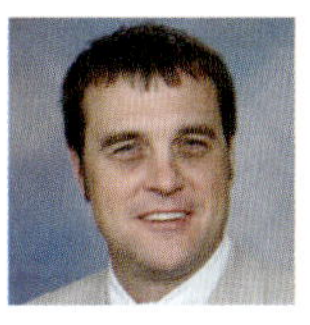

Colin A. McCannel, MD, Los Angeles, California
BCSC Course Chair

Section 9

Faculty for the Major Revision

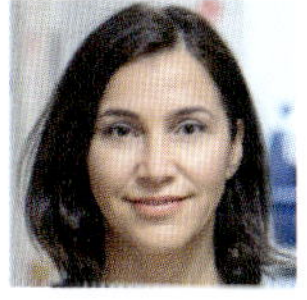

H. Nida Sen, MD, MHSc
Chair
Bethesda, Maryland

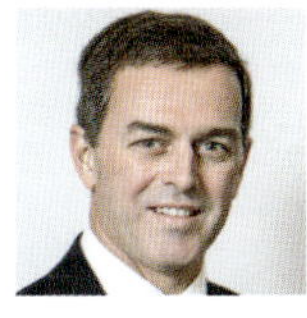

Emilio M. Dodds, MD
Buenos Aires, Argentina

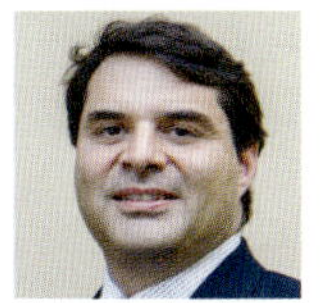

Thomas A. Albini, MD
Miami, Florida

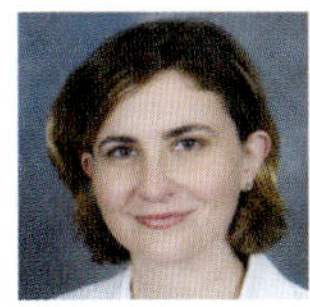

Thellea K. Leveque, MD, MPH
Seattle, Washington

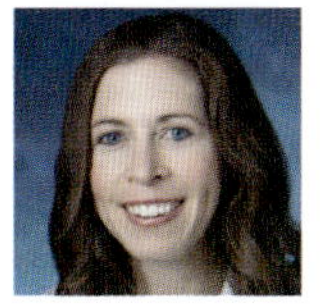

Bryn M. Burkholder, MD
Baltimore, Maryland

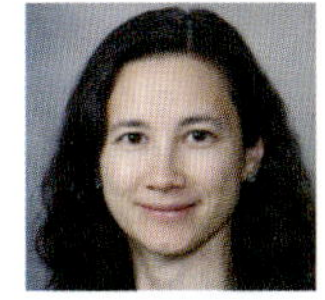

Wendy M. Smith, MD
Rochester, Minnesota

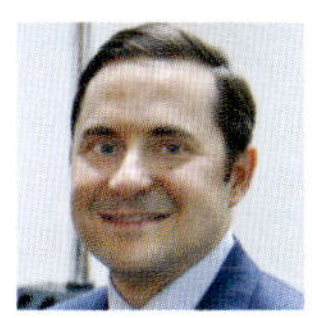

Sam S. Dahr, MD, MS
Oklahoma City, Oklahoma

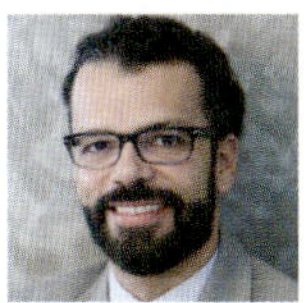

Daniel V. Vasconcelos-Santos
MD, PhD
Belo Horizonte, Brazil

The Academy wishes to acknowledge the American Uveitis Society (AUS) for recommending faculty members to the BCSC Section 9 committee.

The Academy also wishes to acknowledge the following committees for review of this edition:

Committee on Aging: Kelly L. Larkin, MD, Houston, Texas

Vision Rehabilitation Committee: William M. McLaughlin Jr, DO, Allentown, Pennsylvania

Practicing Ophthalmologists Advisory Committee for Education: Michelle S. Ying, MD, MSPH, *primary reviewer,* Ladson, South Carolina; Bradley D. Fouraker, MD, *Chair,* Tampa, Florida; Alice Bashinsky, MD, Asheville, North Carolina; David J. Browning, MD, PhD, Charlotte, North Carolina; Cynthia S. Chiu, MD, Oakland, California; Steven J. Grosser, MD, Golden Valley, Minnesota; Stephen R. Klapper, MD, Carmel, Indiana; Troy M. Tanji, MD, Waipahu, Hawaii

Pan American Association of Ophthalmology BCSC 9 Review Committee: Emilio M. Dodds, MD, *Chair,* Buenos Aires, Argentina; Enzo Castiglione, MD, Santiago, Chile; Cristóbal A. Couto, MD, Buenos Aires, Argentina; Alejandra de la Torre, MD, PhD, Bogotá, Colombia; Ariel Schlaen, MD, Buenos Aires, Argentina; Carlos D. Siverio, MD, Lima, Peru; Daniel V. Vasconcelos-Santos, MD, PhD, Belo Horizonte, Brazil

The Academy also wishes to acknowledge the following committee for assistance in developing Study Questions and Answers for this BCSC Section:

Self-Assessment Committee: John A. Gonzales, MD, San Francisco, California; Michael A. Kapamajian, MD, Los Angeles, California; Humeyra H. Karacal, MD, St Louis, Missouri

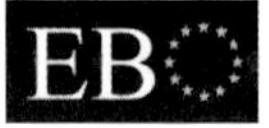

European Board of Ophthalmology: Peter J. Ringens, MD, PhD, *EBO-BCSC Program Liaison,* Maastricht, Netherlands; Joke H. De Boer, MD, PhD, *EBO Chair for BCSC Section 9,* Utrecht, Netherlands

Financial Disclosures

Academy staff members who contributed to the development of this product state that within the 12 months prior to their contributions to this CME activity and for the duration of development, they have had no financial interest in or other relationship with any entity discussed in this course that produces, markets, resells, or distributes ophthalmic health care goods or services consumed by or used in patients, or with any competing commercial product or service.

The authors and reviewers state that within the 12 months prior to their contributions to this CME activity and for the duration of development, they have had the following financial relationships:*

Dr Albini: Abbvie (C), Allergan (C), Bausch + Lomb (C), Clearside Biomedical (C), Genentech (C), Mallinckrodt Pharmaceuticals (C), Novartis Alcon Pharmaceuticals (C), pSivida (C), Santen (C)

Dr Browning: Aerpio Therapeutics (S), Alcon Laboratories (S), Alimera Sciences (C), Emmes (S), Genentech (S), Novartis Pharmaceuticals (S), Ohr Pharmaceutical (S), Pfizer (S), Regeneron Pharmaceuticals (S), Springer (P), Zeiss (O)

Dr Couto: Allergan (L)

Dr Dahr: Novo Nordisk (C)

Dr De Boer: Abbvie (C, L)

Dr de la Torre: Abbvie (C, L)

Dr Fouraker: Addition Technology (C, L), Alcon Laboratories (C, L), OASIS Medical (C, L)

Dr Grosser: InjectSense (O), Ivantis (O)

Dr Klapper: AdOM Advanced Optical Technologies (O)

Dr Larkin: Quark Pharmaceuticals (C)

Dr Schlaen: Abbvie (C, L)

Dr Smith: Inotek Pharmaceuticals (C)

The other authors and reviewers state that within the 12 months prior to their contributions to this CME activity and for the duration of development, they have had no financial interest in or other relationship with any entity discussed in this course that produces, markets, resells, or distributes ophthalmic health care goods or services consumed by or used in patients, or with any competing commercial product or service.

*C = consultant fee, paid advisory boards, or fees for attending a meeting; E = employed by or received a W2 from a commercial company; L = lecture fees or honoraria, travel fees or reimbursements when speaking at the invitation of a commercial company; O = equity ownership/stock options in publicly or privately traded firms, excluding mutual funds; P = patents and/or royalties for intellectual property; S = grant support or other financial support to the investigator from all sources, including research support from government agencies, foundations, device manufacturers, and/or pharmaceutical companies

Recent Past Faculty

Nisha Acharya, MD
Ralph D. Levinson, MD
P. Kumar Rao, MD
Russell W. Read, MD, PhD
Jonathan D. Walker, MD

In addition, the Academy gratefully acknowledges the contributions of numerous past faculty and advisory committee members who have played an important role in the development of previous editions of the Basic and Clinical Science Course.

American Academy of Ophthalmology Staff

Dale E. Fajardo, EdD, MBA, *Vice President, Education*
Beth Wilson, *Director, Continuing Professional Development*
Denise Evenson, *Director, Brand & Creative*
Ann McGuire, *Acquisitions and Development Manager*
Stephanie Tanaka, *Publications Manager*
Susan Malloy, *Acquisitions Editor and Program Manager*
Jasmine Chen, *Manager of E-Learning*
Lana Ip, *Senior Designer*
Beth Collins, *Medical Editor*
Eric Gerdes, *Interactive Designer*
Lynda Hanwella, *Publications Specialist*
Debra Marchi, *Permissions Assistant*

American Academy of Ophthalmology
655 Beach Street
Box 7424
San Francisco, CA 94120-7424

Contents

Introduction to the BCSC

The Basic and Clinical Science Course (BCSC) is designed to meet the needs of residents and practitioners for a comprehensive yet concise curriculum of the field of ophthalmology. The BCSC has developed from its original brief outline format, which relied heavily on outside readings, to a more convenient and educationally useful self-contained text. The Academy updates and revises the course annually, with the goals of integrating the basic science and clinical practice of ophthalmology and of keeping ophthalmologists current with new developments in the various subspecialties.

The BCSC incorporates the effort and expertise of more than 100 ophthalmologists, organized into 13 Section faculties, working with Academy editorial staff. In addition, the course continues to benefit from many lasting contributions made by the faculties of previous editions. Members of the Academy Practicing Ophthalmologists Advisory Committee for Education, Committee on Aging, and Vision Rehabilitation Committee review every volume before major revisions. Members of the European Board of Ophthalmology, organized into Section faculties, also review each volume before major revisions, focusing primarily on differences between American and European ophthalmology practice.

Organization of the Course

The Basic and Clinical Science Course comprises 13 volumes, incorporating fundamental ophthalmic knowledge, subspecialty areas, and special topics:

1 Update on General Medicine
2 Fundamentals and Principles of Ophthalmology
3 Clinical Optics
4 Ophthalmic Pathology and Intraocular Tumors
5 Neuro-Ophthalmology
6 Pediatric Ophthalmology and Strabismus
7 Oculofacial Plastic and Orbital Surgery
8 External Disease and Cornea
9 Uveitis and Ocular Inflammation
10 Glaucoma
11 Lens and Cataract
12 Retina and Vitreous
13 Refractive Surgery

References

Readers who wish to explore specific topics in greater detail may consult the references cited within each chapter and listed in the Basic Texts section at the back of the book. These references are intended to be selective rather than exhaustive, chosen by the BCSC faculty as being important, current, and readily available to residents and practitioners.

Multimedia

This edition of Section 9, *Uveitis and Ocular Inflammation,* includes videos related to topics covered in the book and interactive content, an "activity," developed by members of the BCSC faculty. The videos and the activity are available to readers of the print and electronic versions of Section 9 (www.aao.org/bcscvideo_section09) and (www.aao.org/bcscactivity_section09). Mobile-device users can scan the QR codes below (a QR-code reader may need to be installed on the device) to access the videos and activity.

Videos

Activity

Self-Assessment and CME Credit

Each volume of the BCSC is designed as an independent study activity for ophthalmology residents and practitioners. The learning objectives for this volume are given on page xv. The text, illustrations, and references provide the information necessary to achieve the objectives; the study questions allow readers to test their understanding of the material and their mastery of the objectives. Physicians who wish to claim CME credit for this educational activity may do so by following the instructions given at the end of the book.*

Conclusion

The Basic and Clinical Science Course has expanded greatly over the years, with the addition of much new text, numerous illustrations, and video content. Recent editions have sought to place greater emphasis on clinical applicability while maintaining a solid foundation in basic science. As with any educational program, it reflects the experience of its authors. As its faculties change and medicine progresses, new viewpoints emerge on controversial subjects and techniques. Not all alternate approaches can be included in this series; as with any educational endeavor, the learner should seek additional sources, including Academy Preferred Practice Pattern Guidelines.

The BCSC faculty and staff continually strive to improve the educational usefulness of the course; you, the reader, can contribute to this ongoing process. If you have any suggestions or questions about the series, please do not hesitate to contact the faculty or the editors.

The authors, editors, and reviewers hope that your study of the BCSC will be of lasting value and that each Section will serve as a practical resource for quality patient care.

* This activity meets the Self-Assessment CME requirements defined by the American Board of Ophthalmology (ABO). Please be advised that the ABO is not an accrediting body for purposes of any CME program. ABO does not sponsor this or any outside activity, and ABO does not endorse any particular CME activity. Complete information regarding the ABO Self-Assessment CME Maintenance of Certification requirements is available at https://abop.org/maintain-certification/cme-self-assessment/.

Objectives

Upon completion of BCSC Section 9, *Uveitis and Ocular Inflammation,* the reader should be able to

- describe the immunologic and infectious mechanisms involved in the development of and complications from uveitis and related inflammatory conditions, including acquired immunodeficiency syndrome
- identify general and specific pathophysiologic processes in acute and chronic intraocular inflammation that affect the structure and function of the uvea, lens, intraocular spaces, retina, and other tissues
- differentiate infectious from noninfectious uveitic entities
- formulate appropriate differential diagnoses for ocular inflammatory disorders and identify systemic associations or implications
- based on the differential diagnosis, choose examination techniques and appropriate ancillary studies to differentiate infectious from noninfectious causes
- describe the principles of medical and surgical management of infectious and noninfectious uveitis and related intraocular inflammation, including indications for, adverse effects of, and monitoring of immunosuppressive drugs
- describe the structural complications of uveitis, their prevention, and their treatment
- describe the main principles for differentiating masquerade syndromes from true uveitis and increasing clinical suspicion for these syndromes

CHAPTER 1

Basic Concepts in Immunology: Effector Cells and the Innate Immune Response

Highlights

- An immune response is the process for removing an offending stimulus. The clinical evidence of an immune response is inflammation.
- The immune system is composed of cells, tissues, and molecules that mediate response to infection or foreign material.
- Immune responses are defined as innate or adaptive.
- Innate (natural) immunity provides immediate protection and requires no prior contact with the foreign substance or organism.
- Adaptive (acquired) immunity develops more slowly but provides more specific defense against infections, having a permanent cross talk with the innate immune system.

Definitions

An immune response is a sequence of molecular and cellular events intended to rid the host of a threat: offending pathogenic organisms, toxic substances, cellular debris, or neoplastic cells. There are 2 broad categories of immune responses, *innate* and *adaptive.*

Innate immune responses, or *natural immunity,* require no prior contact with or "education" about the stimulus against which they are directed. Adaptive (or *acquired*) responses are higher-order, more specific responses directed against unique antigens. Chapter 2 discusses these responses in detail. This chapter introduces the crucial cells of the immune system and their functions in innate immunity.

Abbas AK, Lichtman AH, Pillai S. *Basic Immunology: Functions and Disorders of the Immune System.* 5th ed. Philadelphia, PA: Elsevier/Saunders; 2016.

Abbas AK, Lichtman AH, Pillai S. *Cellular and Molecular Immunology.* 9th ed. Philadelphia, PA: Elsevier/Saunders; 2018.

Murphy KM. *Janeway's Immunobiology.* 8th ed. London: Garland Science; 2012.

Components of the Immune System

Leukocytes

White blood cells, or *leukocytes,* include several kinds of nucleated cells that can be distinguished by the shape of their nuclei and the presence or absence of cytoplasmic granules, as well as by their uptake of various histologic stains. They can be broadly divided into 2 subsets:

- myeloid (neutrophils, eosinophils, basophils and mast cells, monocytes and macrophages, and dendritic cells and Langerhans cells)
- lymphoid (T lymphocytes, B lymphocytes, and natural killer cells)

Neutrophils

Neutrophils possess a multilobed nucleus of varying shapes; hence, they are also called *polymorphonuclear leukocytes* (PMNs). Neutrophils also feature cytoplasmic granules and lysosomes and are the most abundant granulocytes in the blood. They are efficient phagocytes that readily clear tissues, degrade ingested material, and act as important effector cells through the release of granule products and cytokines.

During the beginning or acute phases of inflammation, neutrophils are one of the first inflammatory cells to migrate from the bloodstream toward the site of inflammation. This process is called *chemotaxis*. Neutrophils dominate the inflammatory infiltrate in experimental models and clinical examples of active bacterial infections of the conjunctiva (conjunctivitis), sclera (scleritis), cornea (keratitis), and vitreous (endophthalmitis). They are also dominant in many types of active viral infections of the cornea (eg, herpes simplex virus keratitis) and retina (eg, herpes simplex virus retinitis). Neutrophils constitute the principal cell type in ocular inflammation induced by lipopolysaccharides (discussed later) or by direct injection of most cytokines into ocular tissues.

Eosinophils

Eosinophils are characterized by the presence of abundant lysosomes and cytoplasmic granules that consist of more basic protein than other polymorphonuclear leukocytes, (thus acidic dyes, such as eosin, will bind to these proteins.) Eosinophils have receptors for, and become activated by, many mediators; interleukin-5 (IL-5) is especially important. Eosinophilic granule products, such as major basic protein and ribonucleases, destroy parasites efficiently; thus, these cells accumulate at sites of parasitic infection. Eosinophils are also important in allergic immune reactions.

Eosinophils are abundant in the conjunctiva and tears in many forms of allergic conjunctivitis, especially atopic and vernal conjunctivitis. They are not considered major effectors for intraocular inflammation, with the notable exception of helminthic infections of the eye, especially toxocariasis.

Basophils and mast cells

Basophils are the blood-borne equivalent of the tissue-bound mast cell. Mast cells exist in 2 major subtypes, connective tissue and mucosal, both of which can release preformed granules and synthesize certain mediators de novo that differ from those of neutrophils and eosinophils. *Connective tissue mast cells* contain abundant granules with histamine and heparin, and they synthesize prostaglandin D_2 upon stimulation. In contrast, *mucosal mast cells* normally contain low levels of histamine and require T-cell–derived growth-promoting cytokines for stimulation. Stimulated mucosal mast cells primarily synthesize leukotrienes, mainly leukotriene C4. Tissue location can alter the granule type and functional activity, but regulation of these differences is not well understood.

Mast cells act as major effector cells in immunoglobulin E (IgE)–mediated, immune-triggered inflammatory reactions, especially of the allergic or immediate hypersensitivity type. They perform this function through their expression of high-affinity Fc receptors for IgE. *Fc* (from "*f*ragment, *c*rystallizable") refers to the constant region of immunoglobulin that binds cell surface receptors (see Chapter 2). Mast cells may also participate in the induction of cell-mediated immunity, wound healing, and other functions not directly related to IgE-mediated degranulation. Other stimuli, such as complement or certain cytokines, may also trigger degranulation.

The healthy human conjunctiva contains numerous mast cells localized in the substantia propria. In certain atopic and allergic disease states, such as vernal conjunctivitis, the number of mast cells increases in the substantia propria, and the epithelium—usually devoid of mast cells—becomes densely infiltrated. The uveal tract also contains numerous connective tissue–type mast cells, whereas the cornea has none.

Monocytes and macrophages

Monocytes, the circulating cells, and macrophages, the tissue-infiltrating equivalents, are important effectors in innate and adaptive immunity. They are often detectable in acute ocular infections, even if other cell types, such as neutrophils, are more numerous. Mono cytes are relatively large cells (12–20 μm in suspension and up to 40 μm in tissues) that normally travel throughout the body. Most tissues have at least 2 identifiable macrophage populations: tissue resident and blood derived. Although exceptions exist, tissue-resident macrophages are monocytes that migrated into tissue during embryologic development and later acquired tissue-specific properties and cellular markers. Various resident macrophages have tissue-specific names (ie, Kupffer cells in the liver, alveolar macrophages in the lung, and microglia in the brain and retina). Blood-derived macrophages are monocytes that have recently migrated from the blood into a fully developed tissue site.

Macrophages may serve in 3 capacities:

- sentinels that recognize danger signals from pathogens and/or tissue damage
- effectors that induce inflammation and fight pathogens directly
- regulatory/repair cells that conduct tissue repair, regulate the adaptive immune system, and serve as checkpoints during immune cell migration

Various signals can prime resting monocytes into efficient antigen-presenting cells (APCs) and, upon additional signals, activate them into effector cells. Effective activation stimuli include exposure to bacterial products, such as lipopolysaccharide (LPS); phagocytosis of antibody-coated or complement-coated pathogens; or exposure to mediators released during inflammation, such as interleukin-1 (IL-1) or interferon gamma (IFN-γ).

Only after full activation do macrophages become most efficient at the synthesis and release of inflammatory mediators and the killing and degradation of phagocytosed pathogens. Macrophages may undergo activation into *epithelioid cells,* with larger nuclei, abundant cytoplasm, and indistinct cell borders, resembling squamous epithelium. These epithelioid histiocytes are characteristic of granulomatous inflammation, either in infectious uveitis (ie, tuberculosis, syphilis, herpesviruses, fungi, parasitic uveitis) or noninfectious uveitis (ie, sarcoidosis, rheumatoid arthritis, granulomatosis with polyangiitis). Macrophages may also be activated to fuse into multinucleated *giant cells,* which may accompany granulomatous inflammation or occur in the tissue reaction to foreign material.

Dendritic cells and Langerhans cells

Dendritic cells (DCs) are terminally differentiated, bone marrow–derived, mononuclear cells that are distinct from macrophages and monocytes. These specialized cells bridge the innate and adaptive immune systems, but do not directly participate in effector activities. DCs use pattern recognition receptors, such as Toll-like receptors (TLRs), to recognize pathogens. Activated DCs upregulate costimulatory molecules and produce cytokines to drive T-cell priming and effector differentiation as well as activate various types of immune cells. Interestingly, antigen presentation by nonactivated, steady-state DCs might lead to T-cell unresponsiveness, promoting tolerance. All human DCs express high levels of major histocompatibility (MHC) class II (HLA-DR) molecules and may be classified by lineage markers as myeloid/classical or plasmacytoid. Dendritic cells can also be classified functionally and anatomically, as their function is linked to their location:

- Blood DCs are precursors of tissue and lymphoid organ DCs.
- Migratory or tissue DCs reside in most epithelial tissues, where they acquire antigen and migrate via afferent lymphatics to lymph nodes. In tissue sites, DCs are enlarged (15–30 µm), with cytoplasmic veils that form extensions 2–3 times the diameter of the cell and resemble the dendritic structure of neurons.
- Resident or lymphoid DCs arise in lymph nodes directly from blood.
- Inflammatory DCs are in tissues and lymphoid organs during inflammation. Precursors include classical monocytes.

Langerhans cells (LCs) are myeloid cells with dendritic cell function that reside in the epidermis and stratified epithelia of the conjunctival, corneal, buccal, gingival, and genital mucosae. LCs are identified by their many dendrites, electron-dense cytoplasm, and Birbeck granules. Interestingly, they originate from primitive hematopoiesis in the yolk sac and form a stable, self-renewing network that does not require bone marrow–derived precursors in the absence of inflammation. At rest, they are not active APCs, but activity develops after in vitro culture with specific cytokines. On activation, LCs lose their granules and transform to resemble blood and lymphoid DCs. Evidence suggests that LCs migrate along the afferent lymph vessels to the draining lymphoid organs. LCs are important components of the immune system and play roles in antigen presentation, control of lymphoid cell traffic, differentiation of T lymphocytes, and induction of delayed hypersensitivity. Elimination of LCs from skin before an antigen challenge inhibits induction of the contact hypersensitivity response. In the conjunctiva and limbus, LCs are the only cells that constitutively express MHC class II molecules. LCs are present in the peripheral cornea, and any stimulation to the central cornea results in central migration of the peripheral LCs.

Lymphocytes

Lymphocytes are small (10–20 μm) cells with large, round, and dense nuclei. They are also derived from stem cell precursors within the bone marrow; however, unlike other leukocytes, lymphocytes require subsequent maturation in peripheral lymphoid organs. The expression of specific cell-surface proteins (ie, *surface markers*) can subdivide lymphocytes. These markers are in turn related to the functional and molecular activity of individual subsets. Three broad categories of lymphocytes are T lymphocytes; B lymphocytes; and non-T, non-B lymphocytes. Two types of lymphocytes participate in the innate immune response, serving as a bridge between innate and adaptive responses: (1) gamma-delta (γδ) T cells or sentinel T cells, also known as *intraepithelial lymphocytes*, and (2) natural killer (NK) cells, a subset of non-T, non-B lymphocytes. Chapter 2 discusses the roles of lymphocytes in adaptive immunity.

Overview of the Innate Immune System

The innate immune system is a relatively broad-acting rapid reaction force that recognizes "nonself" foreign substances, proteins, or lipopolysaccharides. The innate response can be thought of as a preprogrammed reaction that is immediate, requires no prior exposure to the foreign substance, and is similar for all encountered triggers. The result is the generation of biochemical mediators and cytokines that recruit innate effector cells, especially macrophages and neutrophils, to remove the offending stimulus through phagocytosis or enzymatic degradation. The innate response also alerts the cells of the adaptive immune system to reinforce and refine the attack. In endophthalmitis, bacteria-derived toxins or host cell debris stimulates the recruitment of neutrophils and monocytes, leading to the production of inflammatory mediators and phagocytosis of the bacteria. Responses to *Staphylococcus* organisms are nearly identical to those mounted against any other bacteria.

An array of highly conserved pattern recognition receptors (PRRs) and proteins detect similarly conserved molecular motifs, pathogen-associated molecular patterns (PAMPs), on triggering stimuli. PAMPs include proteins found only in bacterial, fungal, and viral nucleic acids. Cell-associated PRRs may be extracellular, endosomal, or cytoplasmic and include toll-like receptors (TLRs), C-type lectin receptors (CTLRs), nucleotide-binding oligomerization domain-like receptors (NOD-like receptors, or NLRs), and retinoic acid-inducible gene-I-like receptors (RIG-I-like receptors, or RLRs), among others. Since each PRR has evolved to respond to a different PAMP, engagement of a specific PRR subtype conveys information regarding the type of infection (ie, bacterial, fungal, or viral) and the location (ie, extracellular or intracellular). In humans, there are 10 members of the TLR family. Those that respond to bacterial products (TLR1/2, TLR2/6, TLR4, TLR5) are localized in the plasma membrane of innate immune cells and sense extracellular microbes. The TLRs that detect viral nucleic acids (TLR3, TLR7, TLR9) are in endosomal compartments and interact with membrane proteins.

Immunity Versus Inflammation

An immune response is the process for removing an offending stimulus. An immune response that becomes clinically evident is termed an *inflammatory response.* Immunity (innate or adaptive) triggers this response and consists of a sequence of molecular and cellular events resulting in 5 cardinal clinical manifestations: pain, hyperemia, edema, heat, and loss of function. These signs are the consequence of 2 physiologic changes within a tissue: cellular recruitment and altered vascular permeability.

The following pathologic findings are typical in inflammation:

- infiltration of effector cells resulting in the release of biochemical and molecular mediators of inflammation, such as cytokines (eg, interleukins and chemokines) and lipid mediators (eg, prostaglandins, leukotrienes, and platelet-activating factors)
- production of oxygen metabolites (eg, superoxide and nitrogen radicals)
- release of granule products as well as catalytic enzymes (eg, proteases, collagenases, and elastases)
- activation of plasma-derived enzyme systems (eg, complement components and fibrin)

These effector systems are described in greater detail later in this chapter.

Adaptive and innate immune responses are a constant presence, though usually at a subclinical level. For example, ocular surface allergen exposure, which occurs daily in humans, or the nearly ubiquitous event of bacterial contamination during cataract surgery is usually cleared by innate or adaptive mechanisms *without* overt inflammation. The physiologic changes induced by innate and adaptive immunity may be indistinguishable. Compare the hypopyon of bacterial endophthalmitis, which results from innate immunity against bacterial toxins, with the hypopyon of lens-associated uveitis (excluding phacolytic glaucoma), presumably a result of an adaptive immune response against lens antigens. These hypopyons cannot be distinguished clinically or histologically.

Delves PJ, Martin SJ, Burton DR, Roitt IM. *Roitt's Essential Immunology.* 13th ed. Hoboken, NJ: Wiley-Blackwell; 2017.

Triggers of Innate Immunity

Innate immune responses generally use direct triggering mechanisms. Four of the most important are reviewed below and include

- bacteria-derived molecules
- interactions between nonimmune ocular parenchymal cells and toxins or trauma
- recruitment and activation of neutrophils through the activation of vascular endothelial cells
- innate mechanisms for the recruitment and activation of macrophages

Table 1-1 summarizes the effector responses of the ocular innate immune system.

Table 1-1 Innate Immune Response in the Eye

Factor	Description
Triggers	Bacteria-derived molecules that trigger innate immunity Lipopolysaccharide Other cell wall components Exotoxins and secreted toxins Nonspecific soluble molecules that trigger or modulate innate immunity Plasma-derived enzymes Acute-phase reactants Cytokines produced by parenchymal cells within a tissue site
Mechanisms of recruitment and activation	Innate mechanisms for recruitment and activation of neutrophils Neutrophil adhesion to activated vascular endothelium Neutrophil transmigration through vascular endothelium, triggered by chemotactic factors Neutrophil activation (exposure to bacteria and their toxins, chemical mediators) Innate mechanisms for recruitment and activation of macrophages Monocyte adhesion to and transmigration through vascular endothelium Monocyte activation mechanisms Monocyte priming through exposure to certain cytokines

Bacteria-Derived Molecules That Trigger Innate Immunity

Bacterial lipopolysaccharide

Bacterial lipopolysaccharide (LPS), also known as *endotoxin,* is an intrinsic component of the cell walls of most gram-negative bacteria. Among the most important triggering molecules of innate immunity, LPS consists of 3 components:

- lipid A
- O polysaccharide
- core oligosaccharide

The exact structures of each component vary among species of bacteria, but all are recognized by the innate immune system. The primary receptors are the toll-like receptors (TLRs), principally TLR4 and TLR2, which are expressed on macrophages, neutrophils, and dendritic cells, as well as on B cells and T cells. Lipid A is the most potent component, capable of activating effector cells at concentrations of a few picograms per milliliter.

The effects of LPS include activation of monocytes and neutrophils, leading to upregulation of genes for various cytokines (IL-1, IL-6, tumor necrosis factor [TNF]); degranulation; alternative pathway complement activation; and direct impact on the vascular endothelium. LPS is the major cause of shock, fever, and other pathophysiologic responses to bacterial sepsis, making it an important cause of morbidity and mortality during gram-negative bacterial infections. Interestingly, footpad injection of LPS in rodents results in an acute anterior uveitis. This animal model is called *endotoxin-induced uveitis* (EIU; see Chapter 4). See Clinical Examples 1-1 and 1-2.

Other bacterial cell wall components

The bacterial cell wall and membrane are complex. They contain numerous polysaccharide, lipid, and protein structures that can initiate an innate immune response independent of adaptive immunity. Killed lysates of many types of gram-positive bacteria or mycobacteria can directly activate macrophages, making them useful as adjuvants. Some

CLINICAL EXAMPLE 1-1

Lipopolysaccharide-induced uveitis Humans are intermittently exposed to low levels of LPS that the gut releases, especially during episodes of diarrhea and dysentery. Exposure to LPS may play a role in dysentery-related uveitis, arthritis, and reactive arthritis. Systemic administration of a low dose of LPS in rabbits, rats, and mice produces a mild acute uveitis. This effect occurs at doses of LPS lower than those that cause apparent systemic shock. In rabbits, a breakdown of the blood–ocular barrier occurs because of loosening of the tight junctions between the nonpigmented ciliary epithelial cells, which allows leakage of plasma proteins through uveal vessels. Rats and mice exhibit an acute neutrophilic and monocytic infiltrate in the iris and ciliary body within 24 hours.

The precise mechanism of the LPS-induced ocular effects after systemic administration is unknown. One possibility is that LPS circulates and binds to the vascular endothelium or other sites within the anterior uvea. Alternatively, LPS might cause activation of uveal macrophages or circulating leukocytes, leading them to preferentially adhere to the anterior uveal vascular endothelium. Toll-like receptor 2 (TLR2) recognizes LPS, and binding of LPS by TLR2 on macrophages results in macrophage activation and secretion of a wide array of inflammatory cytokines. Degranulation of platelets is among the first histologic changes in LPS uveitis; likely mediators are eicosanoids, platelet-activating factors, and vasoactive amines. The subsequent intraocular generation of several mediators, especially leukotriene B4, thromboxane B2, prostaglandin E2, and IL-6 correlates with the development of the cellular infiltrate and vascular leakage.

Not surprisingly, direct injection of LPS into various ocular sites can initiate a severe localized inflammatory response. For example, intravitreal injection of LPS triggers a dose-dependent neutrophilic and monocytic infiltration of the uveal tract, retina, and vitreous. Injection of LPS into the central cornea results in the development of a ring infiltrate comprised of neutrophils that migrated circumferentially from the limbus.

CLINICAL EXAMPLE 1-2

Role of bacterial toxin production in the severity of endophthalmitis As described in Clinical Example 1-1, intraocular injection of LPS is highly inflammatory and accounts for much of the enhanced pathogenicity of gram-negative infections of the eye. Using clinical isolates or bacteria genetically altered to diminish production of the various types of bacterial toxins, investigators have demonstrated that toxin elaboration in gram-positive or gram-negative endophthalmitis greatly influences inflammatory cell infiltration and retinal cytotoxicity. This effect suggests that sterilization through antibiotic therapy alone, in the absence of antitoxin therapy, may not prevent activation of innate immunity, ocular inflammation, and vision loss in eyes infected by toxin-producing strains.

Booth MC, Atkuri RV, Gilmore MS. Toxin production contributes to severity of *Staphylococcus aureus* endophthalmitis. In: Nussenblatt RB, Whitcup SM, Caspi RR, Gery I, eds. *Advances in Ocular Immunology: Proceedings of the 6th International Symposium on the Immunology and Immunopathology of the Eye.* New York, NY: Elsevier; 1994:269–272.

Jett BD, Parke DW 2nd, Booth MC, Gilmore MS. Host/parasite interactions in bacterial endophthalmitis. *Zentralbl Bakteriol.* 1997;285(3):341–367.

of these components have been implicated in various models for arthritis and uveitis. In many cases, the molecular mechanisms might be similar to those of LPS.

Exotoxins and other secretory products of bacteria

Certain bacteria secrete products known as *exotoxins* into their surrounding microenvironment. Many of these products are enzymes that, although not directly inflammatory, can cause tissue damage and subsequent inflammation and tissue destruction. Examples of these products include

- collagenases
- hemolysins such as streptolysin O, which can kill neutrophils by causing cytoplasmic and extracellular release of their granules
- phospholipases such as the *Clostridium perfringens* α-toxins, which kill cells and cause necrosis by disrupting cell membranes

An intravitreal injection of a purified hemolysin BL toxin derived from *Bacillus cereus* can cause direct necrosis of retinal cells and retinal detachment. In animal studies, as few as 100 *B cereus* can produce enough toxin to cause complete loss of retinal function in 12 hours. In addition to being directly toxic, bacterial exotoxins can also be strong triggers of an innate immune response.

Callegan MC, Jett BD, Hancock LE, Gilmore MS. Role of hemolysin BL in the pathogenesis of extraintestinal *Bacillus cereus* infection assessed in an endophthalmitis model. *Infect Immun.* 1999;67(7):3357–3366.

Murphy K, Travers P, Walport M. *Janeway's Immunobiology.* 8th ed. London: Garland Science; 2012.

Other Triggers or Modulators of Innate Immunity

Another form of innate immunity is the mechanism by which trauma or toxins interact directly with nonimmune ocular parenchymal cells—especially iris or ciliary body epithelium, retinal pigment epithelium, retinal Müller cells, or corneal or conjunctival epithelium. This interaction can result in the synthesis of a wide range of mediators, cytokines, and eicosanoids. For example, phagocytosis of staphylococci by corneal epithelium, microtrauma to the ocular surface epithelium by contact lenses, chafing of iris or ciliary epithelium by an intraocular lens (IOL), or laser treatment of the retina can stimulate ocular cells to produce mediators that assist in the recruitment of innate effector cells such as neutrophils or macrophages. See Clinical Example 1-3.

Innate Mechanisms for the Recruitment and Activation of Neutrophils

Neutrophils are highly efficient effectors of innate immunity. They are categorized as either *resting* or *activated,* according to their secretory and cell membrane activity. Recruitment of resting, circulating neutrophils by the innate immune response occurs rapidly in a tightly controlled process consisting of 2 events:

- neutrophil adhesion to the vascular endothelium through cell-adhesion molecules (CAMs) on leukocytes as well as on endothelial cells primarily in postcapillary venules
- transmigration of the neutrophils through the endothelium and its extracellular matrix, mediated by chemotactic factors

Activation of vascular endothelial cells is triggered by various innate immune stimuli, such as LPS, physical injury, thrombin, histamine, or leukotriene release. *Neutrophil rolling*—a process by which neutrophils bind loosely and reversibly to nonactivated

CLINICAL EXAMPLE 1-3

Uveitis-glaucoma-hyphema syndrome One cause of postoperative inflammation after cataract surgery, uveitis-glaucoma-hyphema (UGH) syndrome, is related to the physical presence of certain IOL styles. Although UGH syndrome was more common when rigid anterior chamber lenses were used during the early 1980s, it has also been reported with posterior chamber lenses, particularly when a haptic of a 1-piece lens is inadvertently placed in the sulcus. The pathogenesis of UGH syndrome appears related to mechanisms for activation of innate immunity. A likely mechanism is cytokine and eicosanoid synthesis triggered by mechanical chafing or trauma to the iris or ciliary body. Plasma-derived enzymes, especially complement or fibrin, can enter the eye through vascular permeability altered by surgery or trauma and can then be activated by the surface of IOLs. Adherence of bacteria and leukocytes to the surface has also been implicated. Toxicity caused by contaminants on the lens surface during manufacturing is rare. Nevertheless, noninflamed eyes with IOLs can demonstrate histologic evidence of low-grade, foreign-body reactions around the haptics.

endothelial cells—involves molecules on both cell types that belong to at least 3 sets of CAM families:

- *selectins,* especially L-, E-, and P-selectin
- *integrins,* especially leukocyte function–associated antigen 1 (LFA-1) and macrophage-1 antigen (Mac-1)
- *immunoglobulin superfamily molecules,* especially intercellular adhesion molecule 1 (ICAM-1) and ICAM-2

The primary events are mediated largely by members of the selectin family and occur within minutes of stimulation (Fig 1-1). Nonactivated neutrophils express L-selectin,

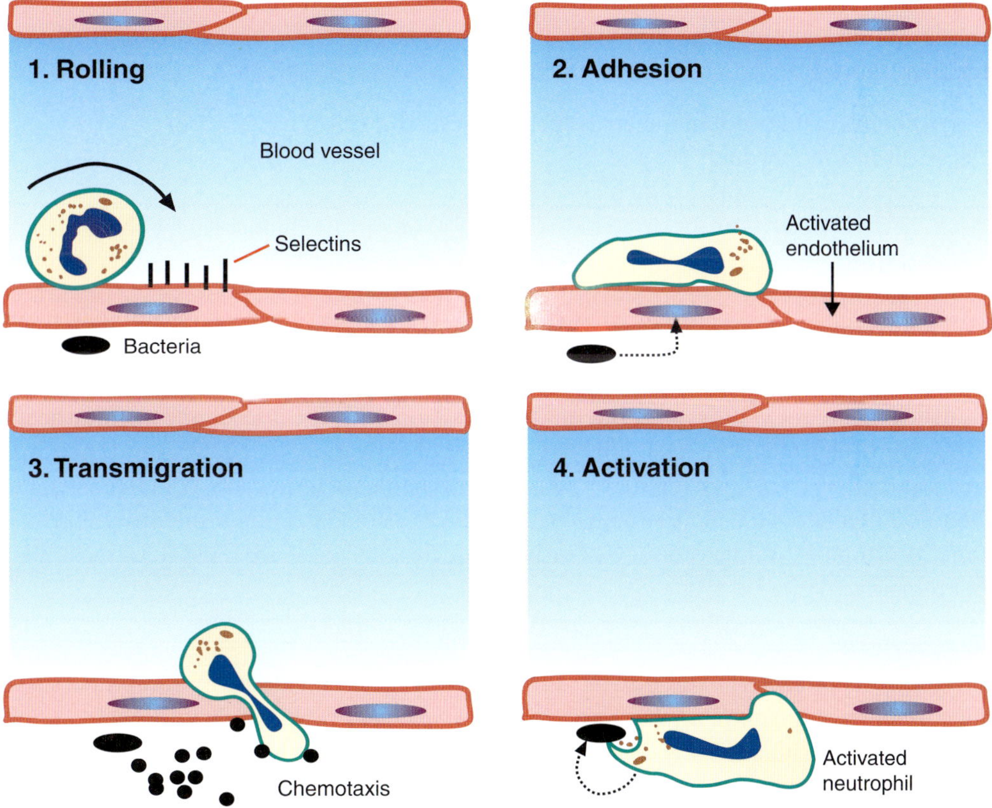

Figure 1-1 Four steps of neutrophil migration and activation. **1,** In response to innate immune stimuli, such as bacterial invasion of tissue, *rolling* neutrophils within the blood vessel bind loosely and reversibly to nonactivated endothelial cells by selectins. **2,** Exposure to innate activating factors and bacterial products *(dotted arrow)* activates endothelial cells, which in turn express E- and P-selectins, β-integrins, and immunoglobulin superfamily molecules to enhance and stabilize the interaction by a process called *adhesion.* **3,** Chemotactic factors triggered by the infection induce *transmigration* of neutrophils across the endothelial barrier into the extracellular matrix of the tissue. **4,** Finally, neutrophils are fully *activated* into functional effector cells upon stimulation by bacterial toxins and phagocytosis. *(Illustration by Barb Cousins, modified by Joyce Zavarro.)*

which mediates a weak bond to endothelial cells by binding to specific selectin ligands. Upon exposure to the triggering molecules described in the previous section, endothelial cells become activated, expressing in turn at least 2 other selectins (E and P) by which they can bind to the neutrophils and help stabilize the interaction in a process called *adhesion.* Subsequently, other factors, such as platelet-activating factor (PAF), various cytokines, and bacterial products can induce upregulation of the β-integrin family. As integrins are expressed, the selectins are shed, and neutrophils then bind firmly to endothelial cells through the immunoglobulin superfamily molecules.

After adhesion, various chemotactic factors are required to induce *transmigration* of neutrophils across the endothelial barrier and extracellular matrix into the tissue site. Chemotactic factors are short-range signaling molecules that diffuse in a declining concentration gradient from the source of production within a tissue to the vessel. Neutrophils have receptors for these molecules and are induced to undergo membrane changes that cause migration in the direction of highest concentration. Numerous such factors include:

- complement products, such as the anaphylatoxin C5a
- fibrin split products
- certain neuropeptides, such as substance P
- bacteria-derived formyl tripeptides, such as *N*-formyl-methionyl-leucyl-phenylalanine (fMLP)
- leukotrienes
- α-chemokines, such as IL-8

Activation of neutrophils into functional effector cells begins during adhesion and transmigration but is fully achieved upon interaction with specific signals within the injured or infected site. The most effective triggers of activation are bacteria and their toxins, especially LPS. Other innate or adaptive mechanisms (especially complement) and chemical mediators (such as leukotrienes and PAF) also contribute to neutrophil activation. Neutrophils, unlike monocytes or lymphocytes, do not leave a tissue to recirculate but remain and die.

Phagocytosis

Phagocytosis of bacteria and other pathogens is a process mediated by receptors. The 2 most important are *antibody Fc receptors* and *complement receptors.* Pathogens in an immune complex with antibody or activated complement components bind to cell-surface-membrane–expressed Fc or complement (C) receptors.

The area of membrane to which the pathogen is bound invaginates and becomes a phagosome, and cytoplasmic granules and lysosomes fuse with the phagosomes. Phagocytes have multiple means of destroying microorganisms, notably, antimicrobial polypeptides residing within the cytoplasmic granules, reactive oxygen radicals generated from oxygen during the respiratory burst, and reactive nitrogen radicals. Although these mechanisms primarily destroy pathogens, released contents, such as lysosomal enzymes, may contribute to the amplification of inflammation and tissue damage.

Innate Mechanisms for the Recruitment and Activation of Macrophages

Monocyte-derived macrophages are the second important type of effector cell (after neutrophils) for the innate immune response that follows trauma or acute infection. The various molecules involved in monocyte adhesion and transmigration from blood into tissues are probably similar to those for neutrophils, although they have not been studied as thoroughly. The functional activation of macrophages, however, is more complex than that of neutrophils. Macrophages exist in different levels or stages of metabolic and functional activity, each representing different "programs" of gene activation and synthesis of macrophage-derived cytokines and mediators. The categories of macrophages include

- resting (immature or quiescent)
- primed
- activated
- stimulated or reparative

Resting and scavenging macrophages

Phagocytosis removes host cell debris in the process called *scavenging*. Resting macrophages are the classic scavenging cell, capable of phagocytosis and uptake of the following:

- dead cell membranes
- chemically modified extracellular protein (ie, acetylated or oxidized lipoproteins)
- sugar ligands, through mannose receptors
- naked nucleic acids
- bacterial pathogens

Resting monocytes express at least 3 types of scavenging receptors but synthesize very low levels of proinflammatory cytokines. Scavenging can occur in the absence of inflammation. See Clinical Example 1-4.

CLINICAL EXAMPLE 1-4

Phacolytic glaucoma Mild infiltration of scavenging macrophages centered around retained lens cortex or nucleus fragments occurs in nearly all eyes with lens injury, including those subjected to routine cataract surgery. This infiltrate is notable for the *absence* of both prominent neutrophil infiltration and significant nongranulomatous inflammation. An occasional giant cell may be present, but granulomatous changes are not extensive.

Phacolytic glaucoma is a variant of scavenging macrophage infiltration in which leakage of lens protein occurs through the intact capsule of a hypermature cataract. Lens protein–engorged scavenging macrophages present in the anterior chamber block the trabecular meshwork outflow channels, resulting in elevated intraocular pressure. Other signs of typical lens-associated uveitis are conspicuously absent. Experimental studies suggest that lens proteins may be chemotactic stimuli for monocytes. See Chapter 8 for further discussion of the clinical presentation.

Primed macrophages

Resting macrophages become primed by exposure to certain cytokines. Upon priming, these cells become positive for MHC class II antigen and capable of functioning as APCs to T lymphocytes (see Chapter 2). Priming involves

- activation of specialized lysosomal enzymes, such as cathepsins D and E, for degrading proteins into peptide fragments
- upregulation of certain specific genes (ie, MHC class II), and costimulatory molecules (ie, B7.1)
- increased cycling of proteins between endosomes and the surface membrane.

Primed macrophages thus resemble dendritic cells. They can exit tissue sites by afferent lymphatic vessels to reenter the lymph node.

Activated and stimulated macrophages

Activated macrophages are classically defined as macrophages producing the full spectrum of inflammatory and cytotoxic cytokines; thus, they mediate and amplify acute inflammation, tumor killing, and major antibacterial activity. *Epithelioid cells* and *giant cells* represent different terminal differentiations of the activated macrophage.

Many different innate stimuli can activate macrophages, including

- cytokines derived from T lymphocytes and other cell types
- chemokines
- bacterial cell walls or toxins from gram-positive or acid-fast organisms
- complement activated through the alternative pathway
- foreign bodies composed of potentially toxic substances, such as talc or beryllium
- exposure to certain surfaces, such as some plastics

Activation of macrophages is also termed *polarization.* Some research classifies activated and stimulated macrophages as M1 or M2, based on the observation that certain stimuli produce distinct patterns of gene or protein expression under experimental conditions. The activation state seems to be somewhat reversible, suggesting that macrophages may switch between subsets (plasticity), depending on environmental signals. In fact, macrophage research suggests there are at least 9 distinct classes of macrophage activation. Consequently, although the M1/M2 model might be oversimplified, it does provide a framework for conceptualizing different levels of macrophage activation in terms of acute inflammation (Fig 1-2).

M1–classically activated macrophage characteristics include

- high production of proinflammatory cytokines and reactive nitrogen and oxygen intermediates
- promotion of T helper-1 (Th1) response
- strong microbicidal and tumoricidal activity

M2–alternatively activated macrophage characteristics include

- parasite containment
- promotion of tissue remodeling

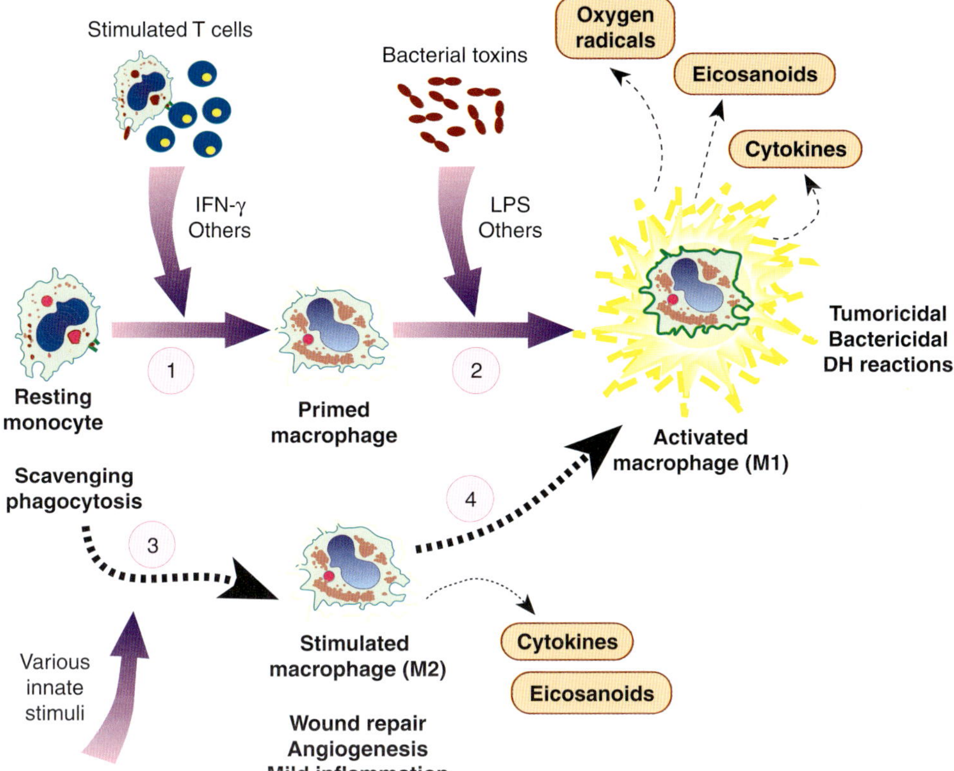

Figure 1-2 Schematic representation of macrophage activation pathway. Classically, *resting monocytes* are thought to be the principal type of noninflammatory scavenging phagocyte. **1,** Upon exposure to low levels of interferon gamma (IFN-γ) from T lymphocytes, monocytes become primed, upregulating major histocompatibility complex (MHC) class II molecules and performing other functions. *Primed macrophages* function in antigen presentation. **2,** *Fully activated macrophages (M1),* after exposure to bacterial lipopolysaccharide and interferon (classical activation), are tumoricidal and bactericidal and mediate severe inflammation. **3,** *Stimulated macrophages (M2)* result from resting monocyte activation by other innate stimuli, without exposure to IFN-γ (alternative activation). These cells are incompletely activated, producing low levels of cytokines and eicosanoids but not reactive oxygen intermediates. These cells participate in wound healing, angiogenesis, and low-level inflammatory reactions. **4,** The activation state seems to be somewhat reversible; macrophages may switch between subsets (plasticity), depending on environmental signals. DH = delayed hypersensitivity; LPS = lipopolysaccharide. *(Illustration by Barb Cousins, modified by Joyce Zavarro.)*

- promotion of tumor progression
- immunoregulatory functions

Activated macrophages synthesize numerous mediators to amplify inflammation such as

- inflammatory or cytotoxic cytokines, such as IL-1, IL-6, and TNF-α
- reactive oxygen or nitrogen intermediates
- lipid mediators

As noted, macrophages that are partially activated to produce some inflammatory cytokines are termed *stimulated* or *reparative* macrophages (M2). Such partially activated macrophages contribute to fibrosis and wound healing through the synthesis of mitogens such as platelet-derived growth factors (PDGFs), metalloproteinases, and other matrix degradation factors as well as to angiogenesis through synthesis of angiogenic factors such as vascular endothelial growth factor (VEGF).

Phagocyte-Killing Mechanisms

Reactive oxygen intermediates

Under certain conditions, oxygen can undergo chemical modification into highly reactive substances with the potential to damage cellular molecules and inhibit functional properties in pathogens or host cells. Three of the most important oxygen intermediates are (1) the superoxide anion, (2) hydrogen peroxide, and (3) the hydroxyl radical:

$O_2 + e^- \rightarrow O_2^-$	superoxide anion
$O_2^- + O_2^- + 2H^+ \rightarrow O_2 + H_2O_2$	superoxide dismutase catalyzes anions to form hydrogen peroxide
$H_2O_2 + e^- \rightarrow OH^- + OH\bullet$	hydroxyl anion and hydroxyl radical

Oxygen metabolites triggered by immune responses and generated by leukocytes, especially neutrophils and macrophages, are the most important source of free radicals during inflammation. A wide variety of stimuli can trigger leukocyte oxygen metabolism, including

- innate triggers, such as LPS or fMLP
- adaptive effectors, such as complement-fixing antibodies or certain cytokines produced by activated T lymphocytes
- other chemical mediator systems, such as C5a, PAF, and leukotrienes

Reactive oxygen intermediates can also be generated as part of noninflammatory cellular biochemical processes, especially by electron transport in the mitochondria, detoxification of certain chemicals, or interactions with environmental light or radiation. These reactive intermediates are highly toxic to living pathogens and damage pathogenic mediators such as exotoxins and lipids.

Reactive Nitrogen Products

Nitric oxide (NO) is a highly reactive chemical species. Like reactive oxygen intermediates, NO is involved in various important biochemical functions in microorganisms and host cells. The formation of NO depends on the enzyme nitric oxide synthetase (NOS), which is in the cytosol and dependent on NADPH (the reduced form of nicotinamide adenine dinucleotide phosphate). Several types of NOS are known, including various forms of constitutive NOS and inducible NOS (iNOS). Activation induces enhanced production of NO in certain cells, especially macrophages, via the calcium-independent, induced synthesis of iNOS. Many innate and adaptive stimuli modulate induction of iNOS, especially cytokines and bacterial toxins.

Mediator Systems That Amplify Immune Responses

Although innate or adaptive effector responses may directly induce inflammation, in most cases this process must be amplified to produce overt clinical manifestations. Molecules generated within the host that induce and amplify inflammation are termed *inflammatory mediators,* and mediator systems include several categories of these molecules (Table 1-2). Most act on target cells through receptor-mediated processes, although some act in enzymatic cascades that interact in a complex fashion.

Plasma-Derived Enzyme Systems

Complement

Complement is an important inflammatory mediator in the eye. Complement components account for approximately 5% of plasma protein and comprise more than 30 different proteins. Complement is activated by 1 of 3 pathways, and this activation generates products that contribute to the inflammatory process (Fig 1-3):

- *Classic pathway activation* occurs upon fixation of complement C1 by antigen–antibody (immune) complexes formed by IgM, IgG1, or IgG3. This pathway results in a connection between innate and adaptive immunity.
- *Alternative pathway activation* occurs continuously but is restricted by host complement regulatory components.
- The *mannose-binding lectin pathway* is activated by certain carbohydrate moieties on the cell wall of microorganisms.

Complement serves the following 4 basic functions during inflammation:

- coats antigenic or pathogenic surfaces with C3b to enhance phagocytosis (opsonization)
- promotes lysis of cell membranes through pore formation by the membrane attack complex (MAC)
- recruits neutrophils and induces inflammation through generation of the anaphylatoxins C3a and C5a
- modulates antigen-specific immune responses through complement activation products, such as iC3b and MACs

Table 1-2 Mediator Systems That Amplify Innate and Adaptive Immune Responses

Plasma-derived enzyme systems: complement, kinins, and fibrin
Vasoactive amines: serotonin and histamine
Lipid mediators: eicosanoids and platelet-activating factors
Cytokines
Neutrophil-derived granule products

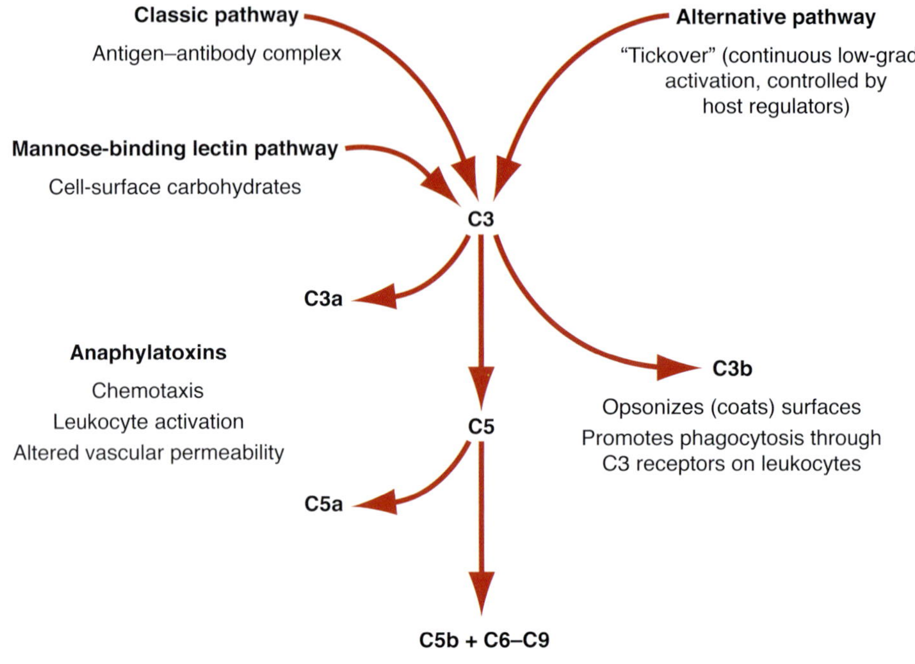

Figure 1-3 Overview of the essential intermediates of the complement pathway. C3a, C3b, C5a, and C5b are complement split products. C5b combines with intact C6, C7, C8, and C9 from the serum.

Anaphylatoxin effects include chemotaxis, changes in cell adhesiveness, and degranulation and release of mediators from mast cells and platelets. C5a stimulates oxidative metabolism and the production and release of toxic oxygen radicals from leukocytes, as well as the extracellular discharge of leukocyte granule contents.

Walport MJ. Complement. First of two parts. *N Engl J Med.* 2001;344(14):1058–1066.
Walport MJ. Complement. Second of two parts. *N Engl J Med.* 2001;344(15):1140–1144.

Fibrin and other plasma factors

Fibrin is the final deposition product of the coagulation pathway. Its deposition during inflammation promotes hemostasis, fibrosis, angiogenesis, and leukocyte adhesion. Fibrin is released from its circulating zymogen precursor, *fibrinogen,* upon cleavage by thrombin. In situ polymerization of smaller units gives rise to the characteristic fibrin plugs or clots. Fibrin dissolution is mediated by *plasmin,* which is activated from its zymogen precursor, *plasminogen,* by plasminogen activators such as tissue plasminogen activator. Thrombin, which is derived principally from platelet granules, is released after any vascular injury that causes platelet aggregation and release. Fibrin may be observed in severe anterior uveitis (the "plasmoid aqueous"), and it contributes to complications such as synechiae, cyclitic membranes, and tractional retinal detachment.

Histamine

Histamine is present in the granules of mast cells and basophils and is actively secreted after exposure to a wide range of stimuli. Histamine acts by binding to 1 of at least 3 known types of receptors that are differentially present on target cells. The best-studied pathway for degranulation is antigen crosslinking of IgE bound to mast-cell Fc IgE receptors, but many other inflammatory stimuli can induce secretion, including complement, direct membrane injury, and certain drugs. Classically, histamine release has been associated with allergy. The contribution of histamine to intraocular inflammation remains subject to debate.

Lipid Mediators

Two groups of lipid molecules synthesized by stimulated cells act as powerful mediators and regulators of inflammatory responses: the arachidonic acid (AA) metabolites, or *eicosanoids,* and the acetylated triglycerides, usually called *platelet-activating factors.* Both groups of molecules may be rapidly generated from the same lysophospholipid precursors by the enzymatic action of cellular phospholipases such as phospholipase A_2 (Fig 1-4).

Eicosanoids

All eicosanoids are derived from AA. It is liberated from membrane phospholipids by phospholipase A_2, which is activated by various agonists; AA is oxidized by 2 major pathways to generate the various mediators:

- the cyclooxygenase (COX) pathway, which produces prostaglandins, thromboxanes, and prostacyclins
- the 5-lipoxygenase pathway, which produces 5-hydroperoxyeicosatetraenoic acid, lipoxins, and leukotrienes

The COX-derived products are evanescent compounds induced in virtually all cells by a variety of stimuli. In general, they act in the immediate environment of their release to directly mediate many inflammatory activities. These include effects on vascular permeability, cell recruitment, platelet function, and smooth-muscle contraction.

Depending on conditions, COX-derived products can either upregulate or downregulate the production of cytokines, enzyme systems, and oxygen metabolites. The 2 forms of COX are COX-1 and COX-2. COX-1 is thought to be constitutively expressed by many cells, especially cells that use prostaglandin for basal metabolic functions, such as cells of the gastric mucosa and renal tubular epithelium. COX-2 is inducible by many inflammatory stimuli, including other inflammatory mediators (eg, PAF and some cytokines) and innate stimuli (eg, LPS).

Prostaglandins may be the cause of uveitic macular edema in association with anterior segment surgery or inflammation. Posterior diffusion of one or more of the eicosanoids through the vitreous is assumed to alter the permeability of the perifoveal capillary network,

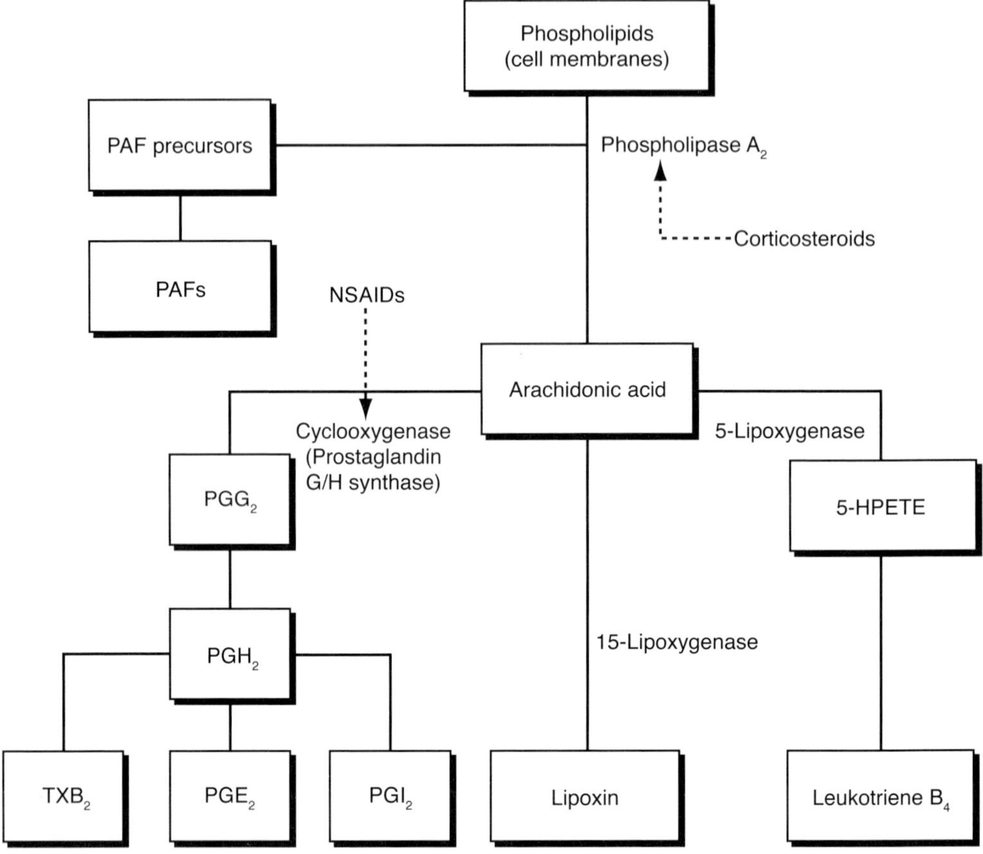

Figure 1-4 Overview of the essential intermediates of the eicosanoid and platelet-activating factor (PAF) pathways. 5-HPETE = 5-hydroperoxyeicosatetraenoic acid; NSAIDs = nonsteroidal anti-inflammatory drugs. *(Modified with permission from Pepose JS, Holland GN, Wilhelmus KR, eds.* Ocular Infection and Immunity. *St Louis, MO: Mosby; 1996.)*

leading to macular edema. Clinical trials in humans suggest that topical treatment with COX inhibitors (eg, NSAIDs) reduces the incidence of macular edema after cataract surgery.

Derivatives of 5-lipoxygenase, an enzyme found mainly in granulocytes and some mast cells, have been detected in the brain and retina. *Leukotrienes* probably contribute significantly to inflammatory infiltration; some leukotrienes have 1000 times the effect of histamine on vascular permeability. Another lipoxygenase product, lipoxin, is a potent stimulator of superoxide anion. Because many of the COX-derived prostaglandins downregulate the lipoxygenase pathway, NSAIDs can tilt AA metabolism toward increased production of inflammatory metabolites, leukotrienes, and lipoxins.

Platelet-activating factors

Platelet-activating factors are a family of phospholipid-derived mediators that appear to be important stimuli in the early stage of inflammation. These factors also serve physiologic functions unrelated to inflammation, especially in reproductive biology, the physiology of secretory epithelium, and neurobiology. In these physiologic roles, a de novo biosynthetic pathway has been identified. However, the *remodeling pathway* is the one implicated in PAF inflammatory actions.

Phospholipase A_2 metabolizes phosphocholine precursors in cell membranes, releasing AA and PAF precursors, which are acetylated into multiple species of PAF. PAF release is stimulated by various innate immune triggers, such as bacterial toxins, trauma, and cytokines. Platelet-activating factors activate not only platelets but also most leukocytes, which in turn produce and release additional PAFs. They function by binding to one or more guanosine triphosphate protein–associated receptors on target cells.

In vitro, PAFs induce an impressive repertoire of responses, including phagocytosis, exocytosis, superoxide production, chemotaxis, aggregation, proliferation, adhesion, eicosanoid generation, degranulation, and calcium mobilization, as well as diverse morphologic changes. PAFs are a major regulator of cell adhesion and vascular permeability in many forms of acute inflammation, trauma, shock, and ischemia.

The precise role of PAFs in intraocular inflammation remains unknown, but synergistic interactions probably exist among PAFs, nitric oxide, eicosanoids, and cytokines. However, intravitreal injection of PAFs in animals induces an acute retinitis and photoreceptor toxicity.

Cytokines

Cytokines are soluble polypeptide mediators synthesized and released by cells for the purposes of intercellular signaling and communication. Table 1-3 lists examples of cytokines associated with ocular inflammation. Various types of intercellular signaling occur, including *paracrine* (signaling of neighboring cells at the same site), *autocrine* (stimulation of a receptor on its own surface, and *endocrine* (action on a distant site through release into the blood).

Traditionally, investigators have subdivided cytokines into families with related activities, sources, and targets, using terms such as *growth factors, interleukins, lymphokines, interferons, monokines,* and *chemokines.* Thus, *growth factor* traditionally refers to cytokines mediating cell proliferation and differentiation. The terms *interleukin* and *lymphokine* identify cytokines thought to mediate intercellular communication among lymphocytes or other leukocytes. Interferons are cytokines that limit or interfere with the ability of a virus to infect a cell. Monokines are immunoregulatory cytokines secreted by monocytes and macrophages. Chemokines are chemotactic cytokines. Although some cytokines are specific for particular cell types, most have such degrees of multiplicity and redundancy of source, function, and target that it is not particularly useful for the clinician to classify cytokines on the basis of the families discussed above. For example, activated macrophages in an inflammatory site synthesize growth factors, interleukins, interferons, and chemokines.

Both innate and adaptive responses result in the production of cytokines. T lymphocytes are the classic cytokine-producing cell of adaptive immunity, but macrophages, mast cells, and neutrophils also synthesize a wide range of cytokines upon stimulation. Cytokine

Table 1-3 Cytokines of Relevance to Ocular Immunology

Family	Example	Major Cell Source	Major Target Cells	Major General Actions	Specific Ocular Actions/ Clinical Relevance
Interleukins	IL-1β	Monocytes Macrophages Neutrophils Dendritic cells T cells	Most leukocytes Various ocular cells	Induce cyclooxygenase type 2 (COX-2) to induce fever, vasodilatation, hypotension (shock) Promote infiltration of inflammatory and immunocompetent cells into extravascular space and tissues Promote angiogenesis Induce IL-6 expression	Altered vascular permeability Neutrophil and macrophage infiltration Langerhans migration to central cornea Targeted by anakinra (IL-1 receptor antagonist) or anti-IL-1β antibody
	IL-2	Th0 or Th1 CD4 T lymphocytes	T lymphocytes B lymphocytes NK cells	Activates CD4 and CD8 T lymphocytes Induces Th1	Detectable levels in some forms of uveitis Targeted by daclizumab (anti-IL2 receptor antibody)
	IL-4	Th2 CD4 T lymphocytes Basophils, mast cells	T lymphocytes B lymphocytes	Induces Th2, blocks Th1 Induces B lymphocytes to make IgE	? Role in atopic and vernal conjunctivitis Increased in serum from patients with Behçet disease
	IL-5	Th2 CD4 T lymphocytes		Recruits eosinophils	? Role in atopic and vernal conjunctivitis
	IL-6	Monocytes Macrophages T lymphocytes Mast cells Endothelium	Most leukocytes Various ocular cells	Many actions on B lymphocytes including enhancement of antibody production Induce T-cell polarization Systematic toxicity (fever, shock, production of acute phase proteins from liver)	Altered vascular permeability Neutrophil infiltration High levels in serum, aqueous, and vitreous in many forms of uveitis and nonuveitic diseases Targeted by tocilizumab (anti-IL6 antibody)

Family	Example	Major Cell Source	Major Target Cells	Major General Actions	Specific Ocular Actions/ Clinical Relevance
	IL-12/23 (IL-12 family)	Macrophages Dendritic cells B lymphocytes (IL-23) Endothelium (IL-23)	Naive CD4 T lymphocytes	Key Th1-inducing cytokine Activates NK cells Mediates chronic inflammation through promotion of Th17 lymphocytes	High expression in aqueous and vitreous from idiopathic uveitis cases High expression in serum from Behçet disease and Vogt-Koyanagi-Harada syndrome Targeted by ustekinumab (binds the p40 subunit of IL-12 and IL-23)
	IL-17A	T lymphocytes (Th17, $\gamma\delta$) NKT lymphocytes	Most leukocytes Various ocular cells	Key cytokine of Th17 response, driving inflammation/tissue damage Induces proinflammatory cytokines, chemokines, and adhesion molecules Important driver of autoimmunity	High expression in patients with active uveitis, noninfectious (Behçet disease, Vogt-Koyanagi-Harada syndrome, birdshot chorioretinopathy, HLA-B27 uveitis) and infectious (viral retinitis, toxoplasmic retinochoroiditis). Leads to disruption of outer blood–retinal barrier (at RPE level)
Alpha chemokines	IL-8/CXCL8	Many cell types	Endothelial cells Neutrophils Many others	Recruits and activates neutrophils Upregulates CAM on endothelium Chemotactic for basophils and T lymphocytes Promotes angiogenesis	High expression in inflamed eye Altered vascular permeability Neutrophil infiltration
Beta chemokines	Macrophage chemotactic protein-1 (MCP-1)/CCL2	Macrophages Endothelium RPE	Endothelial cells Macrophages T lymphocytes	Recruits and activates macrophages, some T lymphocytes	High expression in noninflamed and inflamed eyes Recruits macrophages and T lymphocytes to eye
Tumor necrosis factors	TNF-α or -β	Macrophages (TNF-α) T lymphocytes (TNF-β)	Most leukocytes Various ocular cells	Tumor apoptosis Macrophage and neutrophil activation Cell adhesion and chemotaxis Fibrin deposition and vascular injury Systemic toxicity (fever, shock)	Altered vascular permeability Mononuclear cell infiltration Targeted by adalimumab, infliximab (and other anti-TNF-α antibodies)

(Continued)

Table 1-3 *(continued)*

Family	Example	Major Cell Source	Major Target Cells	Major General Actions	Specific Ocular Actions/ Clinical Relevance
Interferons	Interferon gamma (IFN-γ)	Th1 T lymphocytes NK cells	Macrophages Dendritic cells	Activates macrophages Facilitates Th1 development Mediates delayed-type hypersensitivity reactions	Neutrophil and macrophage infiltration MHC II upregulation on iris and ciliary epithelium, retinal pigment epithelium Can be pathogenic or protective against experimental uveitis depending on the stage at which it is produced
	IFN-α	Most leukocytes	Most parenchymal cells	Prevents viral infection of many cells Inhibits hemangioma, conjunctival intraepithelial neoplasia, and other tumors	Innate protection of ocular surface from viral infection, treatment of ocular surface neoplasms
Growth factors	Transforming growth factor β family (TGF-β)	Many cells Leukocytes, T lymphocytes RPE and NPE of ciliary body Pericytes Fibroblasts	Macrophages T lymphocytes RPE Glia Fibroblasts	Regulates immune response: suppresses T-lymphocyte and macrophage inflammatory functions Regulates wound repair: fibrosis of wounds	High expression in the resting, noninflamed eye Regulator of immune privilege and ACAID
	Platelet-derived growth factors	Platelets Macrophages RPE	Fibroblasts Glia Many others	Fibroblast proliferation	Role in inflammatory membranes, subretinal fibrosis
Neuropeptides	Substance P	Ocular nerves Mast cells	Leukocytes Others	Pain Altered vascular permeability	Altered vascular permeability Leukocyte infiltration, photophobia
	Vasoactive intestinal peptide	Ocular nerves	Leukocytes Others	Suppresses macrophage and T-lymphocyte inflammatory function	Role in ACAID and immune privilege

ACAID = anterior chamber–associated immune deviation; MHC = major histocompatibility complex; NK = natural killer; NPE = nonpigmented epithelium; RPE = retinal pigment epithelium; Th = T helper.

interactions can be additive, combinatorial, synergistic, or antagonistic. Elimination of the action of a single molecule may have an unpredictable outcome; for example, monoclonal antibodies directed against TNF-α result in substantial suppression of immune responses but also increase susceptibility to multiple sclerosis. Finally, not only do innate and adaptive immune responses use cytokines as mediators and amplifiers of inflammation, but cytokines also modulate the initiation of immune responses; the function of most leukocytes is altered by preexposure to various cytokines. Thus, for many cytokines, their regulatory role may be as important as their actions as mediators of inflammation.

Neutrophil-Derived Granule Products

Neutrophils are also a source of specialized products that can amplify immune responses. Many antimicrobial polypeptides are present in neutrophilic granules. The principal ones are bactericidal/permeability-increasing protein, defensins, lysozyme, lactoferrin, and the serine proteases.

In addition to antimicrobial polypeptides, neutrophils contain numerous other molecules that may contribute to inflammation. These compounds include hydrolytic enzymes, elastase, metalloproteinases, gelatinase, myeloperoxidase, vitamin B_{12}–binding protein, cytochrome b_{558}, and others. Granule contents remain inert and membrane-bound when the granules are intact and become active and soluble when granules fuse to the phagocytic vesicles or plasma membrane.

An example of a neutrophil-derived granule product is collagenase. Various forms of collagenase contribute to corneal injury and liquefaction during bacterial keratitis and scleritis, especially in infections with *Pseudomonas* species. Collagenases also contribute to peripheral corneal melting syndromes secondary to rheumatoid arthritis–associated peripheral keratitis.

CHAPTER 2

Immunization and Adaptive Immunity: The Immune Response Arc and Immune Effectors

Highlights

- Adaptive (or acquired) immunity is a "learned" response to specific antigens rather than a response to conserved patterns.
- The adaptive immune system continuously samples antigenic epitopes, determines if they are "self" or "nonself" then mounts an immune response to eliminate foreign antigens.
- Conversion of an antigenic stimulus to an immune response involves activation of immune cells, particularly T and B lymphocytes, and development of memory for that specific antigen.
- The adaptive immune response has two arms/compartments that closely interact with each other, one of humoral defense, employing soluble antibodies secreted by plasma cells and another of cell-mediated defense, coordinated by T lymphocytes.
- The cell-mediated responses (particularly Th1, Th2, and Th17 types) are very relevant to the immunopathology of several intraocular inflammatory conditions.

Definitions

The term *antigen* refers to a substance recognized by the immune system. The term *epitope* refers to each specific portion of an antigen to which the immune system can respond. Antigenic epitopes exist on both native self tissues as well as foreign nonself tissues. A complex, 3-dimensional protein has multiple antigenic epitopes that the immune system can recognize as well as many other sites that remain invisible to the immune system.

The adaptive immune response, unlike the innate immune response discussed in Chapter 1, is a learned response to highly variable but specific antigenic epitopes rather than a response to conserved patterns. The purpose of the adaptive immune system is to continuously sample antigenic epitopes, determine if they are self or nonself, and then mount an immune response to eliminate foreign antigens. Several immunologic concepts, especially those of the immune response arc, the primary adaptive immune response, and the secondary adaptive immune response, are involved in this process. See Clinical Example 2-1.

Analogous to the neural reflex arc, the immune response arc—the interaction between antigen and the adaptive immune system—can be subdivided into 3 phases: afferent, processing, and effector (Fig 2-1).

CLINICAL EXAMPLE 2-1

Primary and secondary response to tuberculosis The afferent phase of the primary response begins after the inhalation of live organisms, which proliferate slowly within the lung. Alveolar macrophages ingest the bacteria and transport the organisms to the hilar lymph nodes, where the processing phase begins. Over the next few days, as T and B lymphocytes are primed, the hilar nodes become enlarged because of the increased number of dividing T and B lymphocytes as well as the generalized increased trafficking of other lymphocytes through the nodes. The effector phase begins when the primed T lymphocytes recirculate and enter the infected lung. The T lymphocytes interact with the macrophage-ingested bacteria, and cytokines are released that activate neighboring macrophages to differentiate into epithelioid cells and to fuse into giant cells, eventually forming caseating granulomas. Meanwhile, some of the effector T lymphocytes home to other lymph nodes throughout the body, where they become inactive memory T lymphocytes, trafficking and recirculating throughout the secondary lymphoid tissue.

A secondary response in the skin is the basis of the tuberculin skin test used to diagnose tuberculosis (TB). The afferent phase of the secondary response begins when a purified protein derivative (PPD) reagent (antigens purified from nontuberculous mycobacteria) is injected into the dermis. These antigens are taken up by dermal macrophages.

The secondary processing phase begins when these PPD-stimulated macrophages migrate into the draining lymph node, where they encounter memory T lymphocytes from the previous lung infection. This leads to reactivation of memory T lymphocytes.

The secondary effector phase commences when the reactivated memory T lymphocytes recirculate and home back into the dermis, where they encounter additional antigen and macrophages at the injection site, causing the T lymphocytes to become fully activated and release cytokines. Within 24–72 hours, the cytokines induce infiltration of additional lymphocytes and monocytes as well as fibrin clotting. This process produces the typical indurated dermal lesion of the TB skin test, called the *tuberculin form* of delayed hypersensitivity (DH). Some individuals, however, are not able to mount a robust DH immune response, explaining the situation of a negative PPD result in the face of active infection (anergy).

A disadvantage of skin testing is the need to examine the injection site 48–72 hours later. The interferon-gamma release assays (IGRAs) eliminate this disadvantage. In this testing method, peripheral blood is collected and exposed to specific *M tuberculosis* antigens. If a patient has been exposed to TB, circulating T lymphocytes that are TB antigen specific should be present. When exposed to TB antigen, the T cells release interferon gamma (IFN-γ), which can be measured either as the concentration of IFN-γ or as the number of cells releasing IFN-γ.

Phases of the Immune Response Arc

Afferent Phase

The afferent phase of the immune response arc comprises the initial recognition, transport, and presentation of antigenic substances to the adaptive immune system. Recognition starts with antigen-presenting cells (APCs), which are specialized cells that bind

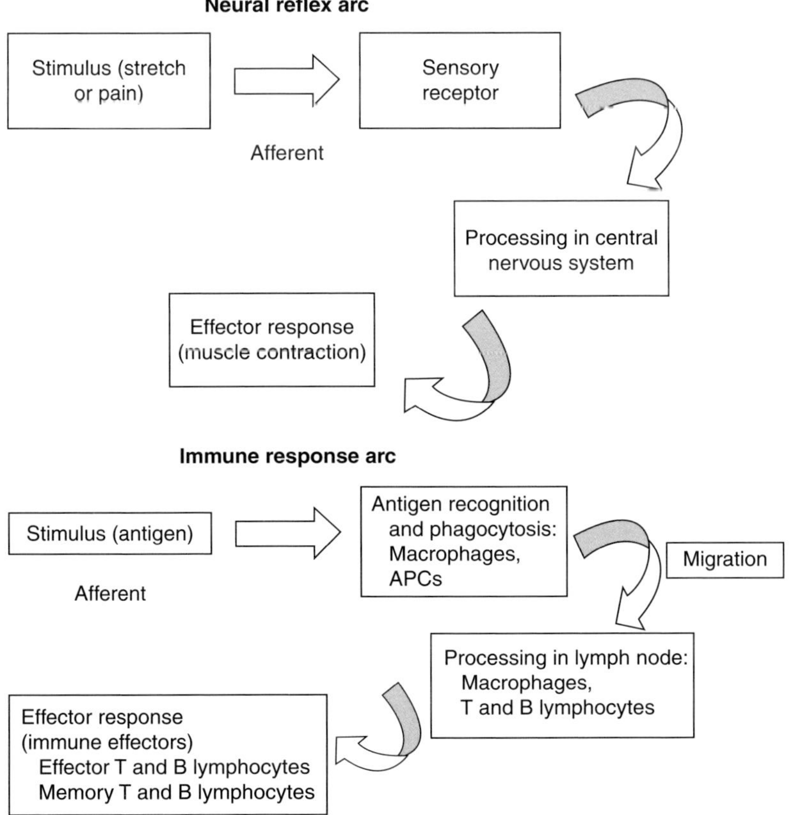

Figure 2-1 Comparison between the neural reflex arc and the immune response arc. APCs = antigen-presenting cells.

antigen at a site. After the APC receives stimulatory signals (ie, complement), phagocytosis of the antigen occurs, as discussed in Chapter 1. Following ingestion of antigen, APCs migrate via afferent lymphatics to lymph nodes. Afferent lymphatic channels, usually simply termed *lymphatics,* are vein-like structures that drain extracellular fluid (ie, lymph) from a site into a regional lymph node. Lymphatics serve 2 major purposes: to convey immune cells and to carry whole antigen from the site of inoculation to a lymph node. In the APCs, enzymatic digestion of proteins within endocytic vesicles produces short chains of 7–11 amino acids: the antigenic epitopic fragments. Each antigenic fragment is combined with a groove-shaped human leukocyte antigen (HLA) peptide residing on the APC surface, and this surface complex contains a unique epitope. The combination of peptide and HLA protein is recognized by the T-lymphocyte receptors CD4 and CD8. HLA molecules vary in their capacity to bind various antigenic peptide fragments within their groove, and thus the HLA type determines the repertoire of peptide antigens capable of being presented to T lymphocytes. Specific HLA alleles are important risk factors for certain forms of uveitis. See Chapter 4 for further discussion of HLA molecules and disease susceptibility.

Major histocompatibility complex (MHC) class I molecules (ie, HLA-A, -B, and -C) serve as the antigen-presenting platform for $CD8^+$ T lymphocytes, which are essentially cytotoxic T cells (Fig 2-2). Class I molecules are present on almost all nucleated cells and generally function to process peptide antigens synthesized by the host cell. If these presented antigens are recognized as self (ie, normal host protein), no immune reaction occurs. However, if there is an alteration of the normal host peptide (termed *altered self*), by tumor or viral peptides after host cell invasion, an immune response is initiated. A viral infection, a neoplasm, or simply a genetic mutation that alters protein structure could also induce autoimmunity by stimulating an inappropriate immune response to normal host proteins.

MHC class II molecules (ie, HLA-DR, -DP, and -DQ) serve as the antigen-presenting platform for $CD4^+$, or *helper,* T lymphocytes (Fig 2–3). The antigen receptor on the helper T lymphocyte can recognize peptide antigens only if the antigens are presented with class II molecules simultaneously. Only certain cell types express MHC class II molecules. Macrophages and dendritic cells are the most important of these types, though B lymphocytes can also function as class II–dependent APCs, especially within a lymph node. Class II–dependent APCs are considered the most efficient APCs for processing extracellular protein antigens; that is, antigens that have been phagocytosed from the external environment (eg, bacterial or fungal antigens).

Processing Phase

The conversion of an antigenic stimulus into an immunologic response occurs through *priming* of naive B and T lymphocytes (lymphocytes that have not yet encountered their specific antigen) within lymph nodes and the spleen. This conversion is also called *activation,* or *sensitization,* of lymphocytes. Processing involves regulation of the interaction between antigen and naive lymphocytes, followed by lymphocyte activation (Fig 2–4).

Preconditions necessary for processing

$CD4^+$ T lymphocytes are the principal cell type for immune processing. These lymphocytes have a receptor that detects antigen only upon formation of a trimolecular complex

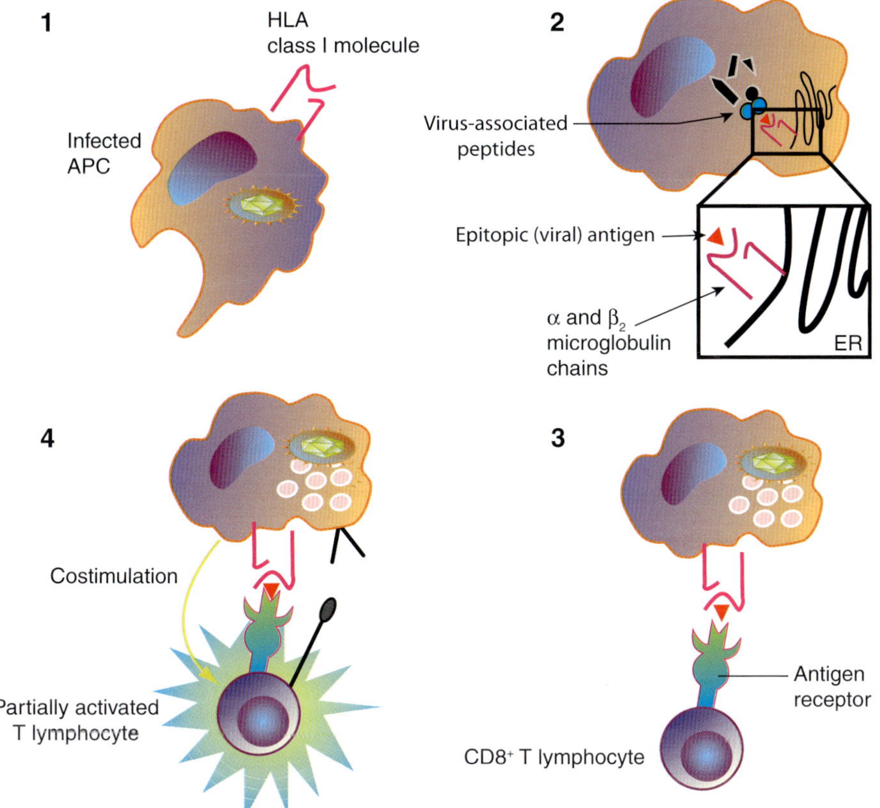

Figure 2-2 Class I–dependent antigen-presenting cells (APCs). **1,** APC is infected by a virus, which causes the cell to synthesize virus-associated peptides that are present in the cytosol. **2,** The viral antigen must be transported (through specialized transporter systems) into the endosomal compartment (endoplasmic reticulum, ER), where the viral antigen encounters human leukocyte antigen (HLA) class I molecules. The fragment is placed into the pocket formed by the α chain of the class I HLA molecule. Unlike class II molecules, the second chain, called β_2-microglobulin, is constant among all class I molecules. **3,** The CD8 T-lymphocyte receptor recognizes the fragment–class I complex displayed on the cell membrane. **4,** With the help of costimulatory molecules such as CD28-B7 and cytokines, the $CD8^+$ T lymphocyte becomes primed, or partially activated. A similar mechanism is used to recognize tumor antigens that are produced by cells after malignant transformation. *(Illustration by Barb Cousins, modified by Joyce Zavarro.)*

consisting of an HLA molecule, a processed antigen fragment, and a T-lymphocyte antigen receptor. The $CD4^+$ molecule stabilizes binding and enhances signaling between the HLA complex on the APC and the T-lymphocyte receptor. When helper T lymphocytes recognize their specific antigen, they become primed and partially activated, acquiring new functional properties, including cell division, cytokine synthesis, and cell membrane expression of *accessory molecules,* such as cell-adhesion molecules and costimulatory molecules. The synthesis and release of immune cytokines, especially interleukin-2 (IL-2), by T lymphocytes is crucial for the progression of initial activation and the functional differentiation of T lymphocytes through autocrine stimulation.

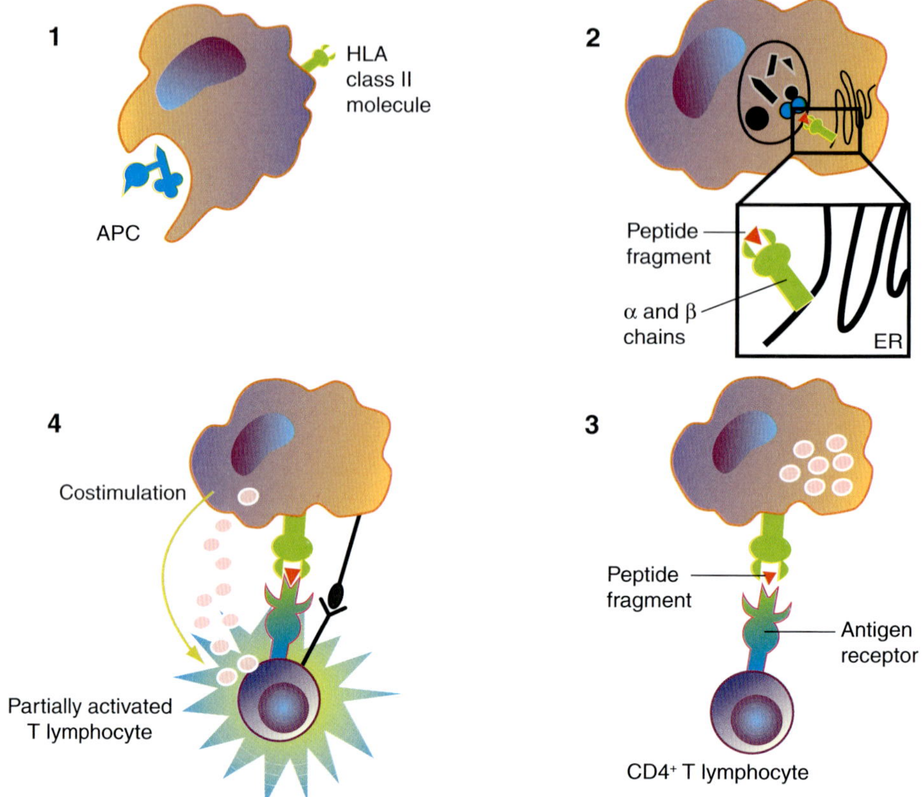

Figure 2-3 Class II–dependent antigen-presenting cells. **1,** APCs endocytose exogenous antigens into the endosomal compartment. **2,** There, the antigen is digested into peptide fragments and placed into the groove formed by the α and β chains of the HLA class II molecule. **3,** The $CD4^+$ T-lymphocyte receptor recognizes the fragment–class II complex. **4,** With the help of costimulatory molecules such as CD28-B7 and cytokines, the $CD4^+$ T lymphocyte becomes primed, or partially activated. *(Illustration by Barb Cousins, modified by Joyce Zavarro.)*

Helper T-lymphocyte differentiation

At the stage of initial priming, $CD4^+$ T lymphocytes are classified as T helper-0 (Th0) cells. These cells can differentiate into functional subsets based on the pattern of cytokines to which they are exposed. Each T-helper (Th) subset produces a characteristic profile of cytokines that is regulated by the expression of subset-specific transcription factors. When the Th subsets were discovered, only 2 were defined: T helper-1 (Th1) and T helper-2 (Th2). Th1 cells secrete interferon gamma (IFN-γ), IL-2, and tumor necrosis factor α and β (TNF-α, TNF-β), whereas Th2 cells produce IL-4, IL-5, and IL-10 but not Th1 cytokines. The T-bet transcription factor directs the Th1 cytokine production. The GATA3 transcription factor regulates Th2 cytokines. The Th2 subset is involved in the clearance of extracellular pathogens and plays an important role in the pathogenesis of allergic conditions such as asthma. Th1 cells participate in the elimination of intracellular pathogens as well as cell-mediated and delayed-type hypersensitivity reactions.

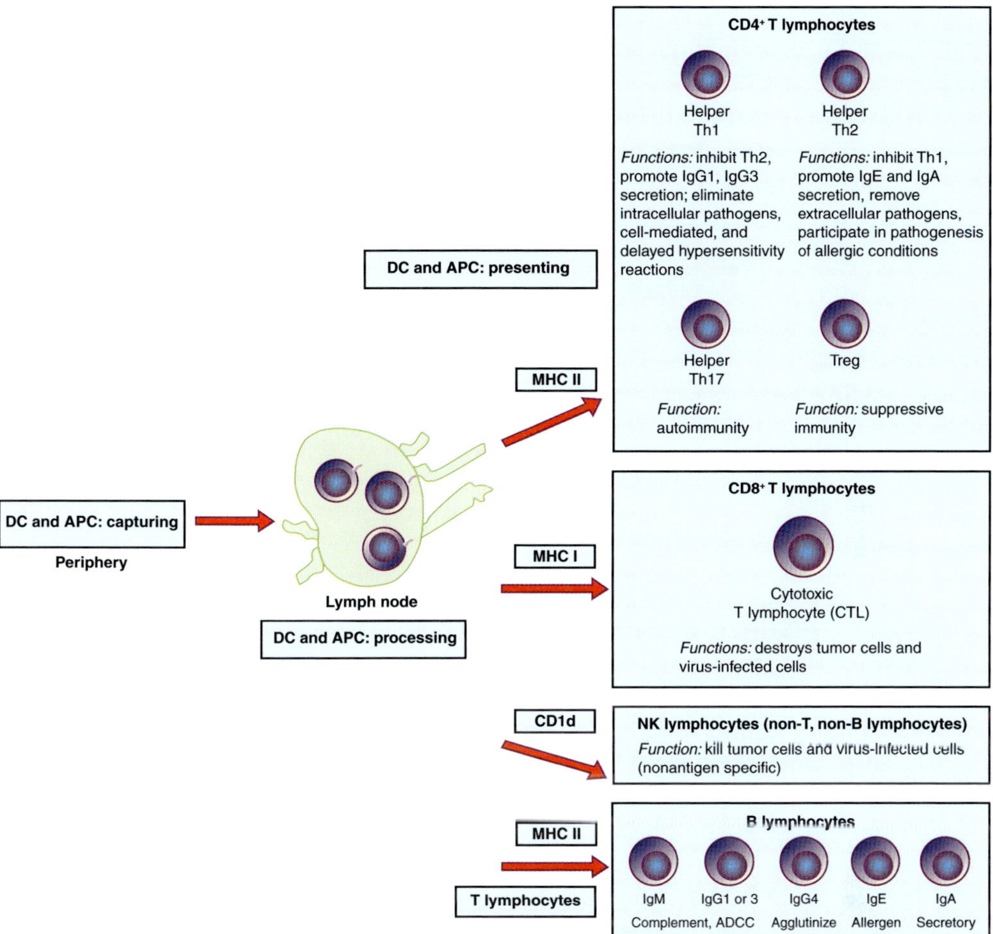

Figure 2-4 Schematic illustration of immune processing of antigen within the lymph node. On exposure to antigen and APCs within the lymph node, the 3 major lymphocyte subsets—B lymphocytes, CD4+ T lymphocytes, and CD8+ T lymphocytes—and NK (non-T, non-B) lymphocytes are activated to release specific cytokines and perform specific functional activities. B lymphocytes are stimulated to produce one of the various antibody isotypes, whose functions include complement activation, antibody-dependent cellular cytotoxicity (ADCC), agglutination, allergen recognition, and release into secretions. CD4+ T lymphocytes become activated into T helper-1 (Th1), T helper-2 (Th2), T regulatory (Treg), or T helper-17 (TH17) subsets. Naive CD8+ T cells become cytotoxic T lymphocytes (CTLs), and non-T, non-B lymphocytes become natural killer (NK) lymphocytes. *(Illustration by Barb Cousins, modified by Joyce Zavarro.)*

Originally, the Th1 subset was thought to be the causal agent in autoimmunity, as transfer of antigen-specific Th1 cells produces autoimmune disease in experimental animal models, and elevated levels of IFN-γ have been detected in areas of inflammation in vivo. Subsequently, research has suggested that other Th subsets, especially Th17 and T regulatory (Treg) cells, play crucial roles in chronic inflammation and autoimmunity, and there is probably plasticity between Th1, Th17, and Treg cells.

Th17 cells produce IL-17, IL-21, IL-22, and IL-24 in association with several transcription factors, including retinoic acid receptor–related orphan receptor-γt and receptor-α, (ROR-γt and -α). Th17 cells contribute to immunity against certain extracellular bacteria and fungi and play a role in the defense of mucosal surfaces. Dysregulation of Th17 proinflammatory cytokines IL-17 and IL-22 has been implicated in systemic inflammatory diseases, such as psoriasis, rheumatoid arthritis, multiple sclerosis, inflammatory bowel disease, Sjögren syndrome, Behçet disease, and systemic lupus erythematosus, as well as in uveitis and scleritis. See Clinical Example 2-2.

T regulatory cells are identified by their simultaneous expression of CD4, CD25, and Foxp3 (a transcriptional regulator protein) and can be divided into 2 types, naturally occurring T regulatory (nTreg) cells and inducible T regulatory (iTreg) or adaptive Treg cells. The nTreg cells appear to be generated in the thymus during development. They are essential to self-tolerance, the process by which autoreactive T cells are minimized

CLINICAL EXAMPLE 2-2

The role of Th17 cells in birdshot chorioretinopathy Birdshot chorioretinopathy (BSCR) is a severe, progressive, posterior uveitis. It is typically characterized by multiple distinctive choroidal lesions in the fundus (not always apparent in the initial phase of the disease), vitritis, and retinal vasculitis leading to diffuse capillary leakage and macular/optic disc edema. Uncontrolled BSCR usually leads to extensive retinal atrophy with visual field loss, floaters, glare, and blurred vision. Significant electroretinographic abnormalities are clinically manifested by poor vision in dim lighting, and loss of color and contrast sensitivity. While the link between HLA-A29 and BSCR is well known, the precise pathogenesis of the disease is still unclear. Histopathologic evidence has demonstrated that BSCR choroidal and vitreal infiltrates are predominantly composed of T cells. Studies of cytokine levels suggest that Th17 cells may play an important role in BSCR. The cytokines IL-1β, IL-6, and TGF-β, which contribute to the differentiation of Th17 cells, have been found to be elevated in ocular fluids and serum of BSCR patients. Elevation of IL-17, the hallmark cytokine of Th17, has also been measured in serum from BSCR patients. Elevations of these cytokines have been demonstrated in other types of noninfectious ocular inflammatory disorders, including idiopathic uveitis, Behçet disease, and even scleritis. Knowledge of the role of Th17 in some types of uveitis may guide treatment with commercially available biologic agents that target Th17 cell activity directly or indirectly. Studies of the efficacy of such agents including secukinumab (anti-IL-17), ustekinumab (anti-IL-12 and 23), and tocilizumab (anti-IL-6) as treatment for uveitis are ongoing.

Kuiper J, Rothova A, de Boer J, Radstake T. The immunopathogenesis of birdshot chorioretinopathy; a bird of many feathers. *Prog Retin Eye Res.* 2015;44:99–110.

and their function downregulated. Treg cells are essential for maintaining peripheral tolerance to self-antigens, thereby preventing autoimmune diseases and limiting chronic inflammatory diseases. Furthermore, Treg cells suppress excessive immune responses deleterious to the host. As a result, these cells play a central role in autoimmune diseases, transplantation tolerance, infectious diseases, allergic disease, and tumor immunity. The suppressive cytokines transforming growth factor β (TGF-β) and IL-10 have been implicated as active players in the effector function of Treg cells as regulators of inflammation. An imbalance between regulatory mechanisms that inhibit the immune system and active proinflammatory mechanisms is thought to be the underlying cause of uveitis and many other immune-mediated diseases.

The cytokine profiles produced by these various Th cell types determine subsequent immune processing, B-lymphocyte antibody synthesis, and cell-mediated effector responses. For example, IFN-γ, produced by Th1 lymphocytes, blocks the differentiation and activation of Th2 lymphocytes, whereas IL-4, produced by Th2 lymphocytes, blocks the differentiation of Th1 lymphocytes. The process determining whether a Th1 or a Th2 response develops consequent to exposure to a specific antigen is not entirely understood, but presumed variables include cytokines preexisting in the microenvironment, the nature and amount of antigen encountered, and the type of APC involved. For example, IL-12, which is produced by macrophage APCs, might preferentially induce Th1 responses.

Abbas AK, Lichtman AH, Pillai S. *Cellular and Molecular Immunology*. 9th ed. Philadelphia, PA: Elsevier/Saunders; 2018.

Amadi-Obi A, Yu CR, Liu X, et al. Th17 cells contribute to uveitis and scleritis and are expanded by IL-2 and inhibited by IL-27/STAT1. *Nat Med.* 2007;13(6):711–718.

Caspi R. Autoimmunity in the immune privileged eye: pathogenic and regulatory T cells. *Immunol Res.* 2008;42(1–3):41–50.

B-lymphocyte activation

A major function of helper T lymphocytes is B-lymphocyte activation. B lymphocytes are responsible for producing antibodies (glycoproteins that bind to a specific antigen, the epitope). These antibodies contain an epitope-specific binding site, termed *paratope,* on the Fab (*f*ragment, *a*ntigen-*b*inding) portion of the molecule. B lymphocytes begin as naive lymphocytes, with immunoglobulins M (IgM) and D (IgD) on their cell surfaces serving as B-lymphocyte antigen receptors. Through these surface antibodies, B lymphocytes detect epitopes on intact antigens *without* the requirement of antigen processing by APCs. After appropriate stimulation of the B-lymphocyte antigen receptor, helper T lymphocyte–B lymphocyte interaction occurs, leading to further B-lymphocyte activation and differentiation. B lymphocytes acquire new functional properties, such as cell division, cell surface expression of accessory molecules, and synthesis of large quantities of antibody. The terminal form of B lymphocyte differentiation is the plasma cell that secretes antibodies. Activated B lymphocytes acquire the ability to change antibody class from IgM to another class (eg, to IgG, IgA, or IgE). This class shift requires a molecular change in the immunoglobulin heavy chain, a process regulated by specific cytokines released by the helper T lymphocyte. For example, treatment of an antigen-primed B lymphocyte with IFN-γ induces a switch from IgM to IgG1 production. Treatment with IL-4 induces a switch from IgM to IgE production.

Effector Phase

The purpose of the adaptive immune response (ie, the elimination or neutralization of foreign antigen) is accomplished during the effector phase. Antigen-specific effectors exist in 2 major subsets:

- T lymphocytes
- B lymphocytes and the antibodies produced by their derived plasma cells

Effector lymphocytes require 2 exposures to antigen for maximum effectiveness. The initial (*priming,* or *activation*) exposure occurs in the lymph node. The second *(restimulation)* exposure occurs in the peripheral tissue from which the antigen originated.

Effector T lymphocytes consist primarily of 2 types, as determined by their different responses on experimental assays and different cell surface molecules (Fig 2-5). *Delayed hypersensitivity* (DH) T lymphocytes usually express CD4 (and thus recognize antigen with MHC class II) and release IFN-γ and TNF-β. They function by encountering antigen presented by APCs in a tissue site, becoming fully activated, and releasing cytokines and mediators that recruit nonspecific, antigen-independent effector cells such as neutrophils, basophils, or monocytes (discussed in Chapter 1). As with helper T lymphocytes, Th1 and Th2 types of DH effector cells have been identified. *Cytotoxic* T lymphocytes express CD8

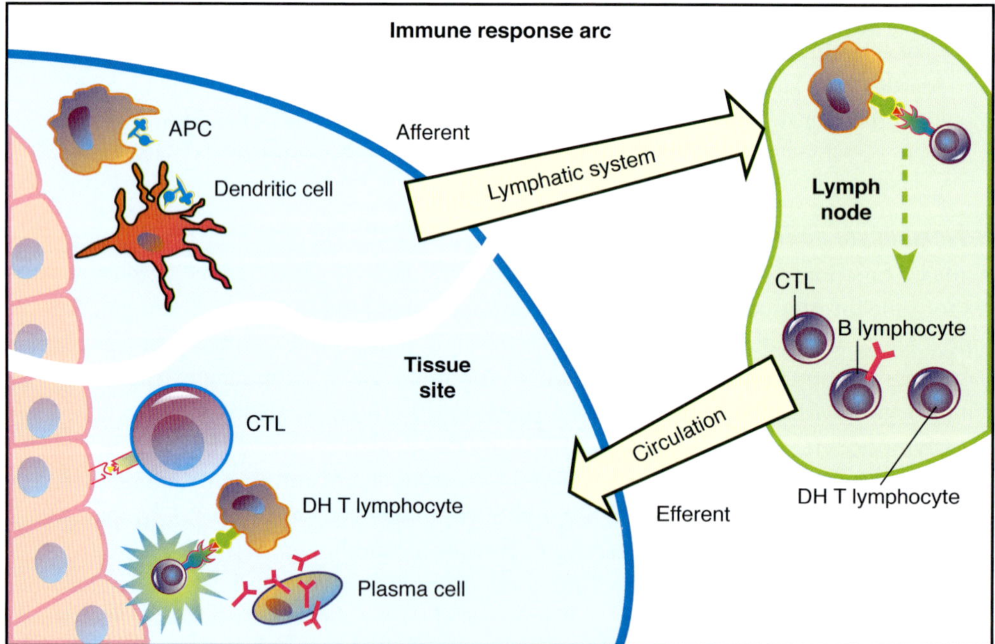

Figure 2-5 Schematic representation of effector mechanisms during adaptive immunity. The tissue site *(left)* is not only where the immune response is initiated but is also ultimately where the immune response arc is completed—when effectors encounter antigen within tissue after their release into the circulation from the lymph node *(right).* The 3 most important effector mechanisms of adaptive immunity are cytotoxic T lymphocytes (CTLs), delayed hypersensitivity (DH) T lymphocytes (CD4-Th lymphocytes), and antibody-plasma cells derived from B lymphocytes. *(Illustration by Barb Cousins, modified by Joyce Zavarro.)*

and serve to kill tumor cells and virus-infected host cells. They accomplish this function through the release of cytokines (eg, IFN-γ, TNF-α, and TNF-β) or specialized cytotoxic pore-forming and apoptosis-activating molecules such as perforin and granzymes. A third subset of effector lymphocytes, grouped as non-T, non-B lymphocytes, includes natural killer cells, lymphokine-activated cells, and killer cells.

Antibodies, or *immunoglobulins,* are produced by plasma cells derived from B lymphocytes after appropriate antigenic stimulation with T-lymphocyte help. Plasma cells initially secrete IgM antibodies, followed later by production of other isotypes after antibody-class switching. Antibodies are released into the efferent lymph fluid (downstream from lymph nodes), draining into the venous circulation. Once bound to their specific epitope, antibodies mediate a variety of immune effector activities, including opsonization for phagocytosis and complement activation via the classical pathway.

Immune Response Arc and Primary or Secondary Immune Response

Immunologic memory is the most distinctive feature of adaptive immunity, with protective immunization the prototypical example of this powerful phenomenon.

Differences Between Primary and Secondary Responses

The idea of an *anamnestic response* posits that the second encounter with an antigen is regulated differently from the first. During the processing phase of the primary response, relatively rare antigen-specific B lymphocytes (perhaps 1 in 100,000 B lymphocytes) and T lymphocytes (perhaps 1 in 10,000 T lymphocytes) must come in contact with appropriately presented antigen. Stimulation of these cells from a completely resting and naive state then occurs, a process that requires days. Following the primary response, various events occur that set the stage for a subsequent rapid and robust secondary response:

- Following stimulation, lymphocytes divide, dramatically increasing the population of antigen-responsive T and B lymphocytes (clonal expansion). In addition, these cells migrate to other sites of potential encounter with antigen.
- Upon removal of antigen, T and B lymphocytes activated during the primary response gradually return to a resting state but are no longer naive. They retain the capacity to become reactivated within 12–24 hours of antigen exposure and thus are termed *memory cells.*
- IgM produced during the primary response is often too large (molecular mass, 900 kDa) to leak passively into a peripheral site. Following antibody-class switching, IgG or other isotypes can leak passively into a site or are already present because they were produced at the site; thus, they can immediately combine with antigen and trigger a very rapid response.
- In some cases, such as in mycobacterial infection, low doses of antigen may remain in the node or site, producing a chronic, low-level, continuous antigenic stimulation of T and B lymphocytes.

Homing

Memory also requires that lymphocytes demonstrate a complex migratory pattern called *homing.* Thus, lymphocytes pass from the circulation into various tissues, from which they subsequently depart, and then pass by way of lymphatics to reenter the circulation. Homing involves the dynamic interaction between lymphocytes and endothelial cells using multiple cell-adhesion molecules. Usually the major types of lymphocytes that migrate into tissue sites are memory lymphocytes that express higher levels of certain cell-adhesion molecules, such as the integrins, than do naive cells. In contrast, naive lymphocytes tend to migrate to lymphoid tissues, where they may meet their cognate antigen. Inflammation, however, changes the rules and breaks down homing patterns. At inflammatory sites, the volume of lymphocyte migration is far greater and selection much less precise, although migration of memory cells or activated lymphocytes still exceeds that of naive cells.

Effector Responses of Adaptive Immunity

Traditionally, 4 mechanisms of adaptive immune-triggered inflammatory responses were recognized:

- anaphylaxis
- antibody-dependent cellular cytotoxicity (ADCC)
- immune complex reactions
- cell-mediated reactions

Coombs and Gell elaborated on these mechanisms in 1962. A fifth category, *stimulatory hypersensitivity,* was described later. This system predated the discovery of T lymphocytes, at a time when understanding was limited to antibody-triggered mechanisms. Familiarity with Coombs and Gell type reactions is important for interpretation of older literature. However, it is more accurate to divide the effector responses of adaptive immunity into 3 main categories (Table 2-1):

- antibody-mediated effector responses
- lymphocyte-mediated effector responses: delayed hypersensitivity, cytotoxic lymphocytes
- combined antibody and cellular mechanisms

Delves PJ, Martin SJ, Burton DR, Roitt IM. *Roitt's Essential Immunology.* 13th ed. Hoboken, NJ: Wiley-Blackwell; 2017.

Owen JA, Punt J, Stranford SA. *Kuby Immunology.* 7th ed. New York, NY: WH Freeman; 2013.

Table 2-1 Types of Effector Responses of Adaptive Immunity

Types of Effector Responses
Antibody-mediated effector responses
Lymphocyte-mediated effector responses
Delayed hypersensitivity
Cytotoxic lymphocytes
Combined antibody and cellular mechanisms

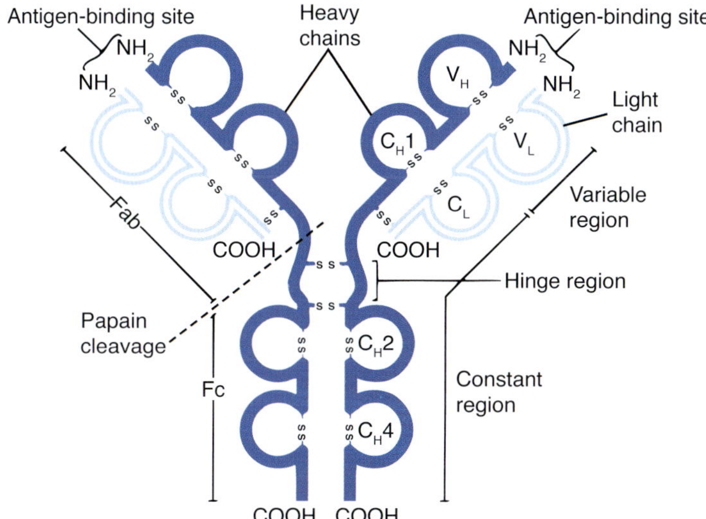

Figure 2-6 Schematic representation of an immunoglobulin (Ig) molecule. The *solid lines* indicate the identical 2 heavy chains; the *light blue double lines* indicate the identical light chains; *-s s-* indicates intrachain and interchain covalent disulfide bonds. Fab = *f*ragment, *a*ntigen-*b*inding region; Fc = *f*ragment *c*rystallizable region (attachment site for effector cells). *(Reprinted with permission from* Dorland's Illustrated Medical Dictionary. *32nd ed. Philadelphia, PA: Elsevier/Saunders; 2012:921.)*

Antibody-Mediated Immune Effector Responses

Structural and functional properties of antibody molecules

Structural features of immunoglobulins Five major classes of immunoglobulin (M, G, A, E, and D) exist, with 9 subclasses or isotypes (IgG1, IgG2, IgG3, IgG4, IgM, IgA1, IgA2, IgE, and IgD). The basic immunoglobulin structure is composed of 4 covalently bonded glycoprotein chains that form a monomer of approximately 150,000–180,000 Da (Fig 2-6). Each antibody monomer contains 2 identical light chains, either kappa (κ) or lambda (λ), and 2 identical heavy chains from 1 of the 9 distinct subclasses of immunoglobulins; the type of heavy chain defines the specific isotype. IgM can form pentamers or hexamers in vivo, and IgA can form dimers in secretions, so the in vivo molecular size of these 2 classes is much larger than that of the others.

Antibodies contain regions called *domains* that carry out the specific functions of the antibody molecule. The Fab region (2 of which are present on each molecule) contains the antigen-binding domain, called the *hypervariable region.* The opposite end of the molecule, on the heavy chain portion, contains the attachment site for effector cells (the *Fc portion,* for *f*ragment *c*rystallizable). It also contains the site of other effector functions, such as complement fixation (for IgG3) or binding to a secretory component for transportation through epithelia and secretion into tears (for IgA). Table 2-2 summarizes the important structural differences among immunoglobulin isotypes.

Functional properties of immunoglobulins Immunoglobulin isotypes differ in how they mediate effector functions of antibody activity. Human IgM and IgG3 are good complement

Table 2-2 Structural and Functional Properties of Immunoglobulin Isotypes

	Structural Properties		Functional Properties		
Immunoglobulin (Ig) Isotype (Heavy Chain)	**% of Total Serum Igs**	**Structural Features**	**Activates Complement**	**Fc Receptor Binding Preferences**	**Other Functions**
IgD δ	<1%	Mostly on surface of B lymphocytes	No	NA	B-lymphocyte antigen receptor
IgM μ	5%	Mostly on B lymphocytes or intravascular	Strong (classic pathway)	NA	B-lymphocyte antigen receptor, agglutination, neutralization, intravascular cytolysis
IgG1 γ	50%	Intravascular, in tissues, crosses placenta	Moderate (classic pathway)	Monocytes	Cytolysis
IgG2 γ	18%	Same as IgG1	Weak (classic pathway)	Neutrophil monocytes, killer lymphocytes	ADCC
IgG3 γ	6%	Same as IgG1	Strong (classic pathway)	Neutrophil monocytes, killer lymphocytes	ADCC, agglutination, cytolysis
IgG4 γ	3%	Same as IgG1	No	NA	Neutralization
IgE ε	<1%	Mostly in skin or mucosa, bound to mast cells	No	Mast cells	Mast-cell degranulation
IgA1 α	15%	In mucosal secretions, binds secretory component in subepithelial tissues for transepithelial transport and protection from proteolysis	Moderate (alternative pathway)	NA	Mucosal immunity, neutralization
IgA2 α	3%	Same as IgA1	Same as IgA1	NA	NA

ADCC = antibody-dependent cellular cytotoxicity; NA = not applicable.

activators, whereas IgG4 is not. Only IgA1 and IgA2 can bind the secretory component and be actively passed into mucosal secretions. The importance of these differences is that 2 antibodies with identical capacity to bind to an antigen—but of different isotype—will produce different effector and inflammatory outcomes.

Terminology

Clonality Each B cell creates, via genetic recombination, a unique Fab fragment that recognizes a single antigenic configuration. Proliferation of an individual B cell via cell division produces daughter cells that contain the same antigenic configuration. Continual clonal expansion results in a population of identical cells that recognize the same epitope, termed a *monoclonal* population. However, a foreign substance has many antigenic epitopes. Thus, many individual B cells will recognize various epitopes on the same substance, and each B cell will undergo simultaneous clonal expansion. The sum reactivity of all these antibodies is a *polyclonal response* that characterizes the typical immune response. Modern molecular biologic techniques allow the amplification of a single B-cell clone and production of large amounts of monoclonal antibodies for therapeutic purposes. Biologic drugs such as infliximab, adalimumab, and rituximab are examples of recombinant monoclonal antibodies.

Idiotypes Because they are proteins, antibodies themselves can be antigenic. Their antigenic sites are called *idiotopes,* as distinguished from *epitopes,* the antigenic sites on foreign molecules. Antibodies to idiotopes are called *idiotypes.* Anti-idiotypic antibodies may function as feedback mechanisms for immune regulation and have clinical significance for modern biologic therapies. Infliximab, for example, is a monoclonal chimeric (mouse and human) antibody to TNF-α that is used to treat some forms of uveitis. Efficacy of this drug may be limited by the development of anti-idiotype antibodies that neutralize the antigen binding site for TNF-α.

Infiltration of B lymphocytes into tissues and local production of antibody

B-lymphocyte infiltration B lymphocytes can infiltrate the site of an immunologic reaction in response to persistent antigenic stimulus. If the process becomes chronic, plasma cell formation occurs, with local production of antibody specific for the inciting antigen(s). If the antigen is known or suspected, as in the case of a presumed infection, assessment of local antibody production can serve as a diagnostic test.

Differentiation between local production of antibody and passive leakage from the blood to the intraocular compartment involves determination of the *Goldmann-Witmer* (GW) *coefficient.* This is calculated by comparing the ratio of specific IgG antibody present in intraocular fluid to the total IgG level in intraocular fluid versus the ratio of specific IgG level in serum to the total IgG level in serum:

GW coefficient = [intraocular specific IgG/intraocular total IgG] /
[serum specific IgG/serum total IgG]

The GW coefficient is used clinically in Europe, where an index of more than 3 indicates intraocular infection by the specific pathogen against which the antibody was produced. The GW coefficient was used to demonstrate that aqueous from eyes with Fuchs uveitis syndrome (FUS) had markedly elevated intraocular IgG titers to rubella virus compared with levels found in controls. The average GW coefficient was 20.6 in FUS patients, compared with less than 1.4 in controls.

Local antibody production within a tissue and chronic inflammation Persistence of antigen within a site, coupled with infiltration of specific B lymphocytes and local antibody formation, can produce a chronic inflammatory reaction called the *chronic Arthus reaction.* The histologic pattern often demonstrates lymphocytic infiltration, plasma cell infiltration, and granulomatous features. This mechanism may contribute to the pathophysiology of certain chronic autoimmune disorders, such as rheumatoid arthritis, which feature formation of pathogenic antibodies.

Abbas AK, Lichtman AH, Pillai S. Cellular and Molecular Immunology. 9th ed. Philadelphia, PA: Elsevier/Saunders; 2018.

Foster CS, Streilein JW, Coma MC. Immune-mediated tissue injury. In: Albert DM, Jakobiec FA, Azar DT, Gragoudas ES, eds. *Principles and Practice of Ophthalmology.* 3rd ed. Philadelphia, PA: WB Saunders; 2008:chap 9.

Lymphocyte-Mediated Effector Responses

Delayed hypersensitivity T lymphocytes

Delayed hypersensitivity (previously termed *Coombs and Gell type IV*) represents the prototypical adaptive immune mechanism for lymphocyte-triggered inflammation. It is especially powerful in secondary immune responses. Previously primed DH $CD4^+$ T lymphocytes leave the lymph node, home into local tissues where antigen persists, and become activated by restimulation with the specific priming antigen and MHC class II–expressing APCs. Fully activated DH T lymphocytes secrete mediators and cytokines, leading to the recruitment and activation of macrophages and/or other nonspecific leukocytes (Fig 2-7). The term *delayed* for this type of hypersensitivity refers to the fact that the reaction becomes maximal 12–48 hours after antigen exposure.

Analysis of experimental animal models and the histologic changes of human inflammation suggest that different subtypes of DH might exist. One of the most important determinants of the pattern of DH reaction is the subtype of DH $CD4^+$ effector T cells that mediate the reaction. Just as helper T lymphocytes can be differentiated into 3 groups—Th1, Th2, and Th17 subsets—according to the spectrum of cytokines secreted, DH T lymphocytes can also be grouped by the same criteria. Experimentally, the Th1 subset of cytokines, especially IFN-γ (also known as *macrophage-activating factor*) and TNF-β, activates macrophages to secrete inflammatory mediators and kill pathogens, thus amplifying inflammation. Th1-mediated DH mechanisms, therefore, are thought to produce the following effects:

- the classic DH reaction (eg, the purified protein derivative [PPD] skin reaction)
- immunity to intracellular infections (eg, to mycobacteria or *Pneumocystis* organisms)
- immunity to fungi
- most forms of severe T-lymphocyte–mediated autoimmune diseases
- chronic transplant rejection

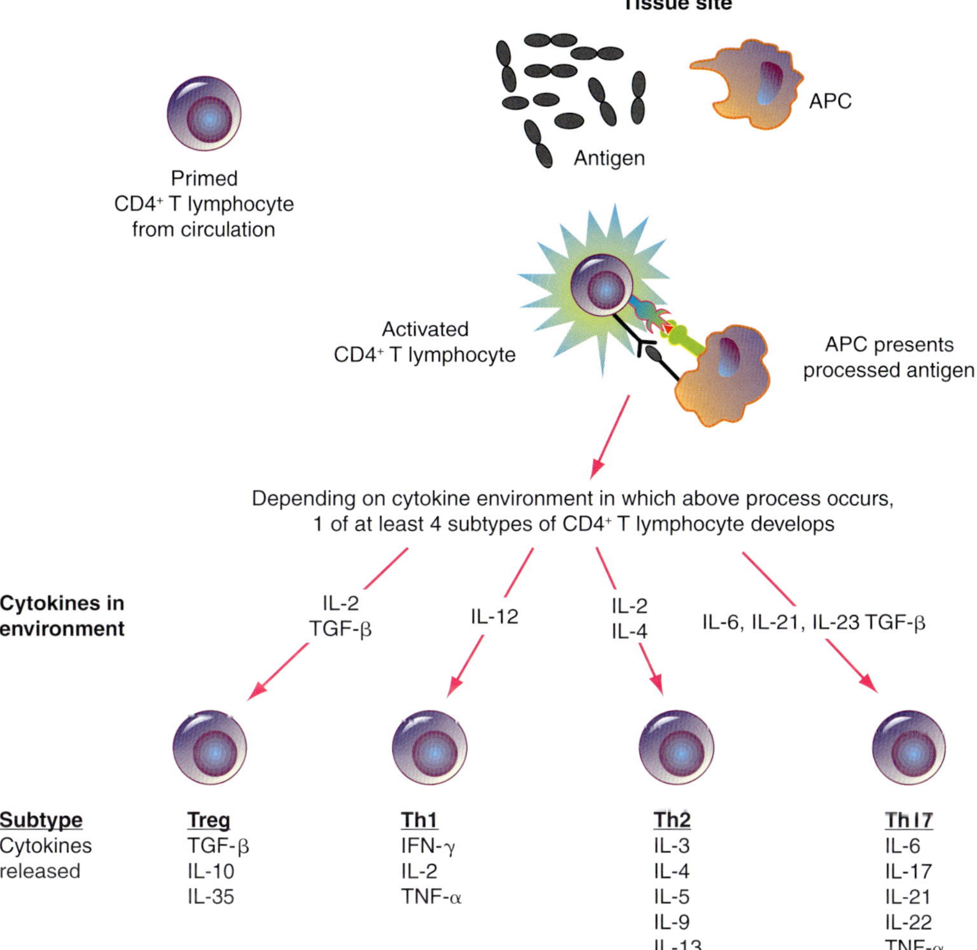

Figure 2-7 Schematic representation of CD4+ T lymphocyte development. After initial priming in the lymph node, CD4+ T lymphocytes enter the tissue site, where they again encounter APCs containing processed antigen. Upon restimulation and depending on the cytokines present in the local environment at the time of restimulation, they become activated into 1 of at least 4 subtypes. T regulatory lymphocytes (Tregs) suppress other T-cell responses. Th1 lymphocytes are the classic delayed-hypersensitivity effector cells and mediate IFN-γ–driven responses. Th2 lymphocytes are thought to be less intensively inflammatory and have been associated with parasite-induced granulomas and atopic diseases. Th17 lymphocytes mediate and sustain inflammation. *(Illustration developed by Russell W. Read, MD, PhD.)*

Table 2-3 summarizes ocular inflammatory diseases thought to require a major contribution of Th1 DH effector mechanisms.

The Th2 subset of DH cells secretes IL-4, IL-5, and other cytokines. IL-4 can induce B lymphocytes to synthesize IgE, and IL-5 can recruit and activate eosinophils within a site. IL-4 can also induce macrophage granulomas in response to parasite-derived antigens.

Table 2-3 Ocular Inflammatory Diseases Likely Involving Th1-Mediated DH Effector Mechanisms

Site	Disease	Presumed Antigen
Conjunctiva	Contact hypersensitivity to contact lens solutions	Thimerosal or other chemicals
	Giant papillary conjunctivitis	Unknown
	Phlyctenulosis	Bacterial antigens
Cornea and sclera	Chronic allograft rejection	Histocompatibility antigens
	Marginal infiltrates of blepharitis	Bacterial antigens
	Disciform keratitis after viral infection	Viral antigens
Anterior uvea	Acute anterior uveitis	Uveal autoantigens, bacterial antigens
	Sarcoidosis-associated uveitis	Unknown
	Idiopathic intermediate uveitis	Unknown
Retina and choroid	Sympathetic ophthalmia	Uveal or retinal autoantigens
	Vogt-Koyanagi-Harada syndrome	Uveal or retinal autoantigens
	Birdshot chorioretinopathy	Retinal or uveal autoantigens
Orbit	Acute thyroid orbitopathy	Probably thyrotropin receptor
	Giant cell arteritis	Unknown

Thus, Th2-mediated DH mechanisms are thought to play a major role in the following:

- response to parasite infections
- late-phase responses of allergic reactions
- asthma
- atopic dermatitis or other manifestations of atopic diseases

The persistence of certain infectious agents, especially bacteria within intracellular compartments of APCs and certain extracellular parasites, can cause destructive induration with granuloma formation and giant cells, termed the *granulomatous* form of DH. However, immune complex deposition and innate immune mechanisms in response to heavy metal or foreign-body reactions can also cause granulomatous inflammation, in which the inflammatory cascade (resulting in DH) is triggered in the absence of specific T lymphocytes. Unfortunately, for most clinical entities in which T-lymphocyte responses are suspected, especially autoimmune disorders such as multiple sclerosis or rheumatoid arthritis, the precise immunologic mechanisms remain highly speculative. See Clinical Example 2-3.

Th17 cells have also been implicated in DH responses. Depending on the local microenvironment, Th cells can also change lineage-specific functions. For example, Th17 cells can gain the ability to secrete Th1 cytokines. They can also switch to a Treg phenotype. This immune plasticity is valuable to homeostasis, minimizing tissue damage associated with DH responses, while maintaining effective microbial clearance.

Cytotoxic lymphocytes

Cytotoxic T lymphocytes Cytotoxic T lymphocytes (CTLs) are a subset of antigen-specific T lymphocytes, usually bearing the CD8 marker, that are especially good at killing tumor cells and virus-infected cells. The CTLs can also mediate graft rejection and some types of autoimmunity. In most cases, the ideal antigen for CTLs is an intracellular protein that

CLINICAL EXAMPLE 2-3

Toxocara granuloma (Th2 DH) *Toxocara canis* is a nematode parasite that infects up to 2% of all children worldwide. It can occasionally produce inflammatory vitreoretinal manifestations. Although the ocular immunology of this disorder is not clearly delineated, animal models and a study of the immunopathogenesis of human nematode infections at other sites suggest the following scenario. The primary immune response begins in the gut after ingestion of viable eggs, which mature into larvae within the intestine. The primary processing phase produces a strong Th2 response, leading to a primary effector response that includes production of IgM, IgG, and IgE antibodies, as well as Th2-mediated DH T lymphocytes. Accidental avoidance of immune effector mechanisms may result in hematogenous dissemination of a few larvae to the choroid or retina, followed by invasion into the retina and/or vitreous. There, a Th2-mediated T-lymphocyte effector response recognizes larva antigens and releases Th2-derived cytokines to induce eosinophil and macrophage infiltration, causing the characteristic eosinophilic granuloma seen in the eye. In addition, antilarval B lymphocytes can infiltrate the eye and are induced to secrete various immunoglobulins, especially IgE. Finally, eosinophils, in part by attachment through Fc receptors, can recognize IgE or IgG bound to parasites and release cytotoxic granules containing the antiparasitic cationic protein directly near the larvae, using a mechanism similar to antibody-dependent cellular cytotoxicity.

Grencis RK. Th2-mediated host protective immunity to intestinal nematode infections. *Philos Trans R Soc Lond B Biol Sci.* 1997;352(1359):1377–1384.

Sympathetic ophthalmia (Th1 DH) Sympathetic ophthalmia is a bilateral panuveitis that follows penetrating trauma to an eye. This disorder represents one of the few human diseases in which autoimmunity can be directly linked to an initiating event. In most cases, penetrating injury activates the afferent phase. It is unclear whether the injury causes a de novo primary immunization to self-antigens—perhaps because of externalization of sequestered uveal antigens through the wound and exposure to the afferent immune response arc of the conjunctiva or extraocular sites—or if the injury instead somehow changes the immunologic microenvironment of the retina, retinal pigment epithelium (RPE), and uvea so that a secondary afferent response is initiated that serves to alter preexisting tolerance to retinal and uveal self-antigens.

The inflammatory effector response is generally thought to be dominated by a Th1-mediated DH mechanism generated in response to uveal or retinal antigens. $CD4^{+}$ T lymphocytes predominate early in the disease course, although $CD8^{+}$ T lymphocytes can be numerous in chronic cases. Activated macrophages are also numerous in granulomas, and Th1 cytokines have been identified in the vitreous or produced by T lymphocytes

(Continued on next page)

(continued)

recovered from the eyes of affected patients. Although the target antigen for sympathetic ophthalmia is unknown, cutaneous immunization in experimental animals with certain retinal antigens (arrestin, rhodopsin, interphotoreceptor retinoid-binding protein), RPE-associated antigens, and melanocyte-associated tyrosinase can induce autoimmune uveitis with physiology or features suggestive of sympathetic ophthalmia. Th1-mediated DH is thought to mediate many forms of ocular inflammation. Table 2–3 lists other examples.

Boyd SR, Young S, Lightman S. Immunopathology of the noninfectious posterior and intermediate uveitides. *Surv Ophthalmol.* 2001;46(3): 209–233.

occurs naturally or is produced because of viral infection. The CTLs appear to require help from $CD4^+$ helper T-lymphocyte signals to fully differentiate. Primed *precursor* CTLs leave the lymph node and migrate to the target tissue, where they are restimulated by the interaction of the CTL antigen receptor and foreign antigens within the antigen pocket of MHC class I molecules (HLA-A, -B, or -C) on the target cell. Additional $CD4^+$ T lymphocytes help at the site, and expression of other accessory costimulatory molecules on the target is often required to obtain maximal killing.

Cytotoxic T lymphocytes kill cells in 1 of 2 ways: "assassination" or "suicide" induction (Fig 2–8). *Assassination* refers to CTL-mediated lysis of targets. A specialized pore-forming protein called *perforin* is released that inserts into cell membranes and causes osmotic lysis of the cell. *Suicide induction* refers to the capability of CTLs to stimulate programmed cell death of target cells, called *apoptosis,* using the CD95 ligand (FasL) to activate the CD95 receptor (Fas) on target cells. Alternatively, CTLs can release cytokines such as TNF to induce apoptosis. The CTLs produce low-grade lymphocytic infiltrate within tumors or infected tissues and usually kill without causing significant inflammation.

Natural killer cells Natural killer (NK) cells are a subset of non-T, non-B lymphocytes. They kill tumor cells and virus-infected cells using the same molecular mechanisms as CTLs. Unlike CTLs, NK cells do not have a specific antigen receptor. Instead, they are triggered by receptors that may be activating or inhibitory. Activating receptors trigger the NK cell to kill target cells that display molecules that should not be present or cells that are missing MHC Class I molecules. Inhibitory NK receptors prevent NK cells from indiscriminately attacking healthy host tissue by recognizing ligands that ought to be present. There are several families of NK receptors, including C-type lectin receptors (CTLRs) and killer immunoglobulin-like receptors (KIRs). Because NK cells are not antigen specific, theoretically the response does not have the time delay associated with induction of the adaptive, antigen-specific CTL immune response. However, NK cells do require some of the same effector activation signals at the tissue site, especially cytokine stimulation. Thus, NK cells are probably most effective in combination with adaptive effector responses.

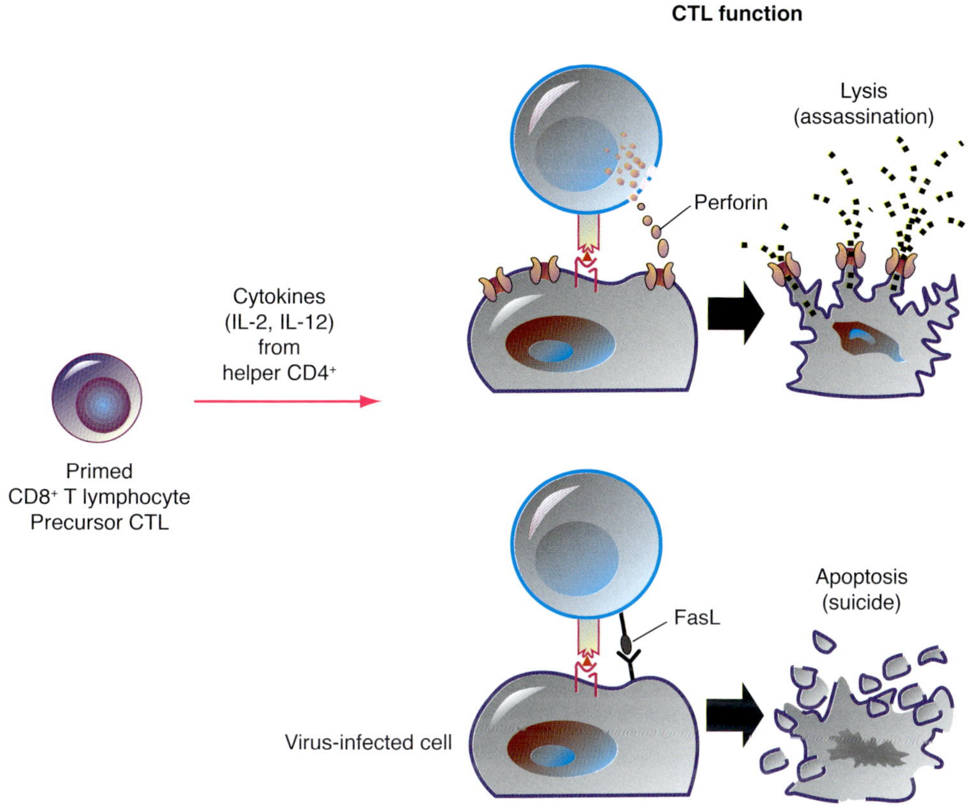

Figure 2-8 Schematic representation of the 2 major mechanisms of CD8+ T-lymphocyte cytotoxicity. CD8+ T lymphocytes, having undergone initial priming in the lymph node, enter the tissue site, where they again encounter antigen in the form of infected target cells. Upon restimulation, usually requiring CD4+ helper T-lymphocyte factors, they become activated into fully cytotoxic T lymphocytes. CTLs can kill by lysing the infected cell using a pore-forming protein called perforin or by inducing programmed cell death, called *apoptosis,* using either FasL or cytokine-mediated mechanisms. *(Illustration by Barb Cousins, modified by Joyce Zavarro.)*

Combined Antibody and Cellular Effector Mechanisms

Antibody-dependent cellular cytotoxicity

An antibody can combine with a cell-associated antigen such as a tumor or viral antigen, but if the antibody is not a subclass that activates complement, it may not induce cytotoxicity. However, because the Fc tail of the antibody is exposed, various leukocytes recognize the Fc domain and are directed to the cell through the antibody. Binding to the antibody then activates various leukocyte cytotoxic mechanisms, including degranulation and cytokine production.

Because human leukocytes express various types of Fc receptors—IgG subclasses have 3 different Fcg receptors, IgE has 2 different Fce receptors, and so on—leukocyte subsets differ in their capacity to recognize and bind different antibody isotypes. Classically, *antibody-dependent cellular cytotoxicity* (ADCC) was observed to be mediated by a subset of large granular (non-T, non-B) lymphocytes, called *killer cells,* that induce cell death in a manner similar to CTLs. The killer cell itself is nonspecific but gains antigen specificity through interaction with specific antibody. Macrophages, NK cells, certain T lymphocytes, and neutrophils can also participate in ADCC using other Fc receptor types. An IgE-dependent form of ADCC may also exist for eosinophils.

ADCC is presumed to be important in tumor surveillance, antimicrobial host protection, graft rejection, and certain autoimmune diseases, such as cutaneous systemic lupus erythematosus. However, this effector mechanism probably does not play an important role in uveitis, although it might contribute to antiparasitic immunity.

Acute IgE-mediated mast-cell degranulation

Mast cells bind IgE antibodies to their surface through a high-affinity Fc receptor specific for IgE molecules, positioning the antigen-recognition site of the bound IgE externally (Fig 2–9). Combining 2 adjacent IgE antibody molecules with a specific allergen causes degranulation of the mast cell and release of preformed and de novo synthesized mediators within minutes. This acute inflammatory reaction is called *immediate hypersensitivity* (previously termed *Coombs and Gell type I,* or *anaphylaxis*).

Preformed mediators include histamine, serotonin, proteoglycans (heparin), neutral proteases (ie, tryptase, chymase), chemotactic factors (eosinophil, neutrophil, or monocyte), and possibly basic fibroblast growth factor. Among the newly generated mediators are the arachidonic acid metabolites prostaglandin D_2, leukotrienes, and thromboxane as well as Th2-type cytokines (IL-4, IL-5, IL-6, IL-9, IL-10, IL-13), TNF-α, IL-1, and CCL2.

The resulting effects include vasodilation, increased capillary permeability, contraction of bronchial and gastrointestinal smooth muscle, and increased mucous secretion in

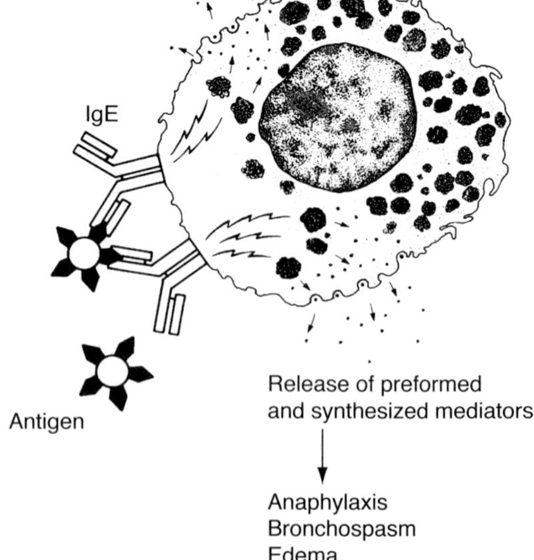

Figure 2-9 Schematic representation of IgE-mediated mast cell degranulation.

mucosal sites. Mast cell-derived cytokines play a role in the late phase of allergic response by activating endothelial cells to recruit eosinophils and other inflammatory cells at the site of hypersensitivity reactions, thus sustaining inflammation. When severe, the immediate hypersensitivity response can produce a systemic reaction, with manifestations ranging from generalized skin lesions, such as erythema, urticaria, or angioedema, to severely altered vascular permeability with plasma leakage into tissues and airway obstruction or hypotensive shock.

Delves PJ, Martin SJ, Burton DR, Roitt IM. *Roitt's Essential Immunology.* 13th ed. Hoboken, NJ: Wiley-Blackwell; 2017.

Muranski P, Restifo NP. Essentials of Th17 cell commitment and plasticity. *Blood.* 2013;121(13):2402–2414.

CHAPTER 3

Ocular Immune Responses

Highlights

- Unique regional immune responses in the eye influence ocular pathology.
- In the context of immune privilege of the eye, several immunoregulatory mechanisms have evolved to modulate the intraocular immune environment.
- Anterior chamber–associated immune deviation (ACAID) is a recognized facet of ocular immune privilege.
- Understanding these ocular immune responses has been valuable to the progress of corneal transplantation, retinal gene therapy, and other developing cell-based therapies.

Regional Immunity and Immunologic Microenvironments

The concept that many organs and tissue sites possess modifications to the classic immune response arc is called *regional immunity.* Regional immunity can affect all 3 phases of the response arc—afferent, processing, and effector. Regional differences in immune response occur because of differences in the immunologic microenvironments of various tissue sites. These regional differences can occur down to the level of specific locations within and around the eye (Table 3-1), such as the

- conjunctiva
- cornea and sclera
- anterior chamber, anterior uvea (iris and ciliary body), and vitreous
- retina, retinal pigment epithelium (RPE), and choriocapillaris
- choroid

A unique feature of the microenvironment of the eye is termed the *ocular immune privilege.* The term was introduced in 1940s by the finding that foreign antigen introduction to the anterior chamber did not elicit inflammatory response. Immune privilege is thought to be an evolutionary adaptation to protect vital structures. Traditionally, central nervous system, eyes, and testicles are considered immune-privileged organs.

Zhou R, Caspi R. Ocular immune privilege. *F1000 Biol Rep.* 2010 Jan 18;2.

Table 3-1 **Comparison of Immune Microenvironments in Various Normal Ocular Sites**

	Conjunctiva	Cornea, Sclera	Anterior Chamber, Anterior Uvea, Vitreous	Subretinal Space, RPE, Choroid
Anatomical features	Lymphatics, follicles	Lymphatics at limbus, none centrally Macromolecules diffuse through stroma	No lymphatics, antigen clearance through trabecular meshwork Partial blood–uveal barrier	No lymphatics Blood–retinal barrier Uveal circulation permeable
Resident APCs	Dendritic and Langerhans cells, macrophages	Langerhans cells at limbus No APCs in central cornea No APCs in sclera Epithelium/endothelium can be induced to express MHC class II	Many dendritic cells and macrophages in iris and ciliary body Hyalocytes are macrophage derived	Microglia in the retina Dendritic cells and macrophages in choriocapillaris RPE expresses TLR and can be induced to express MHC class II
Specialized immune compartments for localized immune processing	?? Follicles	None	None	None
Resident effector cells	Mast cells, T lymphocytes, B lymphocytes, plasma cells, rare neutrophils	Central cornea—none Sclera—none	Rare to no T lymphocytes or B lymphocytes, rare mast cells	Retina—normally no lymphocytes Choroid—mast cells, some lymphocytes
Resident effector molecules	All antibody isotypes, especially IgE, IgG subclasses, IgA in tears Complement and kininogen precursors present	Peripherally—Igs but minimal IgM Centrally—minimal antibody, some complement present Sclera—low antibody concentration, minimal IgM	Kallikrein but not kininogen precursors Some complement present, but less than in blood Minimal Igs in iris, some IgG in ciliary body and aqueous humor	Retina—minimal to no Igs Choroid—IgG and IgM
Immunoregulatory systems	Mucosa-associated lymphoid tissue	Immune privilege—Fas ligand, avascularity, lack of central APCs	Immune privilege—anterior chamber–associated immune deviation, immunosuppressive factors in aqueous, Fas ligand	Immune privilege—?? mechanisms Complement regulator expression

APC = antigen-presenting cell; Ig = immunoglobulin; MHC = major histocompatibility complex; RPE = retinal pigment epithelium; TLR = toll-like receptors.

Immune Responses of the Conjunctiva

Features of the Immunologic Microenvironment

The conjunctiva shares many of the features typical of mucosal sites. It is well vascularized and has good lymphatic drainage to preauricular and submandibular nodes. The tissue contains numerous Langerhans cells, other dendritic cells, and macrophages that serve as potential antigen-presenting cells (APCs). Conjunctival follicles that enlarge after certain types of ocular surface infection or inflammation represent collections of T lymphocytes, B lymphocytes, and APCs. By analogy with similar sites, such as Peyer patches of the intestine, these follicles are likely sites for localized immune processing of antigens that permeate through the thin overlying epithelium.

The conjunctiva, especially the substantia propria, is richly populated with potential effector cells, predominately mast cells. All antibody isotypes are represented, with IgA as the most abundant type in the tear film. Local antibody production presumably occurs as well as passive leakage. Soluble molecules of the innate immune system, especially complement, are also present. The conjunctiva appears to support most adaptive and innate immune effector responses, especially antibody-mediated and lymphocyte-mediated responses, although IgE-mediated mast-cell degranulation is one of the most common and important. See also BCSC Section 8, *External Disease and Cornea,* for further information on conjunctival immune responses.

Immunoregulatory Systems

The conjunctiva contains *mucosa-associated lymphoid tissue* (MALT), an interconnected network of mucosal sites in the body (the epithelial lining of the respiratory tract, gut, and genitourinary tract, and the ocular surface and its adnexae) that share certain immunologic features:

- large number of APCs
- specialized structures for localized antigen processing
- unique effector cells (eg, intraepithelial T lymphocytes and abundant mast cells)

The most distinctive feature of MALT is the homing of effector T and B lymphocytes to all MALT sites after immunization at one site. This migration occurs because of the shared expression of specific cell-adhesion molecules on postcapillary venules of the mucosal vasculature. MALT immune response arcs favor T helper-2 (Th2)–dominated responses that result in the production of predominantly immunoglobulin A (IgA) and IgE antibodies. Processing of soluble antigens through MALT, especially in the gut sites, often produces immune tolerance, presumably by activating Th2-like regulatory T lymphocytes that suppress T helper-1 (Th1)–delayed hypersensitivity (DH) effector cells.

Chodosh J, Kennedy RC. The conjunctival lymphoid follicle in mucosal immunology. *DNA Cell Biol.* 2002;21(5–6):421–433.

Immune Responses of the Cornea

Features of the Immunologic Microenvironment

The cornea is unique in that the peripheral and central portions of the tissue represent distinctly different immunologic microenvironments. In normal eyes, only the limbus is vascularized and richly invested with Langerhans cells. The paracentral and central cornea are normally devoid of APCs and are avascular. Various stimuli, such as mild trauma, certain cytokines (eg, interleukin-1), or infection, can recruit APCs to the central cornea. Plasma-derived proteins (eg, complement, IgM, and IgG) are present in moderate concentrations in the periphery, but only low levels of IgM are present centrally.

Corneal cells also appear to synthesize various antimicrobial and immunoregulatory proteins. Effector cells are absent or scarce in the normal cornea, but neutrophils, monocytes, and lymphocytes can readily migrate through the stroma if appropriate chemotactic stimuli are activated. Lymphocytes, monocytes, and neutrophils can also adhere to the endothelial surface during inflammation, giving rise to keratic precipitates or the classic Khodadoust line of endothelial rejection (Fig 3-1). Localized immune processing probably does not occur in the cornea. See also BCSC Section 8, *External Disease and Cornea.*

Immunoregulatory Systems

The cornea demonstrates a form of immune privilege different from that observed in the anterior uvea. Immune privilege of the cornea is multifactorial. Normal limbal physiology is a major component, especially the maintenance of avascularity and lack of APCs in the mid- and central cornea. The absence of APCs and lymphatic channels partially inhibits afferent recognition in the central cornea. The absence of postcapillary venules centrally can limit the efficiency of effector recruitment, although effector cells and molecules

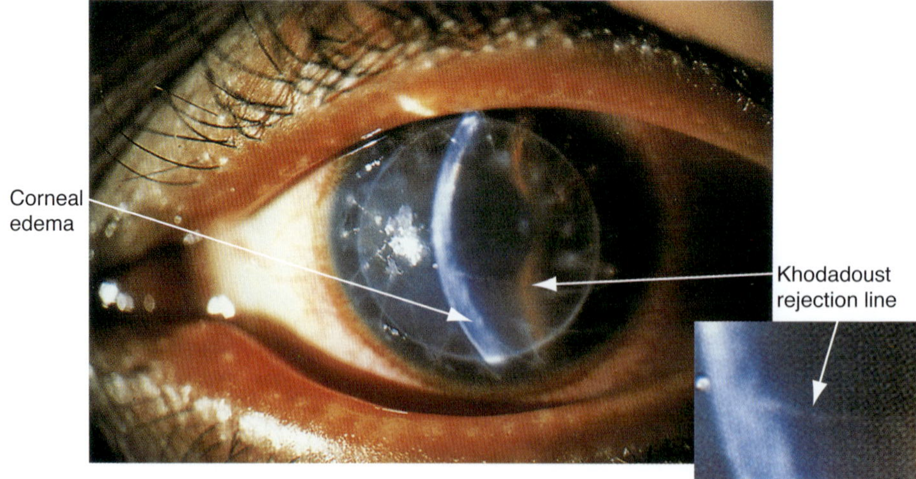

Figure 3-1 Endothelial graft rejection with stromal and epithelial edema on the trailing aspect of the migrating Khodadoust line *(inset)*.

CLINICAL EXAMPLE 3-1

Corneal allograft rejection Penetrating keratoplasty, or the transplantation of corneal allografts, has an extremely high success rate (>90%) even in the absence of systemic immunomodulation. This rate is substantially superior to acceptance rates after transplantation of other donor tissues. The mechanisms of corneal graft survival have been attributed to immune privilege. In experimental models, factors contributing to rejection include the following:

- presence of central corneal vascularization
- induction of MHC molecule expression, which is normally low, by the stroma
- contamination of the donor graft with donor-derived APCs prior to transplantation
- MHC disparity between the host and the donor
- preimmunization of the recipient to donor transplantation antigens

Loss of the immunoregulatory systems of the anterior chamber can influence corneal allograft immunity, and the expression of FasL on corneal endothelium has been observed to be essential for allograft protection in animal models. Rapid replacement of donor epithelium by host epithelium removes this layer as an antigenic stimulus. Once activated, however, antibody-dependent DH and CTL-related mechanisms can target transplantation antigens in all corneal layers.

Klebe S, Coster DJ, Williams KA. Rejection and acceptance of corneal allografts. *Curr Opin Organ Transplant.* 2009;14(1):4–9.

can infiltrate even avascular cornea. Another factor is the presence of intact immunoregulatory systems of the anterior chamber to which the corneal endothelium is exposed. Finally, effector blockade likely provides relative immune privilege to the cornea. (See Clinical Example 3-1.)

Immune Responses of the Anterior Chamber, Anterior Uvea, and Vitreous

Features of the Immunologic Microenvironment

The anterior chamber is a fluid-filled cavity; circulating aqueous humor provides a unique medium for intercellular communication among cytokines, immune cells, and resident tissue cells of the iris, ciliary body, and corneal endothelium. Although aqueous humor is relatively protein depleted compared with serum (containing about 0.1%–1.0% of the total serum protein concentration), even normal aqueous humor contains a complex mixture of biological factors, such as immunomodulatory cytokines, neuropeptides, and complement inhibitors that influence immunologic events within the eye.

A partial blood–ocular barrier is present. Fenestrated capillaries in the ciliary body allow a size-dependent concentration gradient of plasma macromolecules to permeate the interstitial tissue. Smaller plasma-derived molecules are present in higher concentration than larger molecules. The tight junctions between the pigmented and nonpigmented ciliary epithelium provide a more exclusive barrier, preventing interstitial macromolecules from permeating directly through the ciliary body into the aqueous humor. Nevertheless, a small number of plasma macromolecules bypass the nonpigmented epithelium barrier. They can permeate by diffusion anteriorly through the uvea to enter the anterior chamber through the anterior iris surface.

Few resident T lymphocytes and some mast cells are present in the normal anterior uvea. B lymphocytes, eosinophils, and neutrophils are normally not present. Very low concentrations of IgG and complement components occur in normal aqueous humor. The iris and ciliary body contain significant numbers of macrophages and dendritic cells that serve as APCs and possible effector cells. Immune processing is unlikely to occur locally. Rather, because the inner eye does not contain well-defined lymphatic channels, clearance of soluble substances depends on aqueous humor outflow channels; clearance of particulates depends on endocytosis by trabecular meshwork endothelial cells or macrophages. Nevertheless, antigen inoculation into the anterior chamber results in efficient communication with the systemic immune response. Intact soluble antigens gain entrance to the venous circulation, through which they are transported to the spleen.

The vitreous has not been studied as extensively as the anterior chamber. Studies employing proteomics reveal the vitreous as a physiologically active, complex tissue containing diverse proteins originating from inside and outside the eye. An important source for these inflammatory mediators is the retina. The vitreous gel can also electrostatically bind charged protein substances and can serve as an antigen depot as well as a substrate for leukocyte cell adhesion. Hyalocytes are modified resident macrophages. They are important in vitreal immunoregulation/modulation and frequently act as antigen-presenting cells. They also respond to different cytokines, playing a role in the immunopathogenesis of several disorders, including proliferative vitreoretinopathy (PVR). Because the vitreous contains collagen type II, it may also serve as a depot of potential autoantigen.

Immunoregulatory Systems

Relatively mild degrees of inflammation that would be harmless in the skin, for example, can cause severe vision loss if they occur in the eye. A variety of immunoregulatory mechanisms have thus evolved to modulate intraocular immune responses (eg, immune privilege).

Ocular immune privilege has been observed with various antigens, including alloantigens (eg, transplantation antigens), tumor antigens, haptens, soluble proteins, autoantigens, bacteria, and viruses. The best-studied model of immune privilege in the eye is called *anterior chamber–associated immune deviation* (ACAID). Whereas subcutaneous immunization with antigen elicits a strong, delayed-type sensitivity, immunization into the anterior chamber with the identical antigen results in a robust antibody response but a virtual absence of delayed-type hypersensitivity. In fact, preexisting delayed-type hypersensitivity (DH) can be suppressed by the ACAID response.

The ACAID response represents an attenuated effector arc. There are other regulators that contribute to immune privilege of the eye. The eye is further protected from severe inflammation by another modulating system termed *effector blockade,* by which Th1 lymphocytes, cytotoxic T lymphocytes, natural killer cells, and complement activation appear to function less effectively in the anterior uvea than elsewhere. For instance, the anterior uvea is *relatively* resistant to induction of a secondary purified protein derivative DH response after primary immunization with mycobacteria in the skin. There are several mechanisms of effector blockade, but one of the most important and best studied involves the *Fas ligand* (FasL, or CD95 ligand). The FasL is constitutively expressed on the iris and corneal endothelium. It is a potent trigger of programmed cell death, or *apoptosis,* of lymphocytes expressing the Fas receptor. Thus, even if an immune response develops to an ocular antigen, the inflammation can be downregulated by this mechanism of effector blockade.

Note that the immunoregulatory environment can, however, be overcome by sufficient immune stimulation.

Foster CS, Suelves AM. Basic immunology. In: Foster CS, Vitale AT, eds. *Diagnosis and Treatment of Uveitis.* 2nd ed. Philadelphia, PA: WB Saunders; 2013:44–100.

Niederkorn JY. The induction of anterior chamber–associated immune deviation. *Chem Immunol Allergy.* 2007;92:27–35.

Sakamoto T, Ishibashi T. Hyalocytes: essential cells of the vitreous cavity in vitreoretinal pathophysiology? *Retina.* 2011;31(2):222–228.

Skeie JM, Roybal CN, Mahajan VB. Proteomic insight into the molecular function of the vitreous. *PLoS One.* 2015;10(5):e0127567.

Immune Responses of the Retina, Retinal Pigment Epithelium, Choriocapillaris, and Choroid

Features of the Immunologic Microenvironment

The immunologic microenvironments of the retina, RPE, choriocapillaris, and choroid have not been well characterized. The retinal circulation establishes an inner blood–ocular barrier at the level of tight junctions between adjacent endothelial cells, while tight junctions between the cells of the RPE provide an outer barrier between the choroid and the retina. The vessels of the choriocapillaris are highly permeable to macromolecules and allow transudation of most plasma macromolecules into the extravascular spaces of the choroid and choriocapillaris. Well-developed lymphatic channels are absent, although both the retina and the choroid have abundant potential APCs. In the retina, resident microglia (bone marrow–derived cells related to dendritic cells) are interspersed within all layers and can undergo physical changes and migration in response to various stimuli. The choriocapillaris and choroid contain an abundance of certain potential APCs, especially macrophages and dendritic cells.

The RPE can be induced to express major histocompatibility complex (MHC) class II molecules, suggesting that the RPE may interact with T lymphocytes in some circumstances. The presence of T lymphocytes or B lymphocytes within the normal posterior segment has not been carefully studied, but effector cells appear to be absent from the normal retina. Similar to macrophages, RPE cells also express toll-like receptors (TLRs). These special pattern recognition receptors are critical in recognition of pathogens and in the initiation of innate and adaptive immune responses, forming an initial line of defense against invading microorganisms. A moderate density of mast cells is also present in the choroid, especially around the arterioles, but lymphocytes are present only in very low number. Eosinophils and neutrophils appear to be absent. Under various clinical or experimental conditions, however, a large number of T lymphocytes, B lymphocytes, macrophages, and neutrophils can infiltrate the choroid, choriocapillaris, and retina. The RPE and various cell types within the retina and the choroid (eg, pericytes) can synthesize many different cytokines (eg, transforming growth factor-β) that may alter the subsequent immune response. Local immune processing does not seem to occur. (See also BCSC Section 12, *Retina and Vitreous.*)

Detrick B, Hooks JJ. Immune regulation in the retina. *Immunol Res.* 2010;47(1–3):153–161.

CLINICAL EXAMPLE 3-2

Retinal gene therapy Retinal gene therapy is the intentional transfection of neural retina cells or RPE with a replication-defective virus that has been genetically altered to carry a replacement gene of choice. This gene becomes expressed in any cell infected by the virus. Immune clearance of the virus can cause loss of expression of the transferred gene in other body sites. Applications of gene therapy in humans have been successfully completed. The United States Food and Drug Administration has approved treatment of biallelic *RPE65* mutation–associated retinal dystrophy (Leber congenital amaurosis) using adeno-associated virus (AAV) vector to replace the defective *RPE65* gene. The agent (voretigene neparvovec-rzyl) is administered via subretinal injection. Despite the relative immune privilege of the eye, immunogenicity of viral vectors is an ongoing area of investigation. In animal models, intravitreal delivery has lead to a humoral response, while subretinal delivery has not. Intraocular inflammation was observed in approximately 5% of patients receiving voretigene neparvovec-rzy. Use of systemic corticosteroids is recommended, starting 3 days prior to injection of voretigene neparvovec-rzyl. Ocular injection of AAV for the treatment of various inherited retinal dystrophies is under investigation. Areas of study include achromatopsia, choroideremia, Leber hereditary optic neuropathy, X-linked retinoschisis, and X-linked retinitis pigmentosa.

Mancuso K, Hauswirth WW, Li Q, et al. Gene therapy for red-green colour blindness in adult primates. *Nature.* 2009;461(7265):784–787.
Moore NA, Morral N, Ciulla TA, Bracha P. Gene therapy for inherited retinal and optic nerve degenerations. *Expert Opin Biol Ther.* 2018;18(1):37–49.

Immunoregulatory Systems

A form of immune privilege, likely similar to ACAID, is present after subretinal injection of antigen. Iris, ciliary body, and RPE cells all contribute to immune homeostasis of the eye that is mediated by soluble or membrane-bound molecules. This observation may be important because of growing interest in retinal transplantation, stem cell therapies, and gene therapy. (See Clinical Example 3-2.) The RPE can limit activation of T cells and convert effector cells to regulatory cells. The capacity of the choriocapillaris and choroid to function as unique environments for the afferent or effector phases has not yet been evaluated.

Lee RW, Nicholson LB, Sen HN, et al. Autoimmune and autoinflammatory mechanisms in uveitis. *Semin Immunopathol.* 2014;36(5):581–594.

Mochizuki M, Sugita S, Kamoi K. Immunological homeostasis of the eye. *Prog Retin Eye Res.* 2013;33:10–27.

Vogt SD, Barnum SR, Curcio CA, Read RW. Distribution of complement anaphylatoxin receptors and membrane-bound regulators in normal human retina. *Exp Eye Res.* 2006;83(4):834–840.

CHAPTER 4

Special Topics in Ocular Immunology

Highlights

- Examples of animal models of human uveitis include experimental autoimmune uveoretinitis, endotoxin-induced uveitis, equine recurrent uveitis, autoimmune regulator–deficient mice, and interphotoreceptor retinoid-binding protein (IRBP)–specific T-cell receptor transgenic mice.
- All animals with white blood cells express a family of cell-surface glycoproteins called *major histocompatibility complex (MHC) proteins*. In humans, the MHC proteins are called *human leukocyte antigen (HLA) molecules*.
- The presence of many different HLA alleles within a population should ensure that the collective adaptive immune system will be able to respond to a wide range of potential pathogens. However, some individuals might be at increased risk for immunologic diseases.

Animal Models of Human Uveitis

Animal models of uveitis use a variety of species, antigens, adjuvants, and protocols to produce disease that ranges from transient to persistent and mild to severe. None is an exact corollary to human disease, but all have contributed substantially to the understanding of ocular immunology.

Experimental Autoimmune Uveoretinitis

Experimental autoimmune uveoretinitis (EAU) is the most widely used and well-studied animal model of human uveitis. In the original model, a retinal extract administered intradermally with Freund complete adjuvant in rats and rabbits resulted in a panuveitis approximately 1–2 weeks later. Features include inflammation in the anterior segment, vitreous, and choroid. Refinements of the model have occurred over time. Purified arrestin (also called *S-antigen*) has been used in rats, and the model was expanded to include mice, using immunization with IRBP-derived peptides. Depending on the peptide dose used to induce disease, this mouse model can show monophasic active inflammation with vasculitis, papillitis, and intraretinal infiltration that can result in retinal degeneration or a lower grade chronic inflammation with perivascular cuffing and choroidal infiltrates.

Endotoxin-Induced Uveitis

Endotoxin-induced (also termed *experimental immune*) uveitis (EIU) is a transient uveitis model induced by footpad, intraperitoneal, or intravitreal injection of lipopolysaccharide in mice and rats (see Chapter 1). Sixteen to 48 hours after administration, a transient anterior uveitis develops. This model has been especially useful for studies of the dynamics of leukocyte function in the anterior chamber. It is not clear how or even if this model correlates with human disease.

Equine Recurrent Uveitis

This spontaneous uveitis occurs in up to 10% of horses. It is typically a bilateral uveitis featuring anterior and posterior segment inflammation. Immunologic studies have indicated the presence of autoantibodies and autoreactive T cells in this disease.

Autoimmune Regulator–Deficient Mice

The transcription factor AIRE (for *autoimmune regulator*) is used by the thymus in the process of establishing thymic tolerance. Early in life, the thymus expresses many cell-type–specific proteins; T-cell clones reactive to these proteins are deleted. This mechanism is important in the development of self-tolerance. Mice deficient in AIRE do not express these proteins during development; thus, autoreactive T cells escape deletion, and the mice spontaneously develop a posterior uveitis. Recent work has suggested that the major antigen targeted in this autoimmune uveitis is IRBP—the same protein used to generate mouse models of EAU.

Interphotoreceptor Retinoid-Binding Protein–Specific T-Cell Receptor Transgenic Mice

Immunization of mice with a peptide sequence from IRBP induces autoimmune uveitis in mice. Mice bred to be transgenic for an IRBP-specific T-cell receptor develop a spontaneous uveitis that begins around 4 weeks of age and progresses to an incidence of 100% by age 12 weeks. These mice provide a model of spontaneous uveitis that negates the need for peripheral immunization and produces a chronic course, in contrast to the more acute disease of classic EAU.

Chen J, Qian H, Horai R, Chan CC, Caspi RR. Mouse models of experimental autoimmune uveitis: comparative analysis of adjuvant-induced vs spontaneous models of uveitis. *Curr Mol Med.* 2015;15(6):550–557.

Forrester JV, Klaska IP, Yu T, Kuffova L. Uveitis in mouse and man. *Int Rev Immunol.* 2013;32(1)76–96.

HLA Associations and Disease

Normal Function of HLA Molecules

All animals with white blood cells express a family of cell-surface glycoproteins called *major histocompatibility complex* (MHC) proteins. In humans, the MHC proteins are called *human leukocyte antigen* (HLA) molecules. Historically, 6 families of HLA molecules have been identified:

- 3 MHC class I: HLA-A, -B, -C
- 3 MHC class II: HLA-DR, -DP, -DQ

Another category of HLA is HLA-D, whose subset, HLA-DM, is critical for loading and editing of peptides on MHC class II molecules. HLA-E, HLA-F and HLA-G are also relevant in immunity and subsequently in human pathology. Chapter 2 discussed the important role that MHC molecules play in immunologic function. HLA genes are also considered human immune response genes because the HLA type determines the capacity of the antigen-presenting cell (APC) to bind peptide fragments and present it, and thus determines T-lymphocyte immune responsiveness.

Allelic Variation

Within the human population, many alleles exist for each of the 6 HLA types. Because each person has a pair of each HLA type (codominantly expressed), or 1 *haplotype*, an APC expresses pairs of MHC molecules. Thus, except for identical twins, only rarely will all potential haplotypes match between 2 individuals.

Allelic diversity provides protection through *population-wide immunity.* Each HLA haplotype covers a theoretical set of antigens against which an individual can respond. The presence of many different HLA alleles within a population should thus ensure that the collective adaptive immune system can respond to a wide range of potential pathogens. The converse also holds true: some individuals may be at increased risk for immunologic diseases because of either an aberrantly strong immune response to a benign pathogen or an autoimmune disease arising from inappropriate recognition of host peptides in the context of a particular HLA being recognized as foreign. See Clinical Example 4-1.

Clinical detection and classification of different alleles

Determination of HLA type has evolved from prior antisera reactions to molecular techniques that determine the nucleic acid sequence of MHC alleles. Molecules of HLA are composed of 2 chains: the α chain and β chain for class II, and the α chain and the β_2-microglobulin chain for class I. Genotyping specifies the chain, major genetic type, and specific minor molecular variant subtype. For example, genotype DRB1*0408 refers to the HLA-DR4 molecule β chain with the "–08" minor variant subtype. Haplotypes now recognized as a single group will continue to be subdivided into new categories or new subtypes as research progresses.

CLINICAL EXAMPLE 4-1

HLA-B27–associated acute anterior uveitis Approximately 50% of patients with acute anterior uveitis express the HLA-B27 haplotype. Many of these patients also experience other immunologic disorders, such as reactive arthritis, ankylosing spondylitis, inflammatory bowel disease, and psoriatic arthritis (see Chapter 8). Although the immunopathogenesis remains unknown, various animal models permit some informed speculation. Many cases of uveitis or reactive arthritis follow gram-negative gastroenteritis or chlamydial infection. (Chapter 1 discusses the possible role of bacterial lipopolysaccharide and innate mechanisms.) Experiments in rats and mice genetically altered to express human HLA-B27 molecules seem to suggest that bacterial infection of the gut predisposes rats to arthritis and a reactive arthritis–like syndrome, although uveitis is uncommon.

Disease Associations

In 1973, the first association between an HLA haplotype and a disease—ankylosing spondylitis—was identified. Since then, more than 100 other disease associations have been established, including several for ocular inflammatory diseases (Table 4-1). An HLA–disease association is established when there is a statistically increased frequency of an HLA haplotype in persons with that disease compared with the frequency in a disease-free population. The ratio of the probability of the disease occurring in individuals with the HLA haplotype to individuals without the haplotype is termed *relative risk.* A relative risk of 1 denotes no difference in risk, <1 indicates a reduced risk, and >1 an increased risk. Several points are important when considering HLA–disease associations:

- The HLA association identifies individuals at risk, but it is not a diagnostic marker. The associated haplotype is not necessarily present in all people with the disease, nor does its presence in a person ensure the correct diagnosis.
- The association depends on the validity of the haplotyping. Older literature often reflects associations based on HLA classifications (some provisional) that might have changed.
- The association is only as strong as the clinical diagnosis. Diseases that are difficult to diagnose based on clinical features may obscure real associations.
- The concept of *linkage disequilibrium* proposes that if 2 genes are physically close together on a chromosome, they are likely to be inherited together rather than undergo genetic randomization in a population. Thus, HLA genes may be coinherited with a separate gene that confers the actual risk. Sometimes 2 HLA haplotypes can occur together more frequently than predicted by their independent frequencies in the population.

For example, approximately 8% of the Caucasian population in the United States is HLA-A29 positive, but fewer than 1 in 10,000 US residents have birdshot chorioretinopathy

Table 4-1 HLA Associations and Ocular Inflammatory Disease

Disease	HLA Association	Relative Risk (RR), Other Associations
Uveitic diseases with strong HLA associations		
Tubulointerstitial nephritis and uveitis (TINU) syndrome	HLA-DRB1*0102	RR = 167
Birdshot chorioretinopathy	HLA-A29, -A29.2	RR up to 224 for North Americans and Europeans
Reactive arthritis	HLA-B27	RR = 60
Acute anterior uveitis	HLA-B27	RR = 8
Uveitic diseases with weaker HLA associations		
Juvenile idiopathic arthritis	HLA-A2, -DR5, -DR8, -DR11, -DP2.1	Acute systemic disease
Behçet disease	HLA-B51	RR = 4–6; Japanese and Middle Eastern descent
Intermediate uveitis	HLA-B8, -B51, -DR2, -DR15	RR = 6, possibly the DRB1*1501 genotype
Sympathetic ophthalmia	HLA-DR4	Unknown
Vogt-Koyanagi-Harada syndrome	HLA-DR4	RR = 2, Japanese and North Americans RR = 5.3, Mexican Mestizos
Sarcoidosis	HLA-B8 HLA-B13	Acute systemic disease Chronic systemic disease but not for eye
Multiple sclerosis	HLA-B7, -DR2	Unknown
Retinal vasculitis	HLA-B44	British

(although nearly all patients with birdshot chorioretinopathy are HLA-A29 positive). Thus, most individuals who are HLA-A29 positive will never develop birdshot chorioretinopathy. This reinforces that other genetic and environmental factors are implicated. As an example, genes encoding aminopeptidases involved in processing of MHC class I ligands, namely endoplasmic reticulum aminopeptidase (ERAP), have been identified in genome-wide association studies of patients with birdshot chorioretinopathy.

Several mechanisms have been proposed for HLA-disease associations. The most direct theory postulates that HLA molecules act as peptide-binding molecules for etiologic antigens or infectious agents. Thus, individuals bearing a specific HLA molecule might be predisposed to processing certain antigens, such as an infectious agent that cross-reacts with a self-antigen, and other individuals, lacking that haplotype, would not be so predisposed. Specific variations or mutations in the peptide-binding region would greatly influence this mechanism; only molecular typing can detect these variations. Preliminary data in support of this theory is available for patients with type 1 diabetes mellitus.

A second theory proposes molecular mimicry between bacterial antigens and an epitope on the HLA molecule (ie, an antigenic site on the molecule itself). An appropriate antibacterial effector response might inappropriately initiate a cross-reactive effector response with an epitope of the HLA molecule.

A third theory suggests that the T-lymphocyte antigen receptor (gene) might be the true susceptibility factor. Because a specific T-lymphocyte receptor uses a specific HLA haplotype, a strong correlation would exist between an HLA and the T-lymphocyte antigen receptor repertoire.

Kuiper J, Rothova A, de Boer J, Radstake T. The immunopathogenesis of birdshot chorioretinopathy; a bird of many feathers. *Prog Retin Eye Res.* 2015;44:99–110.

Levinson RD. Immunogenetics of ocular inflammatory disease. *Tissue Antigens.* 2007;69(2):105–112.

CHAPTER 5

Diagnostic Considerations in Uveitis

This chapter includes a related video, which can be accessed by scanning the QR code provided in the text or going to www.aao.org/bcscvideo_section09.

This chapter includes a related activity, which can be accessed by scanning the QR code provided in the text or going to www.aao.org/bcscactivity_section09.

Highlights

- *Uveitis* refers to a heterogeneous group of diseases characterized by intraocular inflammation, and accounts for significant visual morbidity worldwide.
- Diseases with similar clinical features can have different prognoses and treatments, making accurate diagnosis imperative.
- A formalized nomenclature is used to describe, categorize, and grade uveitis by clinical and anatomical features.
- The patient history, review of systems, and targeted systemic examination combined with this naming scheme generate the differential diagnosis.
- Laboratory workup and ancillary testing are tailored to the patient and disease characteristics.

Overview

The uvea consists of the middle, pigmented, vascular layer of the eye and includes the iris, ciliary body, and choroid. *Uveitis* is broadly defined as inflammation (ie, *-itis*) of the uvea (from the Latin *uva,* meaning "grape"). Inflammation of the uvea can involve other ocular structures such as the retina, sclera, cornea, vitreous, and optic nerve. The etiology of uveitis is infectious or inflammatory and is variably associated with systemic disease.

Because uveitis can be associated with systemic disease or infection, a careful history and review of systems is an essential first step in diagnosis. A comprehensive physical examination of the eye and pertinent organ systems is performed to characterize the type of inflammation present and to identify any associated systemic findings. The anatomical location of inflammation combined with results from the history and physical examination helps to guide further investigations. Multimodal ophthalmic imaging has an important role in characterizing certain types of intraocular inflammation. Laboratory studies can help determine the etiology of the intraocular inflammation but are never a substitute for a thorough history and physical examination. Determining the specific type of uveitis guides the selection of treatment (see Chapter 6).

Epidemiology

Uveitis is responsible for approximately 10% of all blindness in the United States and Europe and up to 25% of blindness worldwide. In the United States, the prevalence of uveitis is 58–131 per 100,00 and is up to 1070 per 100,000 in the developing world. Anterior uveitis is the most common type of uveitis, representing 70%–80% of cases, followed by panuveitis, posterior uveitis, and intermediate uveitis. Women have slightly higher rates of uveitis overall. Although most surveys show that uveitis incidence peaks between 20 and 60 years of age, recent data suggests that it may also increase over the age of 65. Prevalence is about five- to tenfold lower in children than in adults. Developing countries have higher rates of infectious uveitis and posterior and panuveitis compared to industrialized nations. Certain uveitides have greater distribution by geographic region, such as birdshot chorioretinopathy in western Europe, Behçet disease in Turkey and China, and tuberculous uveitis in India. Chapters 8 and 9 discuss specific uveitic entities in further detail.

Acharya NR, Tham VM, Esterberg E, et al. Incidence and prevalence of uveitis: results from the Pacific Ocular Inflammation Study. *JAMA Ophthalmol.* 2013;131(11):1405–1412.

Gritz DC, Wong IG. Incidence and prevalence of uveitis in Northern California; the Northern California Epidemiology of Uveitis Study. *Ophthalmology.* 2004;111(3):491–500.

Rathinam SR, Krishnadas R, Ramakrishnan R, Thulasiraj RD, Tielsch JM, Katz J, Robin AL, Kempen JH; Aravind Comprehensive Eye Survey Research Group. Population-based prevalence of uveitis in Southern India. *Br J Ophthalmol.* 2011;95:463–467.

Rim TH, Kim SS, Ham D, Yu S, Chung EJ, Lee SC; Korean Uveitis Society. Incidence and prevalence of uveitis in South Korea: a nationwide cohort study. *Br J Ophthalmol.* 2018; 102(1):79–83.

Thorne JE, Suhler E, Skup M, Tari S, et al. Prevalence of noninfectious uveitis in the United States: a claims-based analysis. *JAMA Ophthalmol.* 2016;134(11):123–1245.

Classification of Uveitis

In 2005, the world's major uveitis societies instituted a standard of nomenclature process, termed the Standardization of Uveitis Nomenclature (SUN) system. Uveitis specialists have widely accepted the SUN system of classification as a universal method of describing uveitis entities based on anatomic location of inflammation and specific descriptors of onset, duration, and course.

This text uses an etiologic division of uveitic entities into noninfectious (autoimmune) and infectious conditions and further describes them using the SUN system's basic anatomical classification of uveitis into 4 subcategories: (1) anterior uveitis, (2) intermediate uveitis, (3) posterior uveitis, and (4) panuveitis. When both anterior chamber and vitreous inflammatory cells are present, but the vitritis is more than expected in an isolated anterior uveitis, the classification should be "anterior and intermediate uveitis" and not "panuveitis."

Table 5-1 reviews these 4 groups. The SUN system further refines this anatomical classification of uveitis by defining descriptors based on clinical onset, duration, and course (Table 5-2). In addition, specific terminology for grading and monitoring uveitic activity is described in Table 5-3.

Jabs DA, Nussenblatt RB, Rosenbaum JT; Standardization of Uveitis Nomenclature (SUN) Working Group. Standardization of uveitis nomenclature for reporting clinical data. Results of the First International Workshop. *Am J Ophthalmol.* 2005;140(3):509–516.

Table 5-1 Anatomical Classification of Uveitis Based on Standardization of Uveitis Nomenclature (SUN) Criteria

Type	Primary Site of Inflammation	Includes
Anterior uveitis	Anterior chamber	Iritis Iridocyclitis Anterior cyclitis
Intermediate uveitis	Vitreous	Pars planitis Posterior cyclitis Hyalitis
Posterior uveitis	Retina or choroid	Focal, multifocal, or diffuse choroiditis Chorioretinitis Retinochoroiditis Retinitis Neuroretinitis
Panuveitis	Anterior chamber, vitreous, and retina or choroid	

Reprinted with permission from Jabs DA, Nussenblatt RB, Rosenbaum JT; Standardization of Uveitis Nomenclature (SUN) Working Group. Standardization of nomenclature for reporting clinical data. Results of the First International Workshop. *Am J Ophthalmol.* 2005;140(3):510.

Table 5-2 Descriptors of Uveitis Based on Standardization of Uveitis Nomenclature (SUN) Criteria

Category	Descriptor	Comment
Onset	Sudden Insidious	
Duration	Limited Persistent	≤3 months' duration >3 months' duration
Course	Acute	Episode characterized by sudden onset and limited duration
	Recurrent	Repeated episodes separated by periods of inactivity without treatment ≥3 months' duration
	Chronic	Persistent uveitis with relapse in <3 months after discontinuing treatment

Reprinted with permission from Jabs DA, Nussenblatt RB, Rosenbaum JT; Standardization of Uveitis Nomenclature (SUN) Working Group. Standardization of nomenclature for reporting clinical data. Results of the First International Workshop. *Am J Ophthalmol.* 2005;140(3):511.

Table 5-3 Uveitis Terminology Based on Standardization of Uveitis Nomenclature (SUN) Criteria

Term	Definition
Inactive	Grade 0 cells (anterior chamber)
Worsening activity	Two-step increase in level of inflammation (eg, anterior chamber cells, vitreous haze) or increase from grade 3+ to 4+
Improved activity	Two-step decrease in level of inflammation (eg, anterior chamber cells, vitreous haze) or decrease to grade 0
Remission	Inactive disease for ≥3 months after discontinuing all treatments for eye disease

Reprinted with permission from Jabs DA, Nussenblatt RB, Rosenbaum JT; Standardization of Uveitis Nomenclature (SUN) Working Group. Standardization of nomenclature for reporting clinical data. Results of the First International Workshop. *Am J Ophthalmol.* 2005;140(3):513.

Anatomical Classification

Anterior uveitis

Anterior uveitis produces inflammatory signs predominantly in the anterior chamber, as a result of inflammation of the iris and ciliary body. Inflammation confined to the anterior chamber can be called *iritis*; if there are cells in the retrolental (anterior vitreous) space, it can be called *iridocyclitis*. Inflammatory processes that originate in the cornea with secondary involvement of the anterior chamber are called *keratouveitis*. An inflammatory reaction that involves the sclera and uveal tract is called *sclerouveitis*.

When more than one ocular structure is involved, the convention is that the primary site of inflammation is named first. Severe or chronic anterior uveitis may produce secondary structural complications such as uveitic macular edema, optic disc swelling, cataract, corneal edema, band keratopathy, or iris abnormalities. These complications are not part of the formal classification system but may contribute to disease recognition and therapy. Table 5-4 includes a simplified scheme for patient evaluation in uveitis. (Chapter 8 discusses anterior uveitis in greater detail.)

Intermediate uveitis

In intermediate uveitis, inflammation is most prominent in the vitreous cavity. Inflammation occurs in the ciliary body, pars plana and/or peripheral retina. Clinical signs include vitreous haze and cellular debris that is often associated with peripheral retinal vasculitis. Macular edema is the most common structural complication; severe or chronic disease may cause peripheral exudative or tractional detachments, retinal neovascularization, cataract, or retrolental membrane formation. The diagnostic term, *pars planitis*, refers to the subset of intermediate uveitis in which there are peripheral preretinal collections of exudative and inflammatory debris in the absence of an associated infection or systemic disease (see Table 5-4). (Chapter 8 discusses intermediate uveitis in greater detail.)

Posterior uveitis

Posterior uveitis is defined as intraocular inflammation primarily involving the retina and/or choroid. Inflammatory cells may be observed diffusely throughout the vitreous cavity,

Table 5-4 **Simplified Scheme for Patient Evaluation in Uveitis**

Type of Inflammation	Possible Associated Factors	Suspected Disease[a]	Laboratory Tests, Imaging
Panuveitis			
See entities described below: sarcoidosis, Vogt-Koyanagi-Harada syndrome, sympathetic ophthalmia, Behçet disease, syphilis, toxoplasmosis, endophthalmitis, toxocariasis, cysticercosis			
Anterior Uveitis			
Acute/sudden onset, severe with or without fibrin membrane or hypopyon	Arthritis, back pain, GI/GU symptoms	Seronegative spondyloarthropathies (ankylosing spondylitis, reactive arthritis, inflammatory bowel disease, psoriatic arthritis)	HLA-B27; sacroiliac films; rheumatology, gastroenterology referrals
	Oral and genital ulcers, skin findings	Behçet disease	Clinical diagnosis, screen for other organ involvement; rheumatology referral
	Febrile illness, flank or abdominal pain	Tubulointerstitial nephritis and uveitis (TINU) syndrome	Renal function tests, urinalysis, urine $beta_2$-microglobulin; nephrology referral
	Postsurgical or penetrating eye trauma, or systemic indwelling lines/instrumentation/infection	Infectious endophthalmitis, toxic anterior segment syndrome	B-scan for vitritis, consider vitreous culture, vitrectomy. For endogenous consider blood cultures and systemic infectious workup.
	None	Undifferentiated (idiopathic)	HLA-B27
Moderate severity (red, painful)	Shortness of breath, skin findings, granulomatous inflammation	Sarcoidosis	ACE, lysozyme; CXR; chest CT or gallium scan; biopsy
	Blunt eye trauma	Traumatic iritis	
	Increased IOP	Glaucomatocyclitic crisis, herpetic iritis	Clinical diagnosis; PCR of ocular fluid[b] optional
	Poor response to steroids	Syphilis	Syphilis IgG or FTA-ABS or MHA-TP followed by RPR or VDRL
	Postsurgical	Low-grade endophthalmitis (eg, *Propionibacterium acnes*); IOL-related	Consider vitrectomy, capsulectomy with culture

(Continued)

Table 5-4 *(continued)*

Type of Inflammation	Possible Associated Factors	Suspected Disease[a]	Laboratory Tests, Imaging
		Anterior Uveitis (continued)	
Chronic; minimal redness, pain	Child, especially with arthritis	JIA-related anterior uveitis	ANA, ESR, RF; rheumatology referral
	Heterochromia or small nodules, diffuse KP, unilateral	Fuchs uveitis syndrome	Clinical diagnosis; rubella virus antibody where available
	Postsurgical	Low-grade endophthalmitis (eg, *Propionibacterium acnes*); IOL-related	Consider vitrectomy, capsulectomy with culture
	None	Undifferentiated	
		Intermediate Uveitis	
Mild to moderate	Shortness of breath, skin findings, granulomatous inflammation	Sarcoidosis	ACE, lysozyme; CXR/chest CT or gallium scan; biopsy
	Tick exposure, erythema chronicum migrans rash, endemic area	Lyme disease (can also be anterior, posterior/panuveitis)	ELISA, Western blot for confirmation
	Neurologic symptoms	Multiple sclerosis	MRI of brain and c-spine; LP for oligoclonal bands; neurology referral
	Over age 50 years	Intraocular lymphoma	Vitrectomy; chorioretinal biopsy; cytology; IL-10/IL-6 ratio[b]; genotyping studies; brain MRI, LP
	None	Pars planitis	
		Posterior Uveitis	
Chorioretinitis with vitritis			
Focal	Adjacent scar; raw meat, unwashed vegetable ingestion, endemic area	Toxoplasmosis	Clinical diagnosis; negative serology to rule out the diagnosis; PCR of ocular fluid[b] optional
	Child; history of geophagia	Toxocariasis	Clinical diagnosis; ELISA, complete blood count with differential
	HIV infection or immunosuppressed	CMV retinitis (variable vitritis)	PCR of ocular fluid[b]
Multifocal	Shortness of breath, skin findings	Sarcoidosis	ACE, lysozyme; CXR/chest CT or gallium scan
	Endemic area	Tuberculosis	IGRA or PPD, chest x-ray/chest CT
	Peripheral retinal necrosis with occlusive arteriolar vasculitis	ARN	PCR of ocular fluid[b], possibly vitrectomy/retinal biopsy

Type of Inflammation	Possible Associated Factors	Suspected Disease[a]	Laboratory Tests, Imaging
Posterior Uveitis (continued)			
	HIV infection or immunosuppressed	Syphilis, toxoplasmosis	Syphilis IgG or FTA-ABS or MHA-TP and RPR or VDRL; toxoplasmosis ELISA to rule out
	IV drug use, indwelling lines	*Candida*, *Aspergillus* infection	Blood, vitreous cultures
	Visible intraocular parasite; from Africa or Central/South America	Cysticercosis	ELISA, brain MRI
		Onchocerciasis	Skin snip
	Over age 50 years	Intraocular lymphoma	Vitrectomy; chorioretinal biopsy cytology; IL-10/IL-6 ratio[b] genotyping studies; brain MRI, LP
	None	Birdshot chorioretinopathy	Clinical diagnosis; HLA-A29
		Multifocal choroiditis with panuveitis	Rule out TB, sarcoidosis, syphilis
Diffuse	Dermatologic/CNS symptoms; serous retinal disease	Vogt-Koyanagi-Harada syndrome	Clinical diagnosis; LP to document CSF pleocytosis; consider audiology referral
	Postsurgical/traumatic, bilateral, serous retinal disease	Sympathetic ophthalmia	
	Postsurgical/traumatic, unilateral	Infectious endophthalmitis	Consider vitrectomy, culture
	Child; history of geophagia	Toxocariasis	ELISA, complete blood count with differential
Chorioretinitis *without* vitritis			
Focal	None; history of carcinoma	Neoplastic	Metastatic workup
Multifocal	Ohio/Mississippi Valley	Ocular histoplasmosis	Clinical diagnosis
	Lesions confined to posterior pole	White dot syndromes (eg, APMPPE, MEWDS, PIC)	Clinical diagnosis
	Geographic (maplike) pattern of scars	Serpiginous choroiditis	IGRA or PPD, CXR
Diffuse	From Africa, Central/South America	Onchocerciasis	Skin snip
	Severe immunocompromise (eg, AIDS)	Progressive outer retinal necrosis	Same as for ARN

(Continued)

Table 5-4 *(continued)*

Type of Inflammation	Possible Associated Factors	Suspected Disease[a]	Laboratory Tests, Imaging
Posterior Uveitis (continued)			
Vasculitis			
	Aphthous ulcers, hypopyon	Behçet disease	Clinical diagnosis, screen for other organ involvement; rheumatology referral
	Malar rash, female, arthralgias	Systemic lupus erythematosus	ANA, anti-dsDNA, C3, C4; rheumatology referral
	Chronic sinusitis with hemorrhagic rhinorrhea, dyspnea, renal insufficiency, purpura	Granulomatosis with polyangiitis	c-ANCA (anti–proteinase 3); rheumatology referral

[a] Syphilis may present as any type of uveitis and should be considered in all patients.
[b] Testing where available.
ACE = angiotensin-converting enzyme; AIDS = acquired immune deficiency syndrome; ANA = antinuclear antibody; anti-dsDNA = anti-double-stranded DNA antibody; APMPPE = acute posterior multifocal placoid pigment epitheliopathy; ARN = acute retinal necrosis; C3, C4 = complement 3, complement 4; c-ANCA = c-anti-neutrophil cytoplasmic antibody; CMV = cytomegalovirus; CNS = central nervous system; CSF = cerebrospinal fluid; CT = computed tomography; CXR = chest x-ray; ELISA = enzyme-linked immunosorbent assay; ESR = erythrocyte sedimentation rate; FTA-ABS = fluorescent treponemal antibody absorption; GI = gastrointestinal; GU = genitourinary; HIV = human immunodeficiency virus; IGRA = interferon gamma release assay; IOL = intraocular lens; IOP = intraocular pressure; IV = intravenous; JIA = juvenile idiopathic arthritis; KP = keratic precipitates; LP = lumbar puncture; MEWDS = multiple evanescent white dot syndrome; MHA-TP = microhemagglutination assay–*Treponema pallidum;* MRI = magnetic resonance imaging; PCR = polymerase chain reaction; PIC = punctate inner choroidopathy; PPD = purified protein derivative; RF = rheumatoid factor; RPR = rapid plasma reagin; TB = tuberculosis; VDRL = Venereal Disease Research Laboratory.

overlying foci of active inflammation, or on the posterior vitreous face. Fundoscopy reveals focal, multifocal, or diffuse areas of retinitis and/or choroiditis, often with retinal vasculitis. Entities may have a similar clinical appearance, though some clinical patterns of disease are nearly pathognomonic for diagnosis. Structural complications such as macular edema, epiretinal membrane, and retinal or choroidal neovascularization are not sufficient for the anatomical classification of posterior uveitis (see Table 5-4). (Chapters 9–11 discuss noninfectious and infectious posterior uveitis in greater detail.)

Panuveitis

In panuveitis, inflammation is present diffusely throughout the eye without a predominantly affected site. Inflammation may be associated with an infectious or noninfectious systemic disease (see Table 5-4). (Chapters 9–11 discuss noninfectious and infectious panuveitis in greater depth, and Chapter 12 covers endophthalmitis.)

Retinal vasculitis

Retinal vasculitis is defined by the presence of retinal vascular changes in association with ocular inflammation. The term *retinal vasculitis* is used in distinction to *vasculopathy*, in which there are vessel changes but no visible evidence of inflammation. *Retinal vasculitis* encompasses perivascular sheathing, vascular leakage, or occlusion shown on fluorescein angiography studies. Peripheral vascular sheathing can be observed in intermediate uveitis but is not sufficient for the anatomical classification of posterior/panuveitis. Retinal vasculitis is not considered to be a defining feature for the anatomical classification of uveitis. Table 5-5 summarizes diseases associated with retinal vasculitis.

Classification by Clinical Features

When uveitis symptoms begin quickly, the onset is termed *sudden*; when gradual, the onset is termed *insidious*. The clinical course of uveitis may be acute, chronic, or recurrent. *Acute uveitis* describes episodes of sudden onset and limited duration that usually resolve within 3 months or less. *Chronic uveitis* is persistent, with relapse occurring in less

Table 5-5 Diseases With Retinal Vasculitis

Primarily Arteritis	Primarily Phlebitis	Arteritis and Phlebitis
Systemic lupus erythematosus	Sarcoidosis	Toxoplasmosis
Polyarteritis nodosa	Multiple sclerosis	Relapsing polychondritis
Syphilis	Behçet disease	Granulomatosis with polyangiitis
HSV, VZV (ARN/BARN)	Birdshot chorioretinopathy	Crohn disease
HSV, VZV (PORN)	HIV paraviral syndrome	Frosted branch angiitis
IRVAN	Eales disease	
Churg-Strauss syndrome		
Susac syndrome		

ARN = acute retinal necrosis; BARN = bilateral acute retinal necrosis; HIV = human immunodeficiency virus; HSV = herpes simplex virus; IRVAN = idiopathic retinal vasculitis, aneurysms, and neuroretinitis; PORN = progressive outer retinal necrosis; VZV = varicella-zoster virus.

Adapted with permission from Foster CS, Vitale AT. *Diagnosis and Treatment of Uveitis.* 2nd ed. Jaypee Brothers Medical Publishers, New Delhi, India; 2012:123–128.

than 3 months after discontinuing treatment. *Recurrent uveitis* involves repeated episodes separated by periods of inactivity without treatment that last 3 months or longer.

The severity of the inflammation can influence categorization and prognosis. The inflammatory process may occur in one or both eyes, or it may alternate between them. The distribution of ocular involvement—focal, multifocal, or diffuse—is also helpful to note when classifying uveitis.

The classification of uveitis as either granulomatous or nongranulomatous is still in use. However, the *clinical* appearance of uveitis as granulomatous or nongranulomatous may not necessarily correlate with the *histologic* description and can instead be related to the disease stage, the amount of antigen at presentation, or the patient's state of immunocompromise (eg, a patient being treated with corticosteroids). *Nongranulomatous* inflammation typically has a lymphocytic and plasma cell infiltrate; clinically, cellular deposits (keratic precipitates) tend to be finer and distributed diffusely. *Granulomatous* inflammation also includes epithelioid and giant cells; clinically, cellular deposits with large, clumped, or greasy appearance are predominantly located in a gravity-dependent position on the inferior cornea. Discrete granulomas are characteristic of sarcoidosis and tuberculosis; diffuse granulomatous inflammation appears in Vogt-Koyanagi-Harada syndrome and sympathetic ophthalmia. Zonal granulomatous disease can be observed in lens-induced uveitis.

Symptoms of Uveitis

Symptoms produced by uveitis depend on which part of the uveal tract is inflamed, the rapidity of onset (sudden or insidious), the duration of the disease (limited or persistent), the course of the disease (acute, chronic, or recurrent), and sometimes the underlying etiology.

Anterior uveitis can have a range of presentations, from a quiet asymptomatic white eye to an extremely painful red eye depending on the type of uveitis and/or severity of inflammation. Sudden-onset anterior uveitis usually causes acute pain, photophobia, redness, and blurred vision. Pain results from ciliary spasm associated with inflammation in the region of the iris and may radiate over the larger area served by cranial nerve V (the trigeminal nerve). Intraocular pressure (IOP) elevation due to angle closure or trabeculitis can be another cause of pain.

In contrast, chronic anterior uveitis in patients with juvenile idiopathic arthritis (JIA) may not be associated with any symptoms at all. However, even if initially asymptomatic, chronic or severe anterior uveitis can cause blurred vision because of structural complications such as calcific band keratopathy, cataract, or macular edema.

Isolated intermediate uveitis presents with a white, quiet eye and produces symptoms of floaters and blurred vision. Floaters result from the shadows cast by vitreous cells and debris on the retina. Blurred vision can result from macular edema or vitreous opacities in the visual axis.

Presenting symptoms in patients with posterior uveitis include painless blurred vision, floaters, photopsias, scotomata, metamorphopsia, nyctalopia, or a combination of these symptoms. The blurred vision can be caused primarily by retinitis and/or choroiditis directly affecting macular function, or secondarily by complications of inflammation. Table 5-6 summarizes symptoms of uveitis.

Table 5-6 Symptoms of Uveitis

Redness
Pain
Photophobia
Epiphora
Visual disturbances
  Diffuse blur, caused by
    Refractive shift
    Inflammatory cells
    Cataract, calcific band keratopathy, macular edema, retinochoroiditis
    Corneal, retinal, or optic disc edema
  Floaters
  Photopsias
  Scotomata (central or peripheral)
  Metamorphopsia
  Nyctalopia

Signs of Uveitis

The chemical mediators involved in inflammation (see Chapter 1) result in vascular dilation (ciliary flush), increased vascular permeability (aqueous flare), and chemotaxis of inflammatory cells into the eye (aqueous and vitreous cellular reaction). Table 5-7 summarizes signs of uveitis.

Anterior Segment

Signs of uveitis in the anterior portion of the eye include

- inflammatory cells (Fig 5-1)
- flare (Fig 5-2)
- hypopyon
- fibrin in the anterior chamber
- keratic precipitates (Figs 5-3, 5-4)
- iris nodules (Fig 5-5)
- iris atrophy or heterochromia
- pupillary miosis
- synechiae, anterior and posterior (Fig 5-6)
- pigment dispersion
- cataract*
- band keratopathy*

*Observed in long-standing uveitis

The major finding in anterior uveitis is the presence of inflammatory cells and flare in the anterior chamber, but there may be many additional sequalae. The SUN system grades the intensity of anterior chamber cells according to the number of inflammatory cells observed on slit-lamp examination in a field defined as a 1×1 mm high-power beam at full intensity at a 45°–60° angle in a dark room. Flare is defined by the visibility of the slit-lamp

Table 5-7 Signs of Uveitis

Eyelid and skin
- Vitiligo
- Nodules
- Ptosis/lid edema

Conjunctiva/sclera
- Perilimbal or diffuse injection
- Nodules
- Scleral thinning

Corneal endothelium
- Keratic (cellular) precipitates (diffuse or gravitational)
- Fibrin
- Pigment (nonspecific)

Anterior/posterior chamber
- Inflammatory cells
- Flare (proteinaceous influx)
- Pigment (nonspecific)

Iris
- Nodules
- Posterior synechiae
- Atrophy
- Heterochromia

Angle
- Peripheral anterior synechiae
- Nodules
- Vascularization

Intraocular pressure
- Hypotony
- High pressure
- Trabeculitis or secondary glaucoma

Vitreous
- Inflammatory cells (single/clumped)
- Traction bands

Pars plana
- Snowbanking

Retina
- Inflammatory cells/thickening/whitening
- Inflammatory cuffing of blood vessels
- Neovascularization
- Edema
- Uveitic macular edema
- Epiretinal membranes
- Subretinal fluid
- Retinal pigment epithelium: hypertrophy/clumping/loss

Choroid
- Inflammatory infiltrate/thickening
- Atrophy
- Neovascularization

Optic nerve
- Edema (nonspecific)
- Neovascularization

beam in the anterior chamber. The SUN system adopted the flare grading method described previously by Hogan and colleagues (Table 5-8).

The anterior chamber reaction can be described as

- serous (aqueous flare caused by protein influx)
- purulent (polymorphonuclear leukocytes and necrotic debris causing hypopyon)
- fibrinous (plasmoid, or intense fibrinous exudate)
- sanguinoid (inflammatory cells with erythrocytes, as manifested by hypopyon mixed with hyphema)

Keratic precipitates (KPs) are collections of inflammatory cells on the corneal endothelium. Newly formed KPs tend to be white and smoothly rounded, later transitioning to crenated (shrunken), pigmented, or glassy in nature. Large, yellowish KPs are called *mutton-fat KPs* and are usually associated with granulomatous types of inflammation. Associated corneal edema may be present. Band keratopathy is seen in chronic uveitis (especially JIA associated).

Iris involvement may manifest as either anterior or posterior synechiae, iris nodules (Koeppe nodules at the pupillary border, Busacca nodules within the iris stroma [see Fig 5-5]

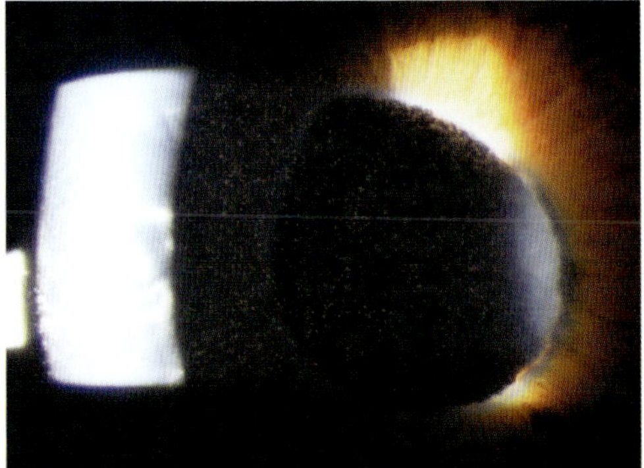

Figure 5-1 Inflammatory cells in the anterior chamber (grade 4+) of a patient with anterior uveitis. *(Courtesy of Emmett T. Cunningham Jr, MD, PhD, MPH.)*

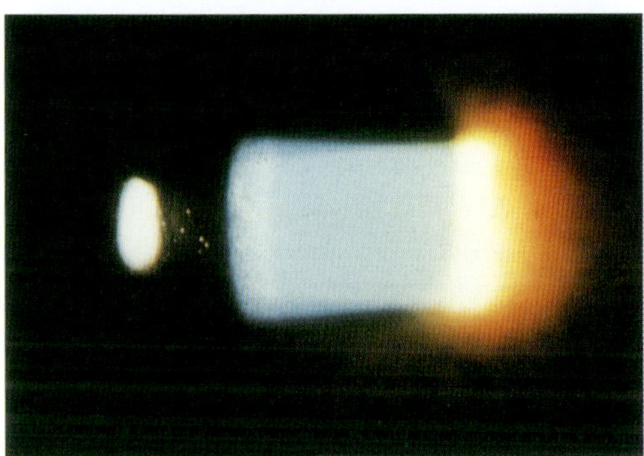

Figure 5-2 Aqueous flare (grade 4+) in a patient with acute anterior uveitis.

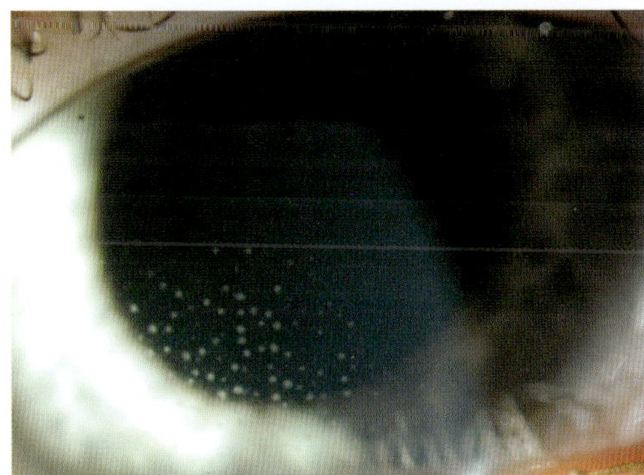

Figure 5-3 Keratic precipitates (medium and small). *(Courtesy of Debra A. Goldstein, MD.)*

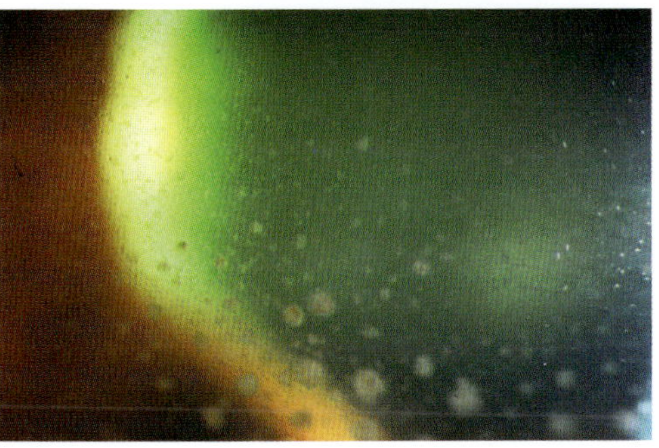

Figure 5-4 Large "mutton-fat" keratic precipitates in a patient with sarcoidosis. Large keratic precipitates such as these generally indicate a granulomatous disease process. *(Courtesy of Debra A. Goldstein, MD.)*

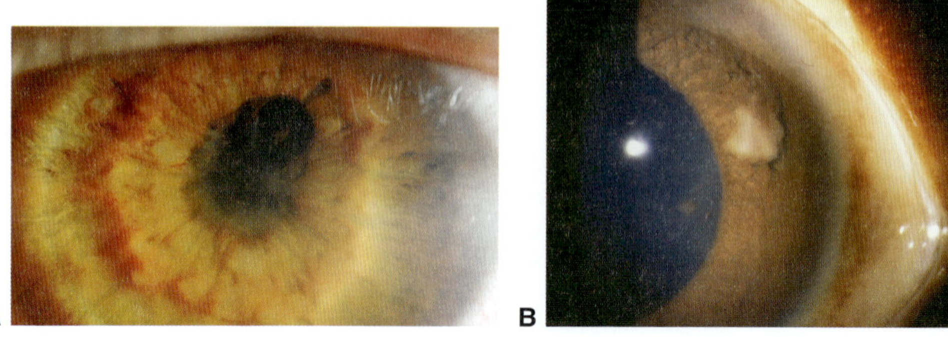

Figure 5-5 Mid-iris nodules (Busacca nodules) in 2 patients **(A, B)** with sarcoidosis. *(Part A courtesy of Debra A. Goldstein, MD. Part B courtesy of Wendy M. Smith, MD.)*

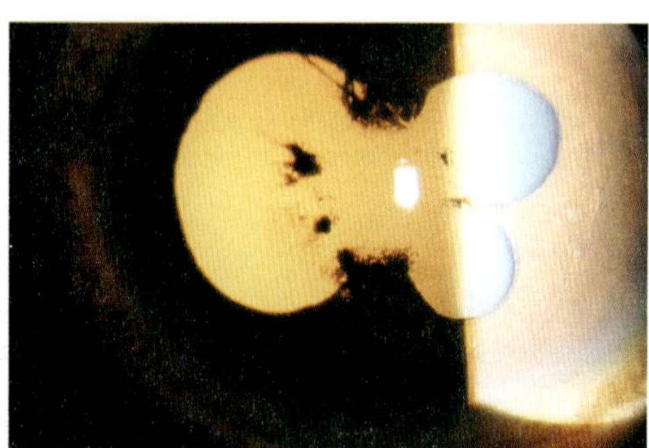

Figure 5-6 Multiple posterior synechiae preventing complete dilation of the pupil. *(Courtesy of David Forster, MD.)*

Table 5-8 Grading Scheme for Anterior Chamber Cells and Flare Based on Standardization of Uveitis Nomenclature (SUN) Criteria

Grade	Number of Cells (High-Intensity 1×1-mm Slit Beam)	Flare
0	<1	None
0.5+	1–5	Not applicable
1+	6–15	Faint
2+	16–25	Moderate (clear iris details)
3+	26–50	Marked (hazy iris details)
4+	>50	Intense (fibrin or plasmoid aqueous)

Reprinted with permission from Jabs DA, Nussenblatt RB, Rosenbaum JT; Standardization of Uveitis Nomenclature (SUN) Working Group. Standardization of nomenclature for reporting clinical data. Results of the First International Workshop. *Am J Ophthalmol.* 2005;140(3):512.

and Berlin nodules in the angle, iris granulomas, heterochromia (eg, Fuchs uveitis syndrome), or stromal atrophy (eg, herpetic uveitis).

With uveitic involvement of the ciliary body and trabecular meshwork, IOP is often low, secondary to decreased aqueous production or increased uveoscleral outflow, but

IOP may increase precipitously if the meshwork becomes clogged by inflammatory cells or debris or if the trabecular meshwork itself is the site of inflammation (trabeculitis). Pupillary block with iris bombé and secondary angle closure may also lead to an acute rise in IOP.

Hogan MJ, Kimura SJ, Thygeson P. Signs and symptoms of uveitis. I. Anterior uveitis. *Am J Ophthalmol.* 1959;47(5, part 2):155–170.

Intermediate Segment

Signs of uveitis in the intermediate portion of the eye include

- inflammatory cells in vitreous
- vitreous haze (Fig 5-7)
- snowballs (clumped vitreous cells)
- snowbanks (exudate over pars plana)
- ciliary body detachment
- retrolental membrane
- vitreous strands or traction band

The hallmark of intermediate uveitis is vitreous cell and haze. Cells may be clumped or individual. The cells make up vitreous haze when viewed in combination with proteinaceous vitreous debris.

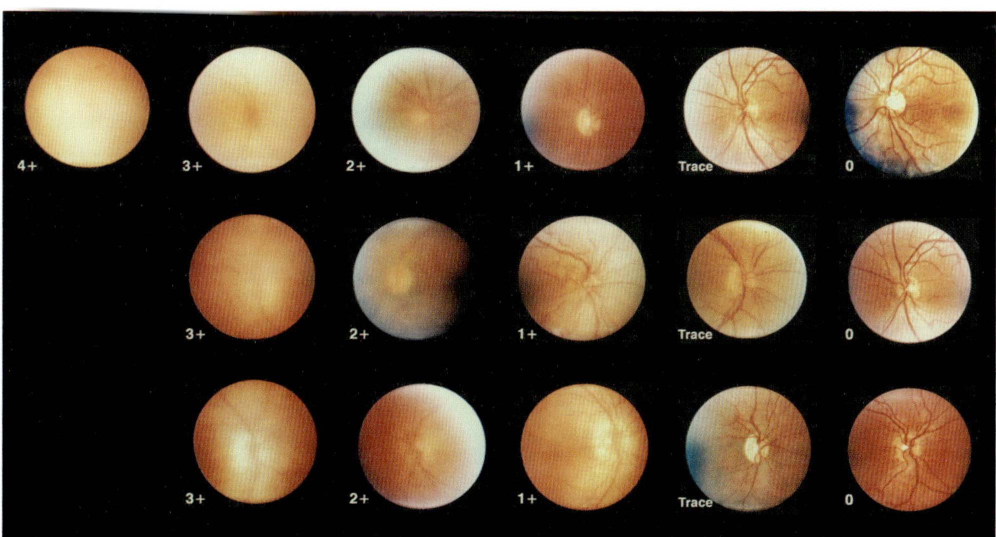

Figure 5-7 Grading scale for vitreous haze: representative standard images. Grade 4: Dense opacity obscuring optic nerve head. Grade 3: Optic nerve visible, borders blurred, no retinal vessels seen. Grade 2: Significant blurring of optic nerve and retinal vessels but still visible. Grade 1: Few opacities, mild blurring of optic nerve and retinal vessels. Trace (0.5+): Trace. Grade 0: Clear. *(Courtesy of NEI, originally published in Nussenblatt RB, Palestine AG, Chan CC, et al. Standardization of vitreal inflammatory activity in intermediate and posterior uveitis.* Ophthalmology. *1985;92(4):467–471.)*

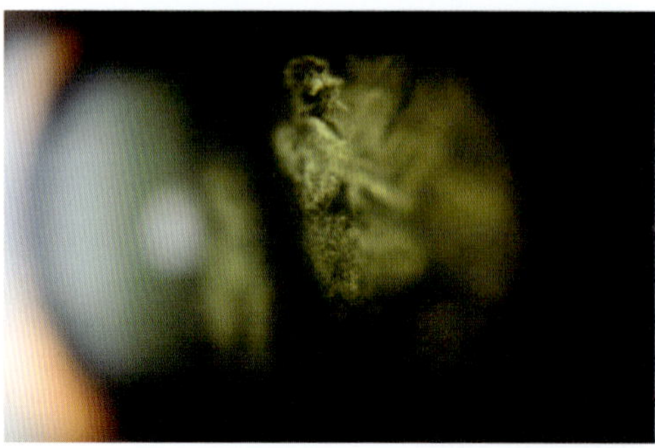

Figure 5-8 Slit-lamp technique for viewing anterior vitreous cells and opacity, demonstrated in a patient with amyloidosis. *(Courtesy of Emilio M. Dodds, MD.)*

Table 5-9 Grading Scheme for Vitreous Chamber Cells and Haze

Grade	Number of Cells in Retrolental Space (High-Intensity 1×0.5-mm Slit Beam)	Vitreous Haze
0	0	Clear view of fundus
0.5+	1–5	Not applicable
1+	6–10	Faint
2+	11–20	Moderate (clear optic nerve details)
3+	21–50	Marked (hazy optic nerve details)
4+	>50	Intense (minimal/no optic nerve detail)

The physician typically grades vitreous cells on a 0–4 numeric scale by observing the retrolental space in a dilated eye using the slit-lamp biomicroscope and a 1×0.5 mm beam (Fig 5-8). The consensus is that cells in the vitreous strands are old, and cells in the syneretic areas are likely new. The SUN system does not specify a grading system for vitreous cells. Table 5-9 shows the vitreous cell grading scale used in the Multicenter Uveitis Steroid Treatment Trial (MUST).

Vitreous haze may be a better indicator of disease activity than cell counts alone. The grading of vitreous haze is based on the clarity of view of the posterior segment on funduscopic examination. The National Institutes of Health grading system for vitreous haze, which the SUN system adopted, employs a standardized set of fundus photographs that defines vitreous haze on a 0–4 scale (see Fig 5-7). Vitreous haze has been used in inclusion criteria in clinical trials for uveitis, and a 2-step improvement has been used as a principal outcome measure.

Additional signs of inflammation in the vitreous include *snowball opacities* (clumps of inflammatory cells in the vitreous) and *snowbanks* (exudates over the pars plana, especially prominent inferiorly). Active snowbanks have a fluffy or shaggy appearance. As pars planitis becomes inactive, the pars plana appears gliotic or fibrotic and smooth; thus, these changes are not referred to as snowbanks. Vitreal strands and snowballs may vary in clinical appearance by disease type. Chronic intermediate uveitis may be associated with cyclitic membrane formation, secondary ciliary body detachment, and hypotony.

Posterior Segment

Signs in the posterior segment of the eye include

- retinal or choroidal inflammatory infiltrates
- inflammatory sheathing of arteries or veins
- exudative, tractional*, or rhegmatogenous* retinal detachment
- retinal pigment epithelial hypertrophy or atrophy*
- atrophy or swelling of the retina, choroid, or optic nerve head*
- preretinal or subretinal fibrosis*
- retinal or choroidal neovascularization*

*Indicates structural complications. Retinal and choroidal signs may be unifocal, multifocal, or diffuse.

Posterior segment inflammation is a result of inflammatory or infectious infiltration and resultant structural damage of the retina and choroid. Retinal and choroidal signs may be unifocal, multifocal, or diffuse. Lesions are described by size, color, and appearance (eg, well demarcated, geographic), and anatomical relationship to posterior pole landmarks (see Table 5-7).

Nussenblatt RB, Palestine AG, Chan CC, Roberge F. Standardization of vitreal inflammatory activity in intermediate and posterior uveitis. *Ophthalmology.* 1985;92(4):467–471.

Review of the Patient's Health and Other Associated Factors

A comprehensive history and review of systems help to narrow the differential diagnosis and guide ancillary testing and treatment options. The patient's personal characteristics, medical history, and social history can help in the classification and identification of uveitis (Table 5-10). Immunocompromise, sexual practices, use of intravenous drugs, hyperalimentation, and certain occupations are just some of the risk factors that can direct the investigation. In this regard, a diagnostic survey for uveitis as shown in the appendix can be very helpful.

Table 5–10 Patient Factors in Diagnosis of Uveitis

Patient Characteristics	Family and Social History	Additional Modifying Factors
Age Sex Race/ethnicity/country of origin	Family or personal history of autoimmune disease/ endemic infection	Immunization history
	Medication or intravenous drug use	Immune system status
	Tobacco exposure	Systemic medications
	Occupation	Trauma history
	Sexual practices	Travel history
	Eating habits	Hospital admissions/surgery
	Pets and animal exposures	Indwelling lines/instrumentation
		Review of systems and existing medical conditions

Although ocular inflammation can be an isolated process involving only the eye, it can also be associated with a systemic condition. However, uveitis frequently does not correlate with inflammatory activity elsewhere in the body and may precede the development of inflammation at other body sites.

Differential Diagnosis of Uveitis

The differential diagnosis of uveitis includes infectious agents (viruses, bacteria, fungi, protozoa, and helminths), noninfectious entities of presumed immunologic origin, and unknown/idiopathic causes (called *undifferentiated uveitis*). In addition, masquerade syndromes such as intraocular lymphoma, retinoblastoma, leukemia, choroidal metastases, and malignant melanoma can be mistaken for uveitis. Other masquerade syndromes include juvenile xanthogranuloma, pigment dispersion syndrome, retinal detachment, vitreous hemorrhage, retinitis pigmentosa, and ocular ischemic syndrome. One should consider each of these entities in the differential diagnosis of uveitis.

A careful history and accurate description of biomicroscopic and fundus findings are extremely helpful in narrowing the differential diagnosis, as certain presentations are characteristic for specific diseases; however, many patients do not present with classic signs and symptoms, or their clinical appearance may evolve with time and treatment. The clinician should consider the differential diagnosis and how well the individual patient's uveitis fits with the various known entities. This system first classifies the type of uveitis based on anatomical criteria and associated factors (eg, acute versus chronic, unilateral versus bilateral, adult versus child) and then matches the pattern of uveitis with a list of potential entities that share similar characteristics. See Table 5-4 for a simplified version of one such system for narrowing the differential diagnosis. Activity 5-1 provides a decision-tree algorithm for the evaluation of a uveitis patient.

ACTIVITY 5-1 Flow chart for clinical diagnosis and treatment of uveitis: simplified interactive tool.
Activity developed by Thellea K. Leveque, MD, MPH.
Access the activity at www.aao.org/bcscactivity_section09.

Ancillary Testing

Medical history, review of systems, thorough ophthalmologic and general physical examination, and formulation of a working differential diagnosis are cornerstones of the workup of a patient with uveitis. They should precede any laboratory testing. Laboratory testing is not a substitute for a thorough, hands-on clinical evaluation.

There is no one standardized battery of tests that fits for all patients with uveitis. Rather, a tailored approach should be based on the most likely causes for each patient. After compiling a list of differential diagnoses based on the anatomical location and clinical characteristics of the inflammation, the ophthalmologist can order appropriate laboratory tests. Many patients require only a few diagnostic tests.

Most uveitis specialists do recommend syphilis testing for all uveitis patients, as syphilis can present as any form of uveitis, and systemic infection is often undiagnosed. In addition, the consequences of treating with steroid in the presence of untreated occult syphilis infection can be disastrous for patient outcomes. In the correct clinical scenario, or where immunomodulatory therapy (IMT) will be used, most uveitis specialists also recommend testing for tuberculosis with a purified protein derivative (PPD) skin test or interferon-gamma release assay. A chest radiograph can screen for sarcoidosis, which is a common cause of uveitis with protean manifestations. Tables 5-4 and 5-11 list some of the laboratory tests and their indications. Later chapters further discuss these tests in context of the various types of uveitis.

It is important to use caution in ordering and interpreting laboratory tests, because even very sensitive and specific tests are not perfect and can yield misleading results if the likelihood of disease in a particular patient is low. In other words, when testing a large group of patients for a very rare disease, a positive test may not actually represent the true presence of disease. The Bayes theorem describes this concept. The theorem is a statistical calculation used to describe the probability of an event based on prior knowledge of conditions that might be related to the event. (See BCSC Section 1, *Update on General Medicine.)*

Ophthalmic Imaging and Functional Tests

Ophthalmic imaging and functional testing are useful both diagnostically and in monitoring the patient's response to therapy. They can provide information not obtainable from biomicroscopic or fundus examination. The use of combined imaging modalities, called *multimodal imaging*, can be complementary and additive in this task. For discussion of ophthalmic imaging modalities and electroretinogram testing, see BCSC Section 12, *Retina and Vitreous.*

Kawali A, Pichi F, Avadhani K, Invernizzi A, Hashimoto Y, Mahendradas P. Multimodal imaging of the normal eye. *Ocul Immunol Inflam.* 2017;25(5):721–731.

Van Gelder RN. Diagnostic testing in uveitis. *Focal Points: Clinical Modules for Ophthalmologists.* San Francisco: American Academy of Ophthalmology; 2013, module 4.

Optical coherence tomography

Optical coherence tomography (OCT) produces a series of high-resolution cross-sectional images of the retina and choroid and is used to identify morphologic changes seen in eyes with uveitis. A noncontact imaging technique, OCT has become the standard-of-care method for objective measurement of uveitic macular edema (Fig 5-9), retinal thickening, subretinal and intraretinal fluid associated with choroidal neovascularization, and serous retinal detachments. Although sometimes useful when the fundus is viewed in eyes with smaller pupils, media opacity can limit the clarity of OCT. OCT is also valuable in monitoring the nerve fiber layer in patients with uveitic glaucoma. Anterior segment OCT may be useful to evaluate an eye for retained lens fragments or IOL chafing in persistent postoperative uveitis. There are ongoing efforts to develop OCT-based objective grading of intraocular cells/inflammation.

Enhanced depth imaging OCT (EDI-OCT; Fig 5-10) provides deeper tissue penetration. This technique allows visualization of the choroid, which can have structural alterations in several uveitic diseases, notably Vogt-Koyanagi-Harada syndrome, sympathetic ophthalmia, and birdshot chorioretinopathy.

Table 5-11 Laboratory Tests and Imaging Studies Used in Uveitis Evaluations

Test	Indications and/or Potential Diagnoses
Hematologic blood tests	
Complete blood count with differential	IMT and select antibiotics/antivirals, leukemia, lymphoma, immune status (eg., neutropenia)
Erythrocyte sedimentation rate	Giant cell arteritis
Interferon-gamma release assay	Latent and active tuberculosis
T-cell subsets	Opportunistic infection, HIV
Serologic tests	
Liver function tests (ALT, AST)	IMT (antimetabolites), sarcoidosis, hepatitis
Serum urea nitrogen, creatinine	IMT (T-cell inhibitors), glomerulonephritis
Angiotensin-converting enzyme, lysozyme, calcium	Sarcoidosis
Antinuclear antibody	Connective tissue disease, juvenile idiopathic arthritis
Antiphospholipid antibodies	Vascular occlusion
Rheumatoid factor, anticitrullinated protein antibody	Rheumatoid arthritis, juvenile idiopathic arthritis
HLA testing	
HLA-B27	Spondyloarthropathy; acute anterior uveitis
HLA-A29	Birdshot chorioretinopathy
HLA-B51 (rarely obtained and of limited value)	Behçet disease
HLA DR, DQ class II	TINU syndrome
ANCA testing—c-ANCA (proteinase 3) and p-ANCA (myeloperoxidase)	Systemic vasculitides
VDRL/RPR (nontreponemal tests); syphilis IgG/FTA-ABS/MHA-TP (treponomal-specific tests)	Syphilis
Lyme disease serology	Lyme disease
Brucella species serology	Brucellosis
Toxoplasma gondii serology	Toxoplasmosis
Fungal serology (complement fixation)	Coccidioidomycosis, typically not obtained for presumed ocular histoplasmosis
Bartonella quintana and *B henselae* serology	Cat-scratch disease
EBV, HSV, VZV, CMV serology	Viral uveitis (little benefit unless negative)
HIV serology/Western blot	HIV/AIDS, opportunistic infections, vascular occlusions
Cerebrospinal fluid (CSF) studies	
Protein, glucose, cell counts/cytology, cultures, Gram stain, CSF VDRL, oligoclonal bands	APMPPE, VKH syndrome, syphilis and other infection, malignancy, primary intraocular lymphoma, MS
Urine studies	
Urinalysis for hematuria, proteinuria, and casts; urinary beta-2 microglobulin	IMT (cyclophosphamide toxicity), ANCA-associated vasculities; TINU syndrome
Radiographic studies	
Chest radiograph	Tuberculosis, sarcoidosis, granulomatosis with polyangiitis
Sacroiliac joint x-rays	HLA-B27–associated ankylosing spondylitis

Test	Indications and/or Potential Diagnoses
CT of chest	Tuberculosis, sarcoidosis, granulomatosis with polyangiitis
CT/magnetic resonance imaging of brain and orbits	Sarcoidosis, central nervous system lymphoma, toxoplasmosis, MS
Intraocular fluid analysis and tissue biopsy	
Intraocular fluid analysis for local antibody production (limited availability)	HSV, VZV, CMV, rubella virus, *Toxoplasma* organisms
Polymerase chain reaction	Viridae: HSV-1, HSV-2, VZV, CMV, EBV, Ebola, Zika, West Nile, rubella Bacteria: universal 16S subunit for pan-bacteria; individual PCR primers available for many individual bacteria, varies by laboratory Protozoa: *Toxoplasma gondii* Fungi: universal 18S or 28S subunit for panfungi: *Candida albicans, Aspergillus* species (28S rRNA gene) Intraocular lymphoma (IgH, TCR, *MYD88*, others)
Endoretinal, subretinal, choroidal biopsy	Necrotizing retinitis, neoplasia (central nervous system lymphoma)
Skin, conjunctival, lacrimal biopsy	Sarcoidosis, infection, lymphoma, amyloidosis
Stool for detection of pathogenic microorganisms	Parasitic diseases; viruses, bacteria, fungi

ALT = alanine aminotransferase; ANCA = antineutrophil cytoplasmic antibody; APMPPE = acute posterior multifocal placoid pigment epitheliopathy; AST = aspartate aminotransferase; c-ANCA = cytoplasmic ANCA; CMV = cytomegalovirus; CSF = cerebrospinal fluid; CT = computed tomography; EBV = Epstein-Barr virus; FTA-ABS = fluorescent treponemal antibody absorption; HIV = human immunodeficiency virus; HLA = human leukocyte antigen; HSV = herpes simplex virus; IgH = immunoglobulin heavy locus; IMT = immunomodulatory therapy; MHA-TP = microhemagglutination assay–*Treponema pallidum;* MS = multiple sclerosis; p-ANCA = perinuclear ANCA; RPR = rapid plasma reagin; TCR = T-cell receptor; TINU = tubulointerstitial nephritis and uveitis syndrome; VDRL = Venereal Disease Research Laboratory; VKH = Vogt-Koyanagi-Harada; VZV = varicella-zoster virus.

OCT angiography (OCT-A) relies on repeated high-resolution scans of the same area to assess differences in blood flow, producing structural images of perfused vessels in ocular tissues. Case reports and case series describing the OCT-A characteristics of active and inactive chorioretinal lesions are emerging. These will have increasing implications for diagnosis and treatment of posterior uveitides over time.

Kim J, Knickelbein J, Jaworski L, et al. Enhanced depth imaging optical coherence tomography in uveitis: an intravisit and interobserver reproducibility study. *Am J Ophthalmol.* 2016;164:49–56.

Pichi F, Sarraf D, Arepalli S, et al. The application of optical coherence tomography angiography in uveitis and inflammatory eye diseases. *Prog Retin Eye Res.* 2017;59:178–201.

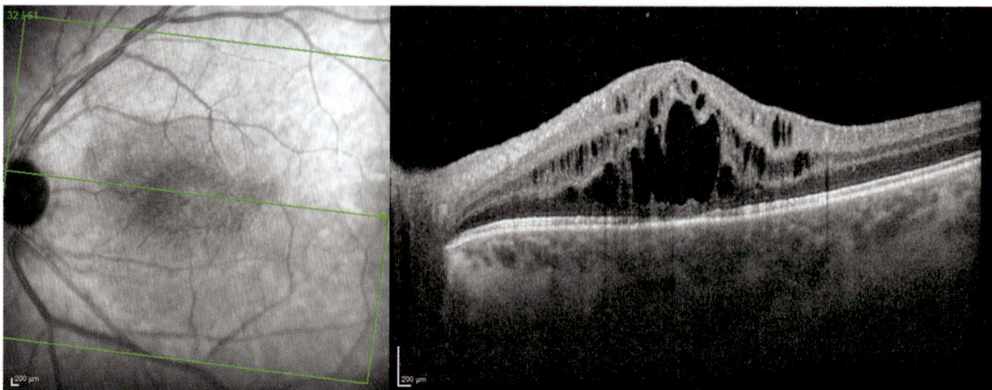

Figure 5-9 Optical coherence tomography image of uveitic macular edema in a patient with juvenile idiopathic arthritis–associated uveitis. *(Courtesy of Thellea K. Leveque, MD, MPH.)*

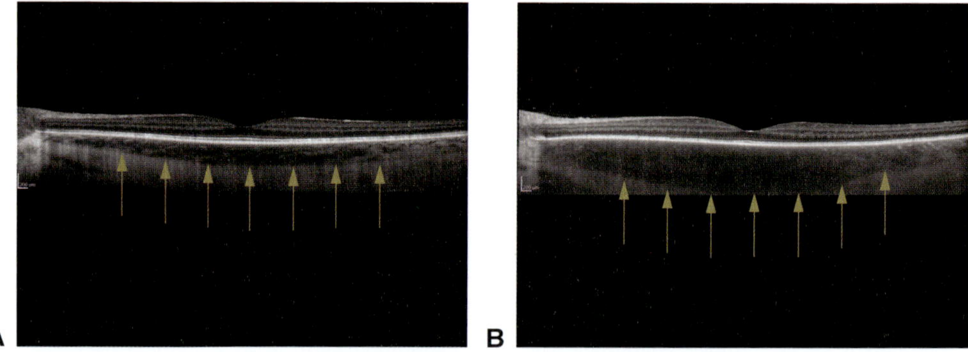

Figure 5-10 Enhanced-depth imaging optical coherence tomography in a patient with Vogt-Koyanagi-Harada syndrome **A,** During quiescence with relatively normal choroidal thickness *(arrows)*. **B,** During uveitis activity with diffuse choroidal thickening *(arrows)*. *(Courtesy of Thellea K. Leveque, MD, MPH.)*

Fluorescein angiography

Fluorescein angiography is an essential imaging modality for evaluating eyes with chorioretinal disease and structural complications caused by posterior uveitis. After intravenous injection of fluorescein sodium, a series of filtered posterior segment images provides a functional and structural view of retinal (and to some degree choroidal) vasculature and anatomy. Fluorescein angiography can detect macular edema (Fig 5-11), retinal vasculitis, secondary choroidal or retinal neovascularization, and areas of optic nerve, retinal, and choroidal inflammation. Several of the retinochoroidopathies, or white dot syndromes, have characteristic appearances on FA. Wide and ultra-wide-field FA can identify retinal vascular pathology not noted on clinical examination.

Laovirojjanakul W, Acharya N, Gonzales JA. Ultra-widefield fluorescein angiography in intermediate uveitis. *Ocul Immunol Inflam.* 2017 Oct 17:1–6.

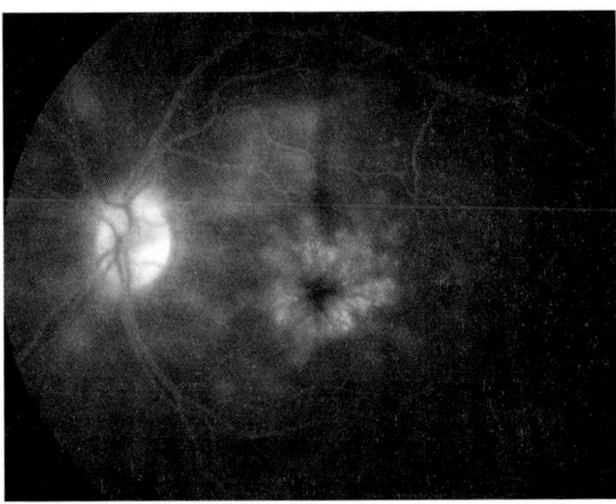

Figure 5-11 Late transit phase fluorescein angiogram of the left eye of a patient with sarcoid-associated anterior uveitis showing a petalloid pattern typical of uveitic macular edema. *(Courtesy of Ramana S. Moorthy, MD.)*

Color photography

Used alone or in conjunction with other imaging, color photographs of the anterior or posterior segment document lesion size, color, location, and morphologic characteristics used to assess clinical progression or regression of disease. These images can be useful in establishing a baseline when assessing a relapsing and remitting inflammatory process (eg, the presence of new posterior synechiae in anterior uveitis, or capturing transitory posterior segment inflammation characteristic of Behçet disease).

Fundus autofluorescence

Fundus autofluorescence (FAF) imaging is another noninvasive imaging technique for analyzing the posterior segment. It maps the fluorescent property of lipofuscin, a breakdown product of retinal proteins, within the retinal pigment epithelium (RPE). Hyperautofluorescence corresponds to increased metabolic activity of the RPE, or window defect due to loss of photoreceptors. Hypoautofluorescence occurs with loss or blockage of RPE cells. Imaging is useful in posterior uveitis that involves the outer retina, RPE, and inner choroid. Autofluorescence patterns vary between the different uveitides, but in many cases, hyperautofluorescence occurs with increased disease activity and fades and darkens as the inflammation subsides.

Indocyanine green angiography

Like FA, indocyanine green (ICG) imaging uses an intravenous injection coupled with serial retinal images to provide data about vasculature and anatomy of the posterior segment; the properties of ICG allow for specialized imaging of the choroidal circulation. In inflammatory diseases involving the outer retina and choroid, findings on ICG often exceed those visible on either fundoscopy or FA, which can have diagnostic and therapeutic implications. Its use is especially beneficial in the evaluation of inflammatory chorioretinopathies of unknown etiology (white dot syndromes), Vogt-Koyanagi-Harada syndrome, sympathetic ophthalmia, and posterior segment sarcoidosis, and in evaluation of choroidal neovascular membrane (see Chapter 9).

Ultrasonography

Anterior segment ultrasound biomicroscopy can be useful in diagnosing pathology of the ciliary body, iris, and iridocorneal angle in uveitis. Posterior segment ultrasound, or

B-scan ultrasound, can be useful in demonstrating vitreous opacities, choroidal thickening or elevation, retinal detachment, and cyclitic membrane formation, as well as in ruling out occult foreign bodies, particularly if media opacities preclude a view of the posterior segment. Retained IOL fragments may be visualized in the anterior or posterior segment. Ultrasonographic imaging may be diagnostic for posterior scleritis (see Chapter 7).

Electroretinography

Full-field electroretinography (ERG) can be used to monitor progression of birdshot chorioretinopathy, diagnose acute zonal occult outer retinopathy (AZOOR) complex diseases, and diagnose autoimmune retinopathy. Electroretinogram findings may also be useful in the uveitis workup when trying to distinguish certain retinal dystrophies from posterior uveitis.

Visual field testing/perimetry

Kinetic and nonkinetic perimetry are used to monitor progression and response to treatment of birdshot chorioretinopathy and AZOOR complex diseases. These techniques are also used to monitor visual field defects in uveitic glaucoma or inflammatory optic neuritis. Microperimetry may be helpful in diseases involving the macula, such as punctate inner choroiditis.

Ocular Fluid and Tissue Sampling

Polymerase chain reaction testing of aqueous and vitreous fluid

Polymerase chain reaction (PCR) testing for diagnosis of infectious uveitis is highly sensitive and specific. It can directly amplify the DNA of a suspected pathogen from a small sample volume of ophthalmic fluid, making it ideal for application in ocular tissue.

Testing of aqueous fluid is an important adjunct in diagnosis of infectious posterior uveitis. Aqueous humor PCR testing that is specific for herpes simplex virus types 1 or 2, varicella-zoster virus, and cytomegalovirus has high diagnostic sensitivity and specificity at levels similar to vitreous biopsy. Anterior chamber paracentesis is generally safer and easier to perform than vitreous sampling. In suspected cases of retinal toxoplasmosis, one can perform anterior chamber paracentesis for PCR, though the diagnostic yield may be lower than vitreous sampling. In toxoplasmosis, a positive anterior chamber PCR result can be more likely in patients with large lesions or immunocompromised patients. Diagnostic utility of isolated aqueous PCR testing for suspected viral anterior uveitis is much lower. In cases for which viral speciation is critical to management, repeat sampling can increase the yield.

Until recently, PCR was not practical for diagnosis of bacterial and fungal uveitis due to the need to specify the selected pathogen of interest for amplification. Now, based on conserved genetic subunits within bacteria (16S) and fungi (5.8S/18S/28S), panbacterial and panfungal PCR tests perform equally or superiorly to culture. The PCR-based techniques for genomic testing of vitreous samples are used in diagnosis of primary intraocular lymphoma. Disadvantages of PCR are cost, limitations in testing for multiple entities due to small fluid sample size, risk of improper amplification of a contaminant, and risk of identification failure when there is a paucity of cellular material.

Doan T, Acharya N, Pinsky BA, et al. Metagenomic DNA sequencing for the diagnosis of intraocular infections. *Ophthalmology.* 2017;124(8):1247–1248.

Harper TW, Miller D, Schiffman JC, Davis JL. Polymerase chain reaction analysis of aqueous and vitreous specimens in the diagnosis of posterior segment infectious uveitis. *Am J Ophthalmol.* 2009;147(1):140–147.

Rothova A, de Boer JH, Ten Dam-van Loon NH, et al Usefulness of aqueous humor analysis for the diagnosis of posterior uveitis. *Ophthalmology.* 2008;115(2):306–311.

Sowmya P, Madhavan HN. Diagnostic utility of polymerase chain reaction on intraocular specimens to establish the etiology of infectious endophthalmitis. *Eur J Ophthalmol.* 2009;19(5):812–817.

Taravati P, Lam D,Van Gelder RN. Role of molecular diagnostics in ocular microbiology. *Curr Ophthalmol Rep.* 2013;1(4).

Ocular serology/local antibody production

European countries consider evaluation of aqueous antibody production based on the Goldmann-Witmer (GW) coefficient to be the gold standard for the diagnosis of toxoplasmosis; however, this is not commercially available in the United States. (Chapter 2 explained calculation of the GW.) Diagnostic yield may increase when PCR and the GW coefficient are used together, especially in viral infections. Aqueous antibody production may persist even in the absence of cellular material, giving it certain advantages over PCR in viral anterior uveitis.

Culture and vital staining

Cell culture and bacterial and fungal staining are useful in cases of suspected bacterial or fungal endophthalmitis. Isolation is time consuming and can lack sensitivity due to the low pathogen load in ocular samples. However, the technique is the traditional first line of testing, widely available, and inexpensive to perform.

Cytology and Pathology

Anterior chamber paracentesis for cytologic studies may be diagnostic in cases involving the anterior or sometimes the posterior segment. Anterior chamber paracentesis in suspected leukemia or lymphoma is sent for cytologic analysis. When there is concern for primary vitreoretinal lymphoma, undiluted vitreous biopsy fluid is sent for cytology and flow cytometry analysis with gene rearrangement studies and cytokine analysis.

Chorioretinal biopsy for pathology is technically challenging and calls for an experienced vitreoretinal surgeon. It may be useful in rapidly progressive posterior uveitic entities for which the etiology is unknown and the therapeutic regimen undetermined. Suspected intraocular lymphoma confined to the subretinal space is also an indication for a chorioretinal biopsy. It is usually performed only if diagnosis cannot be confirmed after all other less-invasive testing. Directed conjunctival biopsy of visible lesions can be useful in lymphoma, cicatricial pemphigoid, and sarcoidosis. Rarely, scleral biopsy can be useful when considering infectious etiologies for scleritis (see Chapter 7). Vitreous biopsy can also be done to identify the etiology of certain uveitides, particularly in suspected cases of infectious chorioretinitis.

Anterior chamber paracentesis technique

Paracentesis involves using sterile technique at the slit lamp or with the patient supine on a treatment gurney or chair. Topical anesthetic drops are instilled; the eye is prepared with topical povidone-iodine solution; and a lid speculum can be placed. A tuberculin (1-mL) syringe is attached to a sterile 30-gauge needle. The syringe is then advanced under direct or slit-lamp visualization into the anterior chamber through the temporal limbus or clear cornea parallel to the iris plane. As much aqueous is aspirated as is safely possible (usually 0.1–0.2 mL), avoiding contact with the iris and lens. Possible complications include anterior chamber bleeding, infection, and damage to the iris or lens.

Vitreous biopsy technique

Vitreous specimens can be obtained either by needle tap or by using a vitrectomy instrument. If a small sample is desired, a needle tap of the vitreous is typically performed with the patient partially reclining in an examination room chair. Topical and subconjunctival anesthesia are administered; the eye is prepared with topical povidone-iodine solution, and a lid speculum is placed. Typically, a 25-gauge, 1-inch needle on a 3mL syringe (to provide greater vacuum) is introduced through the pars plana, directed toward the midvitreous cavity, and used to aspirate the vitreous sample. A diagnostic vitrectomy is performed via a standard 3-port pars plana vitrectomy (see BCSC Section 12, *Retina and Vitreous*). The most common indications for vitreous biopsy include suspected infection, primary intraocular lymphoma or other intraocular malignancy, and infectious etiologies of posterior uveitis or panuveitis. (Endophthalmitis is discussed in detail in Chapter 12, and intraocular lymphoma in Chapter 13.) In addition, chronic uveitis that has an atypical presentation or an inadequate response to conventional therapy may warrant diagnostic vitrectomy.

In all these scenarios, testing typically requires undiluted vitreous specimens. It is possible to obtain 0.5–1.0 mL of undiluted vitreous for evaluation using standard vitrectomy techniques. Complications of diagnostic vitrectomy in uveitic eyes can include retinal tears or detachment, suprachoroidal or vitreous hemorrhage, worsening of cataract or inflammation, and, rarely, sympathetic ophthalmia. Although vitreous surgery can be therapeutic and diagnostic in cases of uveitis, the pharmacokinetics of delivered intravitreal drugs are markedly altered in eyes that have undergone pars plana vitrectomy; the half-life of intravitreal corticosteroids, for example, is significantly reduced in vitrectomized eyes.

Chorioretinal biopsy technique

Video 5-1 demonstrates chorioretinal biopsy.

VIDEO 5-1 Chorioretinal biopsy.
Courtesy of P. Kumar Rao, MD.
Access the video at www.aao.org/bcscvideo_section09.

CHAPTER 6

Therapy for Uveitis

This chapter includes a related video, which can be accessed by scanning the QR code provided in the text or going to www.aao.org/bcscvideo_section09.

Highlights

- The goal of uveitis treatment is to prevent vision loss from structural complications of uncontrolled inflammation, while minimizing the ocular and systemic adverse effects of therapy.
- Medical therapy consists of local or systemic anti-inflammatory and/or antimicrobial agents.
- Anti inflammatory treatments include local and systemic corticosteroids and systemic immunomodulatory therapy.

Therapy for uveitis ranges from simple observation to complex medical or surgical intervention. Many patients with mild, self-limiting anterior uveitis need no referral to a uveitis specialist. However, in uveitis that is chronic or difficult to treat, early referral to a uveitis specialist may be helpful in confirming the diagnosis and determining a therapeutic regimen. Treatment may require coordination with other medical or surgical consultants and detailed informed consent. Discussion with the patient and other specialists about the prognosis and complications of uveitis helps determine the appropriate therapy.

Medical Management of Uveitis

The goal of medical management of uveitis is to effectively control disease activity to eliminate or reduce the risk of vision loss from structural complications of uncontrolled inflammation. It is critical to determine whether the uveitis is related to a systemic or ocular infection, as anti-inflammatory therapy may severely exacerbate an untreated infection. Once infection is properly addressed, any residual inflammation may be cautiously treated with adjuvant anti-inflammatory therapy. Some diseases, such as multiple evanescent white dot syndrome or acute posterior multifocal placoid pigment epitheliopathy, are self-limited and resolve without treatment. Other diseases, such as Fuchs uveitis syndrome and mild pars planitis, are chronic but do not require treatment. However, most patients with chronic uveitis benefit from sustained suppression of the inflammation.

Corticosteroids are the best agents to control inflammation quickly. Route and dose are tailored to each patient, considering any systemic disease involvement and other factors, such as age, immune status, tolerance of adverse effects, local factors to the eye, and response to treatment. Systemic immunomodulatory therapy (IMT) is used widely in the treatment of noninfectious uveitis when a steroid-sparing effect is required. In the correct clinical scenario, cycloplegic agents, nonsteroidal anti-inflammatories (NSAIDs), and carbonic anhydrase inhibitors may be used as adjunctive therapy.

Corticosteroids

Corticosteroids are the mainstay of uveitis therapy. They are used to treat active inflammation in the anterior chamber, vitreous, retina, choroid, or optic nerve, and to treat complications such as macular edema. They may be administered locally (as topical eyedrops, or periocular or intraocular injections) or systemically (orally or intravenously or, less frequently, intramuscularly).

The dose and duration of corticosteroid therapy must be individualized. It is generally preferable to begin therapy with a high dose of corticosteroids (topical or systemic) and taper the dose as the inflammation subsides, rather than to begin with a low dose that may have to be progressively increased to control the inflammation. To reduce the complications of therapy, patients should be maintained on the minimum dosage needed to control the inflammation. Systemic corticosteroids must be tapered gradually (over days to weeks), and not stopped abruptly if utilized for longer than 2–3 weeks to prevent cortisol deficiency, resulting from hypothalamic-pituitary-adrenal (HPA) axis suppression. If surgical intervention to treat uveitis or its complications is required, the dosage may need to be increased to prevent postoperative exacerbation of the uveitis.

For uveitis that is not immediately vision-threatening and that is not known to be chronic, corticosteroids are slowly tapered, and the disease is closely monitored. The corticosteroid dosage at which disease recrudescence occurs determines whether additional treatments are required.

Given enough treatment time and dosage, any route of corticosteroid administration will have adverse effects, so the risk–benefit ratio of their use should be considered carefully and discussed with the patient. Corticosteroids in any form, but particularly local corticosteroids, can cause serious adverse effects in the eye, most notably posterior subcapsular cataract and ocular hypertension. The significant systemic risks of steroids are discussed later in this chapter. (See also BCSC Section 1, *Update on General Medicine,* and Section 2, *Fundamentals and Principles of Ophthalmology*.)

Topical steroid administration

Topical corticosteroid drops are effective primarily for anterior uveitis, although they may have beneficial effects on vitritis or macular edema with some patients. These drops are given at intervals ranging from once daily to hourly. The drugs can also be administered in ointment form for nighttime use. Difluprednate (0.05%), a fluorinated corticosteroid, is highly potent and has deeper tissue penetration than other topical preparations; dosing at 4 times daily is considered the equivalent of 8 or more total drops per day of prednisolone acetate (1%). Clinical studies suggest difluprednate has a similar adverse effect profile to prednisolone but is associated with potentially higher rises and rates of rise in intraocular pressure (IOP), especially in children. Of the topical preparations, loteprednol and fluorometholone produce a smaller ocular hypertensive effect than that of other medications; however, these drugs are not as effective as prednisolone in controlling more severe uveitis. Differences in physical properties of branded versus generic suspensions of prednisolone acetate can affect the bioavailability of the formulations, although some of this discrepancy can be overcome by vigorous agitation of the drug before instillation. (See also BCSC Section 2, *Fundamentals and Principles of Ophthalmology.*)

Slabaugh MA, Herlihy E, Ongchin S, Van Gelder RN. Efficacy and potential complications of difluprednate use for pediatric uveitis. *Am J Ophthalmol.* 2012;153(5):932–938.

Local steroid administration

Sustained-release steroid may be delivered directly into the vitreous cavity or into the periocular space of an eye with noninfectious uveitis when a more posterior effect is needed, or when a patient is nonadherent or only partially responsive to topical or systemic administration. Intermediate- and short-acting local steroid injections may be used intermittently to treat breakthrough inflammation in otherwise well-controlled or mild uveitis. Long-acting intravitreal steroids can be used as alternatives to long-term IMT in certain clinical settings. A limitation of regional therapies is the variable duration of effect, with relapse being the only sign of waning steroid efficacy. Each relapse before reinjection or reimplantation can result in cumulative damage, creating a phenomenon called a "saw-tooth decline." In chronic uveitis, scheduled replacement or reinjection of steroid before the effect wears off may improve long-term prognosis.

Periocular steroid administration

Periocular corticosteroids are generally given as depot injections into the sub-Tenon space or orbital floor. Although systemic absorption is minimal, periocular corticosteroids can cause systemic adverse effects similar to those of oral corticosteroids. Triamcinolone acetonide (40 mg) and methylprednisolone acetate (40–80 mg) are the most commonly used drugs. Short-acting nondepot steroids, such as dexamethasone or betamethasone, may be injected subconjunctivally for a limited duration of effect.

Periocular injections can be performed using either a transseptal or a sub-Tenon (Nozik technique) approach (Fig 6-1). The technique for a sub-Tenon injection given in the superotemporal quadrant is as follows:

- The upper eyelid is retracted, and the patient is instructed to look down and nasally.
- After anesthesia is applied with a cotton swab soaked in proparacaine or tetracaine, a 25- or 27-gauge, ⅝-inch needle on a 3-mL syringe is placed bevel-down against the sclera and advanced through the conjunctiva and Tenon capsule using a gentle side-to-side movement, which allows the physician to determine whether the needle has entered the sclera. If the globe does not torque with the side-to-side movement of the needle, the physician can be reasonably sure that the needle has not penetrated the sclera.
- Once the needle has been advanced to the hub, the corticosteroid is injected into the sub-Tenon space.

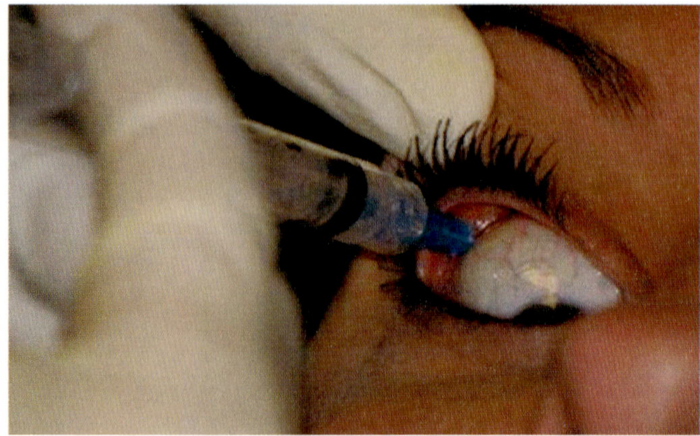

Figure 6-1 Posterior sub-Tenon injection of triamcinolone acetonide demonstrating correct position of the clinician's hands and the needle. The needle is advanced to the hub with a gentle side-to-side motion to detect any scleral engagement and directed caudad and nasally prior to injection of the corticosteroid. The positioning of the tip of the needle in its ideal location is between the Tenon capsule and the sclera. *(Courtesy of Ramana S. Moorthy, MD.)*

Complications of the superotemporal approach include upper eyelid ptosis, periorbital hemorrhage, and globe perforation.

An inferotemporal sub-Tenon injection can also be performed with the Nozik technique, but a transseptal, orbital floor approach (Fig 6-2) using a short 27-gauge needle may be preferred:

- The index finger is used to push the temporal lower eyelid posteriorly and to locate the equator of the globe.
- The needle is inserted inferior to the globe through the skin of the eyelid and directed straight back through the orbital septum into the orbital fat to the hub of the needle.
- The needle is aspirated, and if there is no blood reflux, the corticosteroid is injected.

Complications of the inferior approach can include periorbital and retrobulbar hemorrhage, lower eyelid retractor ptosis, orbital fat prolapse with periorbital festoon formation, orbital fat atrophy, and skin discoloration.

Periocular injections should be avoided in infectious uveitis; their use in necrotizing scleritis should also be avoided due to rare cases of scleral thinning and perforation (see Chapter 7). The physician should be aware that periocular corticosteroid injections have the potential to raise the IOP precipitously or for an extended period, particularly with the longer-acting depot drugs. If this effect occurs, the periocular steroid may be removed surgically if it is located anterior to the septum or in a subconjunctival space.

Leder HA, Jabs DA, Galor A, Dunn JP, Thorne JE. Periocular triamcinolone acetonide injections for cystoid macular edema complicating noninfectious uveitis. *Am J Ophthalmol.* 2011;152(3):441–448.

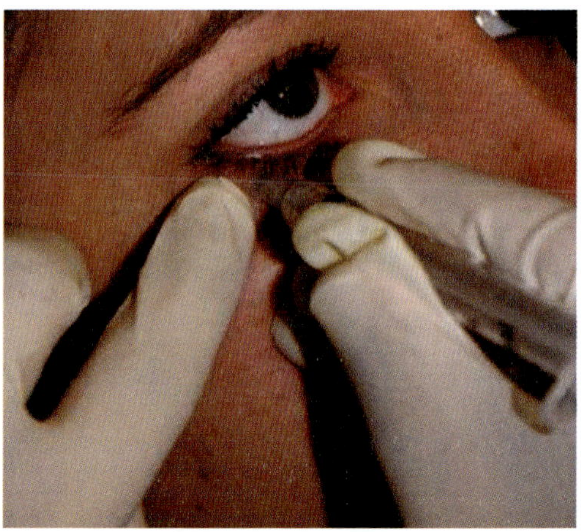

Figure 6-2 Inferior transseptal (orbital floor) injection of triamcinolone acetonide in the right eye. A 27-gauge, ½-inch needle on a 3-mL syringe is inserted through the skin of the lower eyelid and the inferior orbital septum. By using the index finger of the opposite hand, the physician can determine the location of the equator of the globe to prevent perforation and to place the depot corticosteroid as posteriorly as possible. *(Courtesy of Ramana S. Moorthy, MD.)*

Intravitreal steroid administration

Intravitreal therapy achieves a higher, more predictable concentration of steroids in the posterior segment than periocular injection. Intravitreal steroid administration for uveitis currently takes several forms in the United States (US):

- triamcinolone acetonide (4 mg/0.1 mL), preservative free, via pars plana injection with a 30-gauge needle
- fluocinolone acetonide implant (0.59 mg), surgically implantable, via pars plana incision
- fluocinolone acetonide intravitreal insert (0.18 mg), via pars plan injection with integrated 25-gauge injector
- dexamethasone pellet (700 μg), biodegradable, via pars plana injection with an integrated 22-gauge injector

Intravitreal injections of triamcinolone acetonide through the pars plana have been shown to produce sustained visual acuity improvements for 3–6 months in nonvitrectomized eyes; the technique is the same as for standard intravitreal injection (see BCSC Section 12, *Retina and Vitreous*). Published literature on intravitreal triamcinolone administration suggests a definite treatment benefit, although of limited duration, for recalcitrant uveitic macular edema. Intraocular pressure elevation may occur transiently in more than one-half of patients. Up to 25% of patients may require topical medications to control IOP, and 1%–2% may require filtering surgery. Infectious endophthalmitis and rhegmatogenous retinal detachment may occur, but these complications are rare when proper technique is used. This method of treatment is not curative of chronic uveitic conditions and should be used judiciously, as its effects are relatively short lived.

A surgically implantable, sustained-release 0.59-mg fluocinolone acetonide implant is available in the US and is approved by the US Food and Drug Administration (FDA) for the treatment of chronic noninfectious uveitis affecting the posterior segment. The implant is inserted through a small pars plana incision and sutured to the sclera.

Multicenter, controlled clinical studies have shown that the 0.59-mg implant is effective for a median of 30 months, with a mean time of 38 months to first recurrence. At 34 weeks after implantation, inflammation was well controlled in nearly all eyes, and recurrence rates decreased by 90%, with 77% of patients able to discontinue systemic therapy and 96% able to discontinue local corticosteroid injections. However, nearly all phakic eyes developed cataract within 2 years after implantation. Elevated IOP necessitating topical therapy developed in nearly 75% of patients after 3 years, and 37% required filtering surgery.

Postoperative complications (eg, endophthalmitis, wound leaks, hypotony, vitreous hemorrhage, and retinal detachments) have been reported. Reimplantation or exchange may be performed.

The 0.59-mg fluocinolone implant was compared with standard systemic therapy in the Multicenter Uveitis Steroid Treatment (MUST) Trial, which enrolled 255 patients over 3 years. Best-corrected visual acuity was not significantly different between the 2 treatment groups at the 2- and 4.5-year primary endpoints; however, 7-year data published in 2017 showed that the change in vision from baseline favored systemic therapy by 7.1 letters, with the risk of blindness decreasing by 1% in the systemic group but increasing by 8% in the implant group. This difference appeared to be due to retinal damage from relapse of the uveitis before reimplantation (see Table 6-1).

A sustained-release 0.18-mg fluocinolone acetonide injectable intravitreal insert is approved by the US FDA for the treatment of noninfectious posterior uveitis. The nonbioerodible device is injected via a nonshelved wound through the pars plana into the vitreous cavity, where it releases the drug over 36 months. A prospective randomized placebo-controlled clinical trial demonstrated statistically significantly lower uveitis recurrence rates in the implant group compared to sham at 6 months (28% vs 91%) and 12 months (38% vs 98%). Cataract formation was greater in the treatment group, but no significant differences were found in IOP-lowering treatment.

A biodegradable injectable pellet containing 700 µg of dexamethasone is approved by the US FDA and in Europe for the treatment of noninfectious uveitis affecting the posterior segment of the eye and retinal vein occlusion. This implant is injected through the pars plana into the vitreous cavity by creating a shelved wound using the injector (Video 6-1). A prospective randomized controlled clinical trial demonstrated that, at 8 weeks, 47% of eyes treated with a dexamethasone implant had improved vitreous haze, compared to 12% of eyes in the sham group. Statistically significant improvements in visual acuity and macula thickness were reported, and fewer eyes required rescue medication. Intraocular pressure elevation and cataracts were the most commonly reported treatment-related ocular adverse effects in this study.

VIDEO 6-1 Injection of dexamethasone implant.
Courtesy of Thomas A. Albini, MD.
Access the video at www.aao.org/bcscvideo_section09.

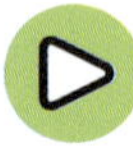

Several longer-term, multicenter retrospective studies have reported relatively positive results on the safety and efficacy of repeated dexamethasone intravitreal implants in uveitic patients with refractory macular edema, with an average time to reinjection of 6 months.

Table 6-1 Selected List of Major Treatment Studies in Uveitis

Study Name	Study Questions	Participants/Method	Results
HURON Chronic Uveitis Evaluation of the Intravitreal Dexamethasone Implant	Efficacy and safety of the injectable dexamethasone intravitreal implant at 2 doses (0.35 mg and 0.70 mg) compared to placebo (sham) Primary endpoint: vitreous haze grade 0 at 8 weeks	Industry-sponsored, randomized, placebo-controlled, double-masked, multicenter clinical trial 229 patients with noninfectious intermediate or posterior uveitis on stable doses of topical or systemic therapy 26-week follow-up	The dexamethasone implant group more likely than the sham group to have vitreous haze grade of 0 at 8 weeks (47% and 36% of eyes treated with 0.70-mg and 0.35-mg dexamethasone implant, respectively, vs 12% of eyes in the sham group; *P*<0.001). <5% of eyes developed IOP ≥35 mm Hg and <10% had IOP ≥25 mm Hg. The proportion of study eyes with IOP elevation of ≥10 mm Hg was not reported. One patient in the 0.35-mg implant group required IOP-lowering surgery. Cataracts developed in 15% (9/62), 12% (6/51), and 7% (4/55) of phakic study eyes in the 0.7-mg and 0.35-mg implant groups and sham group, respectively.
MUST Multicenter Uveitis Steroid Treatment Trial	Efficacy and safety of local therapy using a 0.59-mg fluocinolone acetonide surgically placed intravitreal implant compared to standard therapy (systemic corticosteroid monotherapy or combination steroid-IMT therapy) Primary endpoint: change in BCVA	International, multicenter, prospective, randomized, open-label, parallel-design clinical trial 255 patients (479 eyes) with noninfectious intermediate, posterior or panuveitis severe enough to be treated with corticosteroids 2-, 4.5-, and 7-year follow-up	2- and 4.5-year analysis: There was no significant difference in visual acuity or systemic outcomes between the two groups. There were significantly more local adverse outcomes in the implant group (cataract, IOP elevation requiring medical and surgical intervention, and glaucomatous optic neuropathy). 7-year analysis: Systemic therapy was favored for visual acuity outcome by 7.1 letters, caused by visual decline in the implant group likely due to loss of efficacy of the implant.

(Continued)

Table 6-1 *(continued)*

Study Name	Study Questions	Participants/Method	Results
SITE Systemic Immunosuppressive Therapy for Eye Diseases Cohort Study	To determine overall and cancer-mortality rates in uveitis patients on systemic immunosuppression for ocular inflammatory disease	Retrospective review of 7957 patients with noninfectious ocular inflammatory disease 5 tertiary uveitis referral clinics in the United States from 1979 to 2005	There was no increased cancer mortality in patients treated with oral corticosteroids, AZA, MTX, MMF, or CsA. There was a nonstatistically significant increase in cancer-related mortality rates in patients treated with CP. Cancer-related mortality in tumor necrosis factor inhibitors significantly increased overall, but the association was less robust due to small numbers.
SYCAMORE Adalimumab plus Methotrexate for JIA Uveitis	Efficacy and safety of adding adalimumab in active JIA-associated uveitis treated with MTX Primary endpoint: time to treatment failure	Multicenter, double-blind, randomized, placebo-controlled trial 60 children and adolescents with active uveitis on stable MTX dosage 2-year follow-up	The ADA group was less likely than the placebo group to have treatment failure (hazard ratio, 0.25; 95% confidence interval, 0.12 to 0.49; $P<0.0001$). A significantly greater proportion of patients in the adalimumab group than in the placebo group could eliminate or reduce topical corticosteroids. The rate of adverse events per patient-year was higher in the ADA group than in the placebo group (10.07 vs 6.51 events per patient-year). The number of serious adverse events was also higher in the ADA group than in the placebo group.

Study Name	Study Questions	Participants/Method	Results
VISUAL I, II, III Adalimumab for noninfectious intermediate, posterior, or panuveitis	I: Efficacy and safety in controlling inflammation in active noninfectious uveitis II: Efficacy and safety in preventing flare-up in pharmacologically controlled noninfectious uveitis (10–35 mg prednisone and/or 1 IMT) III: Long-term efficacy and safety in active or controlled noninfectious uveitis Primary endpoint: time to treatment failure	I-II: Industry-sponsored, multicenter, double-masked, randomized placebo-controlled trials in 217 and 226 active and controlled uveitis patients, respectively III: Industry-sponsored, multicenter open-label extension study in 371 uveitis patients from VISUAL I or II who completed study or met treatment failure criteria	I: The ADA group was less likely than the placebo group to have treatment failure (hazard ratio, 0.50; 95% confidence interval, 0.36 to 0.70; $P < 0.001$). Adverse events and serious adverse events were more common in the ADA group (1052.4 vs 971.7 adverse events and 28.8 vs 13.6 serious adverse events per 100 person-years). II: The ADA group was less likely than the placebo group to have treatment failure (hazard ratio, 0.57; 95% confidence interval, 0.39–0.84; $P = 0.004$). The incidence of adverse and serious adverse events was similar between treatment groups. III: 60% of patients with active uveitis (145/242) achieved quiescence at week 78, 66% of whom were corticosteroid free. 74% of patients with inactive uveitis (96/129) achieved quiescence at week 78, 93% of whom were corticosteroid free. Adverse events and serious adverse events were comparable to those in previous VISUAL trials.

ADA = adalimumab; AZA = azathioprine; BCVA = best-corrected visual acuity; CsA = cyclosporine; CP = cyclophosphamide; IOP = intraocular pressure; IMT = immunomodulatory therapy; JIA= juvenile idiopathic arthritis; MMF = mycophenolate mofetil; MTX = methotrexate.

Relative contraindications to the dexamethasone implant are aphakia, prior vitrectomy, and absence of lens capsule because of the risk of implant migration into the anterior chamber (see Table 6.1).

Androudi S, Letko E, Meniconi M, Papadaki T, Ahmed M, Foster CS. Safety and efficacy of intravitreal triamcinolone acetonide for uveitic macular edema. *Ocul Immunol Inflamm.* 2005;13(2–3):205–212.

Goldstein DA, Godfrey DG, Hall A, et al. Intraocular pressure in patients with uveitis treated with fluocinolone acetonide implants. *Arch Ophthalmol.* 2007; 125(11):1478–1485.

Jaffe GJ. Reimplantation of a fluocinolone acetonide sustained drug delivery implant for chronic uveitis. *Am J Ophthalmol.* 2008;145(4):667–675.

Jaffe GJ, Foster S, Pavesio C, Paggiarinno D, Riedel GE. Effect of an injectable fluocinolone acetonide insert on recurrence rates in noninfectious uveitis affecting the posterior segment: 12-month results. *Ophthalmology.* 2018 Oct 24. pii: S0161-6420(18)31715-9.

Khurana RN, Appa SN, McCannel CA, et al. Dexamethasone implant anterior chamber migration: risk factors, complications, and management strategies. *Ophthalmology.* 2014;121(1):67–71.

Lowder C, Belfort R Jr, Lightman S, et al; Ozurdex HURON Study Group. Dexamethasone intravitreal implant for noninfectious intermediate or posterior uveitis. *Arch Ophthalmol.* 2011;129(5):545–553.

Tomkins-Netzer O, Taylor SR, Bar A, et al. Treatment with repeat dexamethasone implants results in long-term disease control in eyes with noninfectious uveitis. *Ophthalmology.* 2014;212(8):1649–1654.

Writing Committee for the Multicenter Uveitis Steroid Treatment (MUST) Trial and Follow-up Study Research Group; Kempen JH, Altaweel MM, Holbrook JT, et al. Association between long-lasting intravitreous fluocinolone acetonide implant vs systemic anti-inflammatory therapy and visual acuity at 7 years among patients with intermediate, posterior, or panuveitis. *JAMA.* 2017;317(19):1993–2005.

Zarranz-Ventura J, Carreno E, Johnston RL, et al. Multicenter study of intravitreal dexamethasone implant in noninfectious uveitis: indications, outcomes and reinjection frequency. *Am J Ophthalmol.* 2014;158(6):1136–1145.

Systemic steroid administration

Systemic corticosteroids are used for vision-threatening chronic uveitis when local corticosteroids are insufficient or contraindicated or when systemic disease also requires therapy. Of the many oral corticosteroid formulations that are available, prednisone is the most commonly used. The readily available blister packages of methylprednisolone, which contain predetermined taper schedules, have no role in the treatment of uveitis. Most patients require 1–1.5 mg/kg/day of oral prednisone (usually no higher than 60–80 mg/day), which is gradually tapered every 1–2 weeks. Doses >60 mg/day are associated with an increased risk of ischemic necrosis of bone and should be avoided if possible. The lowest possible dose that will effectively quiet the ocular inflammation and minimize adverse effects is desired. If corticosteroid therapy at a dose of more than 7.5 mg/day is required for longer than 3 months, IMT is indicated. Long-term use at 7.5 mg or less per day shows no increased risk of steroid adverse effects over months to years, although there are data to suggest increased cardiovascular risks with large cumulative doses of prednisone (eg, 5 mg/day over 20 years).

In cases of an explosive onset or severe noninfectious uveitis, therapy with intravenous, high-dose, pulse methylprednisolone (1 g/day infused over 1 hour) may be administered for 3 days, followed by a gradual taper of oral prednisone starting at 1–1.5 mg/kg/day. Although this mode of therapy may control intraocular inflammation, it should only be administered by a physician experienced with this approach, as there are multiple adverse effects, some of which can be life-threatening.

The many adverse effects of both short- and long-term use of systemic corticosteroids must be discussed with patients, whose general health must be closely monitored, often with the assistance of an internist. Short-term risks include ocular hypertension, hyperglycemia, systemic hypertension, gastric reflux, insomnia, emotional lability, weight gain, fluid retention, and others. Intermediate-term risks include cataract, osteoporosis, avascular necrosis of joints, diabetes mellitus, and others. If possible, corticosteroids should be avoided in patients at high risk for corticosteroid-induced exacerbations of existing conditions (eg, diabetes mellitus, hypertension, peptic ulcer or gastroesophageal reflux disease, psychiatric conditions, or a history of immune compromise).

Patients taking systemic corticosteroids and NSAIDs concomitantly have a higher risk of gastric ulcers; therefore, this combination is best avoided. If necessary, these and other at-risk patients should receive a histamine-H_2 receptor antagonist or proton-pump inhibitor. Patients receiving long-term systemic corticosteroid maintenance therapy should supplement their diets with calcium and vitamin D to lessen the risk of osteoporosis.

The following tests can be used to evaluate patients at risk for corticosteroid-induced bone loss:

- serial height measurements
- serum calcium and phosphorus levels
- serum 25-hydroxycholecalciferol levels (if vitamin D stores are uncertain)
- follicle-stimulating hormone and testosterone levels (if gonadal status is uncertain)
- bone-mineral-density screening (for anyone receiving corticosteroid therapy for more than 3 months)

The US FDA has approved several drugs for the prevention and treatment of corticosteroid-induced osteoporosis in men and women. These medications may be administered to at-risk patients receiving prednisone.

The systemic adverse effects and potency of commonly used corticosteroids are discussed in BCSC Section 1, *Update on General Medicine*. See also BCSC Section 2, *Fundamentals and Principles of Ophthalmology*.

Systemic Immunomodulatory Therapy

The use of systemic immunomodulatory therapy (IMT; sometimes referred to as *immunosuppressive* or *disease-modifying antirheumatic drugs, DMARDs*) may greatly benefit patients with chronic, severe, or steroid-dependent noninfectious uveitis. These drugs can modify or regulate one or more immune functions, and work by different mechanisms, depending on the class of the medication (see Chapter 1, Table 1-3).

Immunomodulatory medications may be loosely divided into nonbiologic-IMT agents and biologic agents. Nonbiologic-IMT agents are further divided into antimetabolites, T-cell inhibitors, and alkylating agents. Biologic agents, a newer and rapidly expanding group of genetically engineered proteins targeting specific immune mechanisms, include drugs that inhibit tumor necrosis factor α (TNF inhibitors) and drugs inhibiting other pro-inflammatory immune mediators. In clinical practice, alkylating agents and biologic agents are more likely to be used for severe inflammation. However, use of alkylating agents has decreased due to the growing body of evidence on the relative safety and efficacy of biologic agents. Currently, the use of IMT for treating uveitis is considered off-label in the US, except for adalimumab, a TNF inhibitor, which is approved for noninfectious uveitis affecting the posterior segment.

Although many case series have been published, the largest amount of data on use of nonbiologic-IMT agents in uveitis comes from the Systemic Immunosuppressive Therapy for Eye Diseases (SITE) Cohort Study, a standardized retrospective study that evaluated each drug's safety, adverse effect profile, and effectiveness in clinical practice (see Table 6-1 and further discussion later in this section). There are limited comparative effectiveness data on the immunomodulatory medications for uveitis.

Indications

The use of IMT in treatment of uveitis is warranted for consideration in the following settings:

- vision-threatening intraocular inflammation
- inadequate response to corticosteroid treatment
- corticosteroids contraindicated because of systemic problems or intolerable adverse effects
- long-term corticosteroid dependence

Certain ocular inflammatory entities warrant the early use of IMT, including ocular cicatricial pemphigoid, serpiginous choroiditis, Behçet disease, sympathetic ophthalmia, Vogt-Koyanagi-Harada (VKH) syndrome, and necrotizing scleritis associated with systemic vasculitis. Although these disorders may initially respond well to corticosteroids, the initial treatment of these entities with IMT has been shown to improve long-term prognosis and lessen visual morbidity. Several expert-panel recommendations have been published to establish consensus on how and when to select, initiate, modify, and withdraw nonbiologic-IMT or biologic agents.

Treatment

Before initiation of IMT, the physician should evaluate the following:

- absence of infection
- absence of recent live vaccine administration
- absence of hepatic, renal, and hematologic contraindications
- absence of pregnancy or breastfeeding
- family planning and contraception

- meticulous follow-up available from a physician who is, by virtue of training and experience, qualified to counsel, prescribe, and safely monitor such medications and personally manage their potential toxicities
- objective longitudinal evaluation of the disease process
- informed consent

There may be a delay in therapeutic response for weeks to months after initiation of nonbiologic-IMT; biologic agents typically have a more rapid onset. Most patients need to be maintained on corticosteroids until the immunomodulatory agent begins to take effect, at which time the corticosteroid dose may be gradually tapered.

Because of the potentially serious complications associated with the use of IMT, patients must be monitored closely by a practitioner experienced with IMT. Blood monitoring, including complete blood count with differential and liver and renal function tests, should be performed regularly. Serious complications of nonbiologic-IMT include renal and hepatic toxicity and bone marrow suppression. Alkylating agents may cause sterility and are associated with an increased risk of malignancies, such as leukemia or lymphoma. Certain biologic agents may promote an infusion or injection reaction; TNF inhibitors increase the risk of multiple sclerosis and lymphoma. All IMT increases the risk of opportunistic and secondary infection.

However, the SITE cohort study of 7957 patients (66,802 patient-years) with noninfectious uveitis treated with IMT showed that patients who took azathioprine, methotrexate, mycophenolate mofetil, cyclosporine, or systemic corticosteroids had overall cancer mortality rates similar to those who never took those medications; the study confirmed that TNF inhibitors were associated with increased overall (twofold) and cancer (3.8-fold) risk of mortality. While there is no direct evidence in uveitis patients, IMT may be associated with an increased risk of nonmelanoma skin cancer, warranting sunscreen counseling. Trimethoprim–sulfamethoxazole prophylaxis against *Pneumocystis jirovecii* infection should be considered in patients receiving alkylating agents, or in those on intermediate-term high-dose steroids and IMT. The physician should obtain thorough informed consent prior to initiating IMT.

Male and female patients require counseling regarding fertility, birth control, and family planning prior to initiation of IMT. Many IMT medications have absolute contraindications in pregnancy. Generally, IMT should be discontinued 3 months prior to trying to conceive.

Dick AD, Rosenbaum JT, Al-Dhibi HA, et al; Fundamentals of Care for Uveitis International Consensus Group. Guidance on noncorticosteroid systemic immunomodulatory therapy in noninfectious uveitis: Fundamentals Of Care for UveitiS (FOCUS) initiative. *Ophthalmology.* 2018;125(5):757–773.

Jabs DA. Immunosuppression for the uveitides. *Ophthalmology.* 2018;125(2):193–202.

Jabs DA, Rosenbaum JT, Foster CS, et al. Guidelines for the use of immunosuppressive drugs in patients with ocular inflammatory disorders: recommendations of an expert panel. *Am J Ophthalmol.* 2000;130(4):492–513.

Kempen JH, Daniel E, Dunn JP, et al. Overall and cancer related mortality among patients with ocular inflammation treated with immunosuppressive drugs: retrospective cohort study. *BMJ.* 2009;339:b2480.

Leroy C, Rigot J-M, Leroy M, et al. Immunosuppressive drugs and fertility. *Orphanet J Rare Dis.* 2015;10:136.

Levy-Clarke G, Jabs DA, Read RW, Rosenbaum JT, Vitale A, Van Gelder RN. Expert panel recommendations for the use of anti-tumor necrosis factor biologic agents in patients with ocular inflammatory disorders. *Ophthalmology.* 2014;121(3):785–796.

Nguyen QD, Callanan D, Dugel P, Godfrey DG, Goldstein DA, Wilensky JT. Treating chronic noninfectious posterior segment uveitis: the impact of cumulative damage. Proceedings of an expert panel roundtable discussion. *Retina.* 2006;26(8)1–16.

Wakefield D, McCluskey P, Wildner G, et al. Inflammatory eye disease: pre-treatment assessment of patients prior to commencing immunosuppressive and biologic therapy: recommendations from an expert committee. *Autoimmun Rev.* 2017;16(3):213–222.

Yates WB, Vajdic CM, Na R, McCluskey PJ, Wakefield D. Malignancy risk in patients with inflammatory eye disease treated with systemic immunosuppressive therapy: a tertiary referral cohort study. *Ophthalmology.* 2015;122(2):265–273.

Nonbiologic Immunomodulatory Therapy

Antimetabolites

The antimetabolites include azathioprine, methotrexate, and mycophenolate mofetil. Clinical trials are lacking, but retrospective series report that, compared with the other antimetabolites, azathioprine has a slightly higher incidence of adverse effects and mycophenolate mofetil has a significantly shorter time to treatment success. Antimetabolites are often the first IMTs used when corticosteroid sparing is desired. A head-to-head randomized prospective study of 80 uveitis patients assigned to methotrexate or mycophenolate reported similar efficacy of the 2 medications. While generally effective, ongoing low-dose systemic corticosteroid therapy is often necessary to achieve complete inflammatory control. When initiated, these medications require long-term use, as disease control continues to improve between 6 and 12 months of follow-up.

Azathioprine, a purine nucleoside analogue, interferes with DNA replication and RNA transcription. Azathioprine is administered orally at a dose of up to 2 mg/kg/day in adults. Nausea, vomiting, and upset stomach are the most common adverse effects. Bone marrow suppression is unusual at the doses of azathioprine used to treat uveitis. However, patients taking allopurinol and azathioprine concomitantly are at higher risk for bone marrow suppression. Mild hepatic toxicity can usually be reversed by dose reduction. On average, 25% of patients discontinue therapy due to adverse effects. Complete blood counts and liver function tests must be closely monitored. The variability of clinical response to azathioprine among patients is probably caused by genetic variability in the activity of thiopurine S-methyltransferase (TPMT), an enzyme responsible for the metabolism of 6-mercaptopurine (6-MP). A genotypic test is available that can help determine patient candidacy for azathioprine therapy before treatment and can help clinicians individualize patient doses. Evaluation of TPMT activity has revealed 3 groups of patients:

- low/no TPMT activity (0.3% of patients); azathioprine therapy not recommended
- intermediate TPMT activity (11% of patients); azathioprine therapy at reduced dosage
- normal/high TPMT activity (89% of patients); azathioprine therapy at higher doses than in patients with intermediate TPMT activity

Azathioprine is beneficial in many types of noninfectious ocular inflammatory diseases, including Behçet disease, intermediate uveitis, VKH syndrome, sympathetic ophthalmia, and necrotizing scleritis. Overall, nearly 50% of patients treated with azathioprine achieve inflammatory control and can taper the prednisone dosage to 10 mg/day or less.

Methotrexate is a folic acid analogue and inhibitor of dihydrofolate reductase; it inhibits DNA replication, but its anti-inflammatory effects result from extracellular release of adenosine. Treatment with this medication is unique in that it is given either orally or subcutaneously as a *weekly* dose of up to 15–25 mg/week in adults. The dosage is variable in children and depends on body surface area. Methotrexate can be given orally, subcutaneously, intramuscularly, or intravenously and is usually well tolerated. It has greater bioavailability when given parenterally. Folate is given concurrently at a dose of 1–2 mg/day to reduce adverse effects. Methotrexate may take up to 6 months to produce its full effect in controlling intraocular inflammation. Gastrointestinal distress and anorexia may occur in 10% of patients. Reversible hepatotoxicity occurs in up to 15% of patients, and cirrhosis occurs in fewer than 0.1% of patients receiving methotrexate long-term. Methotrexate is teratogenic; mixed data exist on safety of male conception while on methotrexate therapy. Complete blood counts and liver function tests should be conducted regularly. Numerous studies have shown methotrexate to be effective in treating various types of uveitis, including juvenile idiopathic arthritis (JIA)–associated anterior uveitis, sarcoidosis, panuveitis, and scleritis. It has been a first-line choice for IMT in children. Uncontrolled clinical trials have shown that it can enable corticosteroid sparing in two-thirds of patients with chronic ocular inflammatory disorders. Intravitreal methotrexate is used for primary intraocular lymphoma; its role in uveitis and macular edema is being investigated.

Mycophenolate mofetil inhibits both inosine monophosphate dehydrogenase and DNA replication. It is given orally at a dosage of 1–1.5 g twice daily in adults. Median time to successful control of ocular inflammation (in combination with less than 10 mg/day of prednisone) is approximately 4 months. Fewer than 20% of patients receiving mycophenolate mofetil have adverse effects—reversible gastrointestinal distress and diarrhea are common—and these can usually be managed by dose reduction. Very few patients find the drug intolerable. Regular laboratory monitoring is required to check for adverse effects. Two large, retrospective studies found mycophenolate mofetil to be an effective corticosteroid-sparing agent in up to 85% of patients with chronic uveitis. It has similar efficacy in children (88%) and can be a safe alternative to methotrexate in patients with pediatric uveitis.

Doycheva D, Deuter C, Stuebiger N, Biester S, Zierhut M. Mycophenolate mofetil in the treatment of uveitis in children. *Br J Ophthalmol.* 2007;91(2):180–184.

Gangaputra S, Newcomb CW, Liesegang TL, et al; Systemic Immunosuppressive Therapy for Eye Diseases Cohort Study. Methotrexate for ocular inflammatory diseases. *Ophthalmology.* 2009;116(11):2188–2198.

Malik AR, Pavesio C. The use of low dose methotrexate in children with chronic anterior and intermediate uveitis. *Br J Ophthalmol.* 2005;89(7):806–808.

Pasadhika S, Kempen JH, Newcomb CW, et al. Azathioprine for ocular inflammatory diseases. *Am J Ophthalmol.* 2009;148(4):500–509.

Rathinam SR, Babu M, Thundikandy R, et al. A randomized clinical trial comparing methotrexate and mycophenolate mofetil for noninfectious uveitis. *Ophthalmology.* 2014;121(10):1863–1870.

Siepmann K, Huber M, Stübiger N, Deuter C, Zierhut M. Mycophenolate mofetil is a highly effective and safe immunosuppressive agent for the treatment of uveitis: a retrospective analysis of 106 patients. *Graefes Arch Clin Exp Ophthalmol.* 2006;244(7):788–794.

Teoh SC, Hogan AC, Dick AD, Lee RW. Mycophenolate mofetil for the treatment of uveitis. *Am J Ophthalmol.* 2008;146(5):752–760.

Thorne JE, Jabs DA, Qazi FA, Nguyen QD, Kempen JH, Dunn JP. Mycophenolate mofetil therapy for inflammatory eye disease. *Ophthalmology.* 2005;112(8):1472–1477.

T-cell inhibitors

Cyclosporine, a macrolide product of the fungus *Beauveria nivea,* and tacrolimus, a product of *Streptomyces tsukubaensis,* are calcineurin inhibitors that eliminate T-cell receptor signal transduction and downregulate interleukin-2 (IL-2) gene transcription and receptor expression of $CD4^+$ T lymphocytes.

Cyclosporine is available in 2 oral preparations. One is a microemulsion (Neoral, Novartis) and has better bioavailability than the standard formulation (Sandimmune, Novartis). These 2 formulations are not bioequivalent. The microemulsion is initiated at 2 mg/kg/day, and the standard formulation at 2.5 mg/kg/day in adults. Dosing is adjusted based on trough levels, toxicity, and clinical response to 1–5 mg/kg/day. The most common adverse effects with cyclosporine are systemic hypertension and nephrotoxicity. Additional adverse effects include paresthesia, gastrointestinal upset, fatigue, hypertrichosis, and gingival hyperplasia. Blood pressure, serum creatinine levels, and complete blood counts must be assessed regularly. If serum creatinine levels rise by 30%, dose adjustment is required; sustained elevation requires medication cessation. Cyclosporine was shown to be effective in a randomized, controlled clinical trial for the treatment of Behçet uveitis, with control of inflammation in 50% of patients. However, the dose used in this study was 10 mg/kg/day—substantially higher than current dosing (5 mg/kg/day)—and led to substantial nephrotoxicity. Even at standard dosages, toxicity necessitating cessation of therapy is more common in patients over the age of 55 years. Overall, cyclosporine is modestly effective in controlling ocular inflammation (33.4% and 51.9% of patients by 6 and 12 months, respectively). As with antimetabolites, the need for ongoing low-dose systemic corticosteroid therapy is often necessary to achieve complete inflammatory control.

Tacrolimus is given orally at 0.10–0.15 mg/kg/day in adults. Because of its lower dose and increased potency, its main adverse effect, nephrotoxicity, is less common than with cyclosporine. Serum creatinine level and complete blood counts are monitored regularly. The dose is escalated until a therapeutic trough blood level is reached. A prospective trial of cyclosporine and tacrolimus suggested equal efficacy in controlling chronic posterior and intermediate uveitis, with tacrolimus demonstrating greater safety (lower risk of hypertension and hyperlipidemia). Long-term tolerability and efficacy are excellent as well, with an 85% chance of reducing prednisone dosage to less than 10 mg/day. A randomized uveitis trial of tacrolimus monotherapy versus tacrolimus plus prednisone showed no difference, confirming that steroid discontinuation can be achieved in many cases.

Hogan AC, McAvoy CE, Dick AD, Lee RW. Long-term efficacy and tolerance of tacrolimus for the treatment of uveitis. *Ophthalmology.* 2007;114(5):1000–1006.

Kaçmaz RO, Kempen JH, Newcomb C, et al. Cyclosporine for ocular inflammatory diseases. *Ophthalmology.* 2010;117(3):576–584.

Lee RW, Greenwood R, Taylor H, et al. A randomized trial of tacrolimus versus tacrolimus and prednisone for the maintenance of disease remission in noninfectious uveitis. *Ophthalmology.* 2012;119(6):1223–1230.

Murphy CC, Greiner K, Plskova J, et al. Cyclosporine vs tacrolimus therapy for posterior and intermediate uveitis. *Arch Ophthalmol.* 2005;123(5):634–641.

Alkylating agents

Alkylating agents include cyclophosphamide and chlorambucil. These drugs are generally used only if other immunomodulators fail to control uveitis, and their use may now be partially supplanted by the targeted efficacy and preferred safety profile of the biologic agents. The most worrisome adverse effect of alkylating agents is an increased risk of malignancy. Use of alkylating agents for a limited duration may be justifiable for severe, vision- or life-threatening recalcitrant disease, but otherwise cancer risk may be a relevant constraint on use of this approach. Patients with polycythemia rubra vera treated with chlorambucil had a 13.5-fold-greater risk of leukemia. Patients with granulomatosis with polyangiitis treated with cyclophosphamide had a 2.4-fold-increased risk of cancer and a 33-fold-increased risk of bladder cancer. With the doses and durations used for the treatment of uveitis, the risk is probably lower. Nonetheless, these drugs should be used with great caution and only by clinicians experienced in the management of their dosing and potential toxicity. Patients may wish to consider sperm or embryo banking before beginning cyclophosphamide or chlorambucil therapy because of the high rate of sterility if the cumulative dose exceeds certain limits. Alkylating agents may be used as first-line therapy for necrotizing scleritis associated with systemic vasculitides, such as granulomatosis with polyangiitis or relapsing polychondritis. These drugs have been found beneficial as well in patients with intermediate uveitis, VKH syndrome, sympathetic ophthalmia, and Behçet disease.

Cyclophosphamide is an alkylating agent whose active metabolites alkylate purines in DNA and RNA, resulting in impaired DNA replication and cell death. It is probably more effective in controlling ocular inflammation when given orally at a dose of 2 mg/kg/day in adults than when administered as intermittent intravenous pulses. The dose is adjusted to maintain leukocyte counts between 3000 and 4000 cells/μL after the patient has been tapered off corticosteroids. Myelosuppression and hemorrhagic cystitis are the most common adverse effects. Hemorrhagic cystitis is more common when cyclophosphamide is administered orally, but fluid intake of more than 2 L/day reduces the risk. Complete blood counts and urinalysis are monitored weekly to monthly. Microscopic hematuria is a warning for the patient to increase hydration, and gross hematuria is an indication to discontinue therapy. If the leukocyte count falls below 2500 cells/μL, cyclophosphamide should be discontinued until the cell count recovers. Other toxicities include teratogenicity, sterility, and reversible alopecia. Opportunistic infections such as *Pneumocystis jirovecii* pneumonia occur more commonly in patients receiving cyclophosphamide; trimethoprim–sulfamethoxazole prophylaxis is recommended for these patients. Inflammation control is achieved in three-fourths of patients within 12 months; disease remission occurs in two-thirds of patients within 2 years; and one-third of patients discontinue therapy within 1 year because of reversible adverse effects.

Chlorambucil is a very long-acting alkylating agent that also interferes with DNA replication. It is absorbed well when administered orally. The drug is traditionally given as a single daily dose of 0.1–0.2 mg/kg in adults. It may also be administered as short-term, high-dose therapy. Because chlorambucil is myelosuppressive, complete blood counts should be monitored closely. Like cyclophosphamide, it is associated with increased hematologic malignancy risk. It is also teratogenic and causes sterility. Uncontrolled case series suggest that chlorambucil is effective, providing long-term, drug-free remissions in 66%–75% of patients with recalcitrant sympathetic ophthalmia, Behçet disease, and other vision-threatening uveitic syndromes.

Faurschou M, Sorensen IJ, Mellemkjaer L, et al. Malignancies in Wegener's granulomatosis: incidence and relation to cyclophosphamide therapy in a cohort of 293 patients. *J Rheumatol.* 2008;35(1):100–105.

Patel SS, Dodds EM, Echandi LV, et al. Long-term, drug-free remission of sympathetic ophthalmia with high-dose, short-term chlorambucil therapy. *Ophthalmology.* 2014;121(2):596–602.

Pujari SS, Kempen JH, Newcomb CW, et al. Cyclophosphamide for ocular inflammatory diseases. *Ophthalmology.* 2010;117(2):356–365.

Biologic agents

Inflammation is driven by a complex series of cell–cell and cell–cytokine interactions. Inhibitors of various cytokines and inflammatory mechanisms have been labeled *biologic agents* or, occasionally, *biologic response modifiers.* They play an important role in the treatment of uveitis, as these drugs result in targeted immunomodulation, thereby theoretically reducing the short-term systemic adverse effects that are common with the previously discussed nonbiologic immunomodulatory drugs. Biologic agents are considerably more expensive and may carry higher long-term risks of serious infections or secondary malignancies than antimetabolites and T-cell inhibitors. Therefore, biologic agents are reserved for specific conditions, such as Behçet disease or situations in which nonbiologic-IMT agents have failed.

Tumor Necrosis Factor Inhibitors

The best-studied inhibitors of TNF-α for uveitis are adalimumab and infliximab; their emergence over the last decade has changed the management of some types of uveitis. There is expert consensus that the TNF inhibitors should be considered first-line for Behçet disease. Other TNF inhibitors include certolizumab and golimumab, which have far fewer uveitis data, and etanercept, which is not effective for ocular inflammatory diseases. TNF-α is believed to play a major role in the pathogenesis of JIA, ankylosing spondylitis, and other spondyloarthropathies. These drugs are generally prescribed and administered by uveitis specialists and rheumatologists experienced with their use, adverse effects, and toxicities. TNF inhibitors have been associated with central nervous system demyelination (promoting or unmasking multiple sclerosis), increased risk of malignancy (such as lymphoma), hepatitis B reactivation, and deep fungal and other serious atypical infections. Their use may be contraindicated in congestive heart failure, and latent tuberculosis must be ruled out or completely treated with oversight of a specialist in infectious diseases prior to use. Live vaccines should not be administered to a patient taking TNF inhibitors. Although individual case reports have been made for intravitreal TNF inhibitors, their intravitreal use is untested, potentially retinotoxic, and should not be used without further study.

Adalimumab, a fully human monoclonal immunoglobulin G1 (IgG1) antibody directed against TNF-α is the first US FDA–approved systemic medication for noninfectious uveitis. Self-administered via subcutaneous injection, the initial dosage is 80 mg, followed by a maintenance dose of 40 mg/0.8 mL every other week starting 1 week after the initial dosage. Because it is a fully human antibody, risk of antidrug–antibody formation is lower than in infliximab, a mouse/human chimeric antibody. Injection site reactions may occur and are usually mild. An industry-sponsored, randomized, double-masked controlled trial in adults with noninfectious uveitis (VISUAL I/II), with an open label extension arm (VISUAL III) demonstrated that adalimumab was associated with significant reductions in treatment failure compared to placebo for both active and controlled uveitis. Also, significantly higher rates of quiescence and steroid-free quiescence were achieved and maintained through 52 weeks compared to placebo, regardless of disease status at entry. Adverse events and serious adverse events were reported more frequently among patients who received adalimumab compared to placebo.

Adalimumab has been shown to be as effective as infliximab in controlling inflammation, with success rates of up to 88% without relapse in pediatric patients with uveitis and 100% in adult patients with Behçet uveitis, posterior uveitis, and panuveitis. However, uveitis relapses requiring local corticosteroid injections may occur.

Adalimumab has been shown to reduce the rate of anterior uveitis flares and recurrences in HLA-B27–associated uveitis. Another randomized, placebo-controlled trial—involving patients with JIA-associated uveitis (SYCAMORE) comparing methotrexate alone to methotrexate plus adalimumab—demonstrated that the addition of adalimumab reduced time to treatment failure and increased likelihood of reducing topical steroid usage. Adverse events in this pediatric study were seen in 5% of the adalimumab group, 22% of which were considered serious adverse events. (See also Table 6-1.)

Infliximab is a mouse/human-chimeric, immunoglobulin G1 kappa (IgG1κ) monoclonal antibody directed against TNF-α. It is administered through infusions at weeks 0, 2, and 4 and every 4–8 weeks thereafter for maintenance. It is effective in controlling current inflammation and decreasing the likelihood of future attacks in Behçet uveitis, undifferentiated uveitis, sarcoidosis, VKH syndrome, and many other entities in more than 75% of patients. Similar favorable effects have been reported in patients with HLA-B27–associated anterior uveitis treated with infliximab. However, one study showed that despite treatment success, nearly one-half of patients could not complete the 50 weeks of therapy because of adverse events, including drug-induced lupus, systemic vascular thrombosis, congestive heart failure, new malignancy, demyelinating disease, and vitreous hemorrhage. As many as 75% of patients receiving more than 3 infusions developed antinuclear antibodies; greater likelihood of antibody formation may occur with higher doses and more frequent infusions. Increasing the dose and frequency may benefit the most severe ocular inflammatory diseases, however. Low-dose methotrexate (5–7.5 mg/week) may be administered concomitantly to reduce the risk of drug-induced lupus syndrome and the formation of human antichimeric antibodies, which can lead to reduced efficacy of infliximab.

Biester S, Deuter C, Michels H, et al. Adalimumab in the therapy of uveitis in childhood. *Br J Ophthalmol.* 2007;91(3):319–324.

Giganti M, Beer PM, Lemanski N, et al. Adverse events after intravitreal infliximab (Remicade). *Retina.* 2010;30(1):71–80.

Ramanan AV, Dick AD, Jones AP, et al; SYCAMORE study group. Adalimumab plus methotrexate for uveitis in juvenile idiopathic arthritis. *N Engl J Med.* 2017;376(17):1637–1646.

Sfikakis PP, Markomichelakis N, Alpsoy E, et al. Anti-TNF therapy in the management of Behçet's disease—review and basis for recommendations. *Rheumatology (Oxford).* 2007;46(5):736–741.

Suhler EB, Adán A, Brézin AP, et al. Safety and efficacy of adalimumab in patients with noninfectious uveitis in an ongoing open-label study: VISUAL III. *Ophthalmology.* 2018;125(7):1075–1087.

Tugal-Tutkun I, Mudun A, Urgancioglu M, et al. Efficacy of infliximab in the treatment of uveitis that is resistant to treatment with the combination of azathioprine, cyclosporine, and corticosteroids in Behçet's disease: an open-label trial. *Arthritis Rheum.* 2005;52(8):2478–2484.

Other Biologic Agents

Rituximab, a chimeric monoclonal antibody directed against $CD20^+$ cells (mainly B lymphocytes) given as an intravenous infusion, may be useful in the treatment of Behçet retinal vasculitis, granulomatosis with polyangiitis-associated necrotizing scleritis or other scleritis, and mucous membrane pemphigoid. Case series have reported success in refractory JIA-associated uveitis.

Interferon alfa-2a/2b (IFN-α2a/2b), administered subcutaneously, has been reported to be beneficial in some patients with uveitis. IFN-α2a has antiviral, immunomodulatory, and antiangiogenic effects. Reports in the European literature indicate that IFN-α2a is efficacious and well tolerated in patients with Behçet uveitis, controlling inflammation in almost 90%; it is somewhat less effective in non-Behçet uveitis, with inflammation control in 60%. There are also reports of IFN-α2b successfully treating uveitic macular edema. Prior to initiation of IFN-α2a therapy, patients discontinue any other immunomodulatory drugs. A flu-like syndrome has been observed, most frequently during the first weeks of therapy; however, symptoms may be reduced through prophylactic administration of acetaminophen. Despite the use of low interferon doses, leukopenia or thrombocytopenia may occur. Depression is another important adverse effect of interferon therapy.

Abatacept, a T-cell costimulation inhibitor given as an intravenous infusion, has been used in JIA uveitis with mixed results, including one small study suggesting only 14% sustained inflammation control; another study suggested a 49% success rate at 1 year.

Gueudry J, Wechsler B, Terrada C, et al. Long-term efficacy and safety of low-dose interferon alpha2a therapy in severe uveitis associated with Behçet disease. *Am J Ophthalmol.* 2008;146(6):837–844.

Kötter I, Zierhut M, Eckstein AK, et al. Human recombinant interferon alfa-2a for the treatment of Behçet's disease with sight threatening posterior or panuveitis. *Br J Ophthalmol.* 2003;87(4):423–431.

Other Therapeutic Agents

Topical mydriatic and cycloplegic drugs are beneficial for breaking or preventing the formation of posterior synechiae and for relieving photophobia secondary to ciliary spasm. Short-acting cycloplegics, such as tropicamide and cyclopentolate hydrochloride (1%) or phenylephrine (2.5%), allow the pupil to remain mobile and permit rapid recovery when discontinued.

Oral NSAIDs are used in treatment of mild-to-moderate nonnecrotizing anterior scleritis (see Chapter 7) and may have limited utility in treatment of chronic anterior uveitis (eg, JIA-associated anterior uveitis) and possibly macular edema. Oral NSAIDs may also allow the patient to be maintained on a lower dose of topical corticosteroids. Potential complications of prolonged systemic NSAID use include cardiovascular, gastrointestinal, renal, and hepatic toxicity. (See also BCSC Section 1, *Update on General Medicine,* for more information.) Topical NSAIDs may be used in mild cases of diffuse episcleritis, as well as in macular edema. In rare cases, severe corneal complications, such as keratitis and corneal perforations, may occur with the use of topical NSAIDs. (For further discussion of NSAIDs and corneal complications, refer to BCSC Section 8, *External Disease and Cornea.*)

The use of oral *carbonic anhydrase inhibitors* as an adjunct in treatment of uveitic macular edema is supported by a small but significant body of literature spanning several decades. These agents may be particularly useful in diffuse leakage from the retinal pigment epithelium, rather than in leakage from retinal vessels.

Intravenous immunoglobulin has been reported to be effective in some patients with uveitis that is otherwise refractory to IMT, as well as in patients with mucous membrane pemphigoid.

Surgical Management of Uveitis

Surgery is performed in patients with uveitis for diagnostic and/or therapeutic reasons. Therapeutic surgical procedures for uveitis and its complications are discussed in Chapter 14.

CHAPTER 7

Scleritis

Highlights

- Scleritis is characterized by primary inflammation of the sclera, typically leading to marked pain and congestion of the deep episcleral plexus.
- Underlying systemic inflammatory conditions are frequently associated with scleritis. It is important to properly investigate and treat these conditions.
- Treatment of scleritis requires systemic administration of anti-inflammatory and/or immunomodulatory drugs.
- Worse prognosis is associated with infectious, posterior, or necrotizing scleral inflammation.

Introduction

Scleritis, inflammation of the sclera, is a typically painful, destructive condition that carries a potential risk of permanent ocular structural damage with visual compromise. Scleritis often manifests with an acute episode of marked ocular pain, swelling, and redness. It can also evolve with decreased vision, mainly in the presence of necrotizing disease or when inflammation involves the posterior sclera, threatening the central choroid and retina. Scleritis can be immune mediated or can be associated with infection, trauma, surgery, and medications. Approximately 40% of scleritis cases are associated with a systemic disease, especially rheumatoid arthritis. Early and accurate diagnosis is critical, as scleral inflammation can be the first sign of a treatable sight- or life-threatening disease.

Classification of Scleritis

Scleral inflammation is classified based on the site (anterior vs posterior), severity (necrotizing vs nonnecrotizing), and pattern of scleral inflammation (diffuse vs nodular). This classification system is useful in the clinical setting, helping to predict the clinical course, systemic disease association, treatment, and prognosis (Table 7-1). An underlying inflammatory systemic disorder can be identified in nearly 40% of individuals with scleritis. In those with necrotizing scleritis, this association rises to up to 50%–60%.

Although infrequent, the onset of features of necrotizing scleritis in a case of initially nonnecrotizing disease can occur in up to 15% of cases, prompting further investigation and adequate therapy.

Table 7-1 Classification of Scleritis

Type	Subtype
Anterior scleritis	Diffuse scleritis
	Nodular scleritis
	Necrotizing scleritis
	With inflammation (granulomatous, vaso-occlusive, postsurgical)
	Without (overt) inflammation *(scleromalacia perforans)*
Posterior scleritis	

Reprinted with permission from Watson PG, Hayreh SS. Scleritis and episcleritis. *Br J Ophthalmol.* 1976;60(3):163–191.

Similar to uveitis, scleritis can also be classified as *noninfectious* or *infectious.* The latter is frequently associated with surgery or trauma. This distinction is critical since aggressive inadvertent use of corticosteroids or immunomodulatory therapy in cases of an underlying infectious etiology can lead to devastating consequences.

Pathophysiology

Noninfectious scleritis is an immune-mediated condition frequently involving the small blood vessels of the sclera. Pathophysiologic mechanisms vary according to the type of scleritis and underlying associated systemic disease. Onset is usually with infiltration of inflammatory cells in the sclera and episclera, mediated by proinflammatory cytokines and intercellular adhesion molecules.

The diffuse anterior subtype of scleritis is associated with a nongranulomatous response involving macrophages, lymphocytes, and plasma cells, which often assume a perivascular distribution.

In nodular scleritis, and particularly in necrotizing scleritis, the inflammatory response is more significant and specific, involving direct antibody-mediated damage (type II hypersensitivity), deposition of immune complexes triggering a type III hypersensitivity reaction, or a delayed (type IV) hypersensitivity response mainly characterized by granulomatous inflammation of the sclera. Inflammation may progress to an essentially vasculitic response, culminating in fibrinoid necrosis of the vessel wall and, eventually, necrosis of the sclera, episclera, conjunctiva, and cornea. Proinflammatory cytokines and activated metalloproteinases may play a role in local scleral and corneal damage.

Fong LP, Sainz de la Maza M, Rice BA, Kupferman AE, Foster CS. Immunopathology of scleritis. *Ophthalmology.* 1991;98(4):472–479.

Usui Y, Parikh J, Goto H, Rao NA. Immunopathology of necrotising scleritis. *Br J Ophthalmol.* 2008;92(3):417–419.

Epidemiology

Scleritis does not show geographic or racial differences. The incidence of scleritis is estimated at 3.4–4.1 per 100,000 persons and prevalence at 5.2 per 100,000 persons in the United States (US). Scleritis is more common in females. In tertiary centers, however, scleritis comprises 0.1%–2.6% of newly referred cases. Nonnecrotizing anterior scleritis is the most common form of the disease. While noninfectious scleritis is more common in the US, it is important to consider infectious scleritis, including herpetic, nocardial, mycobacterial, and fungal infection, in patients with risk factors based on medical and surgical history and geography.

Homayounfar G, Nardone N, Borkar DS, et al. Incidence of scleritis and episcleritis: results from the Pacific Ocular Inflammation Study. *Am J Ophthalmol.* 2013;156(4):752–758.

Honik G, Wong IG, Gritz DC. Incidence and prevalence of episcleritis and scleritis in Northern California. *Cornea.* 2013;32(12):1562–1566.

Williamson J. Incidence of eye disease in cases of connective tissue disease. *Trans Ophthalmol Soc UK.* 1974;94(3):742–752.

Clinical Presentation

Individuals with scleritis usually present with tenderness and dull pain in the affected eye and periocular area. The pain may worsen with eye movements and radiate to the face, cheek, and jaw. When cornea or posterior sclera is involved, vision may be affected.

The eye with scleritis typically shows scleral edema and intense hyperemia (Fig 7-1), leading to a characteristic violaceous hue on external examination. Slit-lamp examination characteristically discloses marked dilation of deep episcleral plexus, which is displaced outward by scleral edema/inflammatory infiltration. This is important in the distinction from episcleritis, in which no scleral edema is found and only superficial episcleral plexus is affected. Careful utilization of a topical vasoconstrictor (eg, phenylephrine drops) to bleach superficial blood vessels may facilitate this assessment and help distinguish episcleritis, in which the redness would blanch with phenylephrine, from scleritis. Close

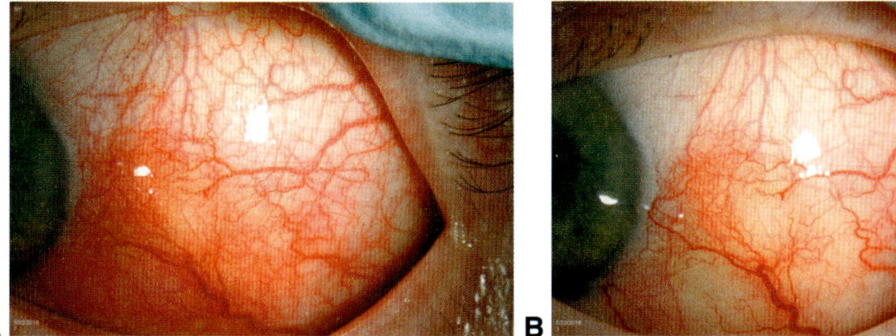

Figure 7-1 Diffuse anterior scleritis, with dilation of deep episcleral vessels before **(A)** and after **(B)** instillation of phenylephrine. *(Courtesy of H. Nida Sen, MD/National Eye Institute.)*

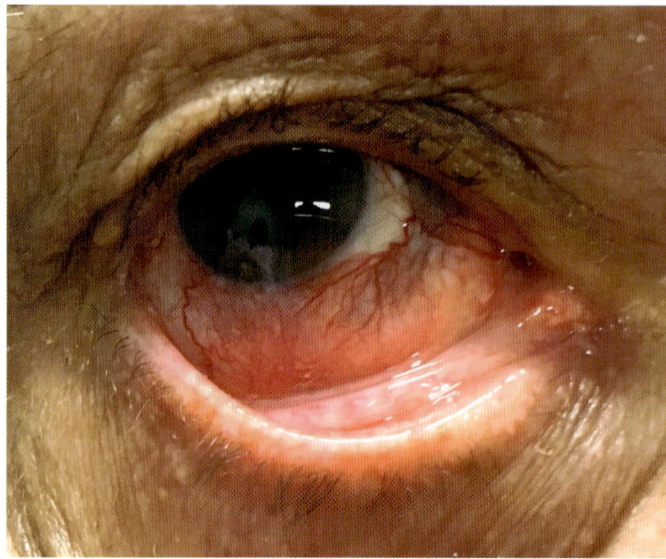

Figure 7-2 Anterior necrotizing scleritis, showing active scleral inflammation associated with an avascular area close to the limbus, adjacent to an area of scleral thinning. *(Courtesy of Daniel V. Vasconcelos-Santos, MD, PhD.)*

biomicroscopic inspection is also very important to assess the presence of signs of necrotizing disease (Fig 7-2).

Sainz de la Maza M, Molina N, Gonzalez-Gonzalez LA, Doctor PP, Tauber J, Foster CS. Clinical characteristics of a large cohort of patients with scleritis and episcleritis. *Ophthalmology*. 2012;119(1):43–50.

Sainz de la Maza M, Vitale AT. Scleritis and episcleritis. *Focal Points: Clinical Modules for Ophthalmologists*. San Francisco: American Academy of Ophthalmology; 2009, module 4.

Diffuse Anterior Scleritis

Anterior scleritis is defined as scleral inflammation anterior to the recti muscles. This is the most common and least severe type of scleritis, with a less than 10% risk of complications in most individuals. Onset is frequently insidious, with severe pain and diffuse or sectoral deep episcleral vascular congestion. Scleral swelling/infiltration is more diffuse (see Fig 7-1), so that no nodule is formed. Recurrences are very common. The main systemic associations include rheumatoid arthritis, systemic lupus erythematosus, and relapsing polychondritis. Inflammatory bowel disease, reactive arthritis, and, less frequently, ankylosing spondylitis can also be implicated.

Nodular Anterior Scleritis

Features of nodular anterior scleritis include a tender and typically immobile scleral nodule, in addition to the local or diffuse violaceous hue associated with markedly engorged, deep episcleral vessels. Up to 10% of patients with nodular anterior scleritis initially can progress to necrotizing disease, particularly in the setting of an underlying systemic inflammatory condition. It is important to rule out infectious etiologies in cases of nodular anterior scleritis, especially in the presence of necrosis (Fig 7-3). This necrotic change often manifests as an avascular area in the center of the nodule (eventually with superficial ulceration) or as a new independent lesion, extending circumferentially. After resolution of scleral inflammation, increased scleral translucency may be seen, eventually with thinning (Fig 7-4) and even formation of a staphyloma.

Necrotizing Scleritis

Necrotizing scleritis is the most severe and destructive type of scleral scleritis and is more likely to lead to vision loss. It is more frequently associated with systemic disease (approximately 50%–60%), some being life-threatening systemic vasculitic diseases. Necrotizing scleritis more frequently affects older individuals and is more prevalent in women. In the past, patients with necrotizing scleritis suffered from mortality rates as high as 30%; however, this improved significantly with the evolution of biologic therapies. Necrotizing scleritis can be further subdivided into 2 groups: (1) necrotizing scleritis with inflammation and (2) necrotizing scleritis without (overt) inflammation (scleromalacia perforans).

Doshi RR, Harocopos GJ, Schwab IR, Cunningham ET Jr. The spectrum of postoperative scleral necrosis. *Surv Ophthalmol.* 2013;58(6):620–633.

Lin CP, Su CY. Infectious scleritis and surgical induced necrotizing scleritis. *Eye (Lond).* 2010;24(4):740.

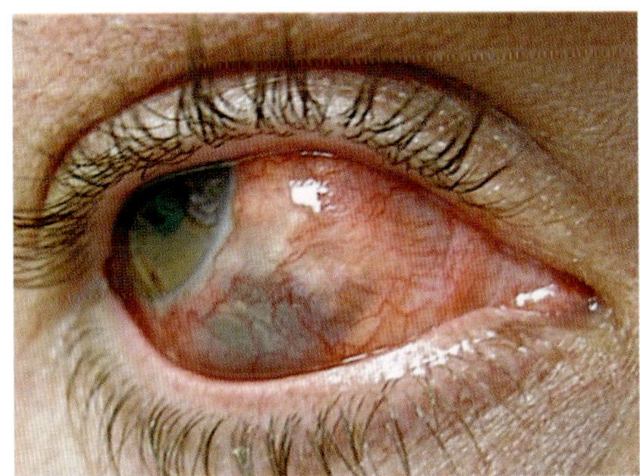

Figure 7-3 Infectious scleritis by actinomycetes, with a nodule superiorly and a large area of scleral thinning inferiorly. *(Courtesy of Daniel V. Vasconcelos-Santos, MD, PhD.)*

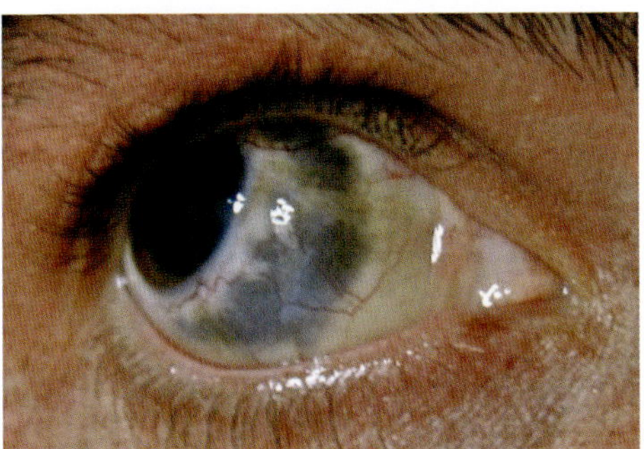

Figure 7-4 Infectious scleritis by actinomycetes (same patient as in Fig 7-3). Inflammation resolved after antibiotic treatment, but an arch of scleral thinning remained. *(Courtesy of Daniel V. Vasconcelos-Santos, MD, PhD.)*

Sainz de la Maza M, Molina N, Gonzalez-Gonzalez LA, Doctor PP, Tauber J, Foster CS. Clinical characteristics of a large cohort of patients with scleritis and episcleritis. *Ophthalmology*. 2012;119(1):43–50.

Necrotizing scleritis with inflammation

Necrotizing scleritis with inflammation is characterized by overt signs and symptoms of scleral inflammation. It may be subdivided into 3 types: (1) vaso-occlusive, (2) granulomatous (Fig 7-5), and (3) postsurgical.

The vaso-occlusive type progressively displays plaques of nonperfusion of episclera/conjunctiva, associated with scleral edema/infiltration and severe congestion of adjacent episcleral/conjunctival vessels (Fig 7-6). The limbal area and peripheral cornea are often spared. These cases are usually associated with infection or with an underlying systemic immune-mediated disease.

The granulomatous type typically starts with necrotizing inflammation of the limbal area, further extending anteriorly to the cornea and posteriorly to the sclera. The inflamed area assumes a "lumpy" aspect, associated with inflammatory infiltration and edema. Subsequently, necrosis and ulceration of the affected tissues (cornea,

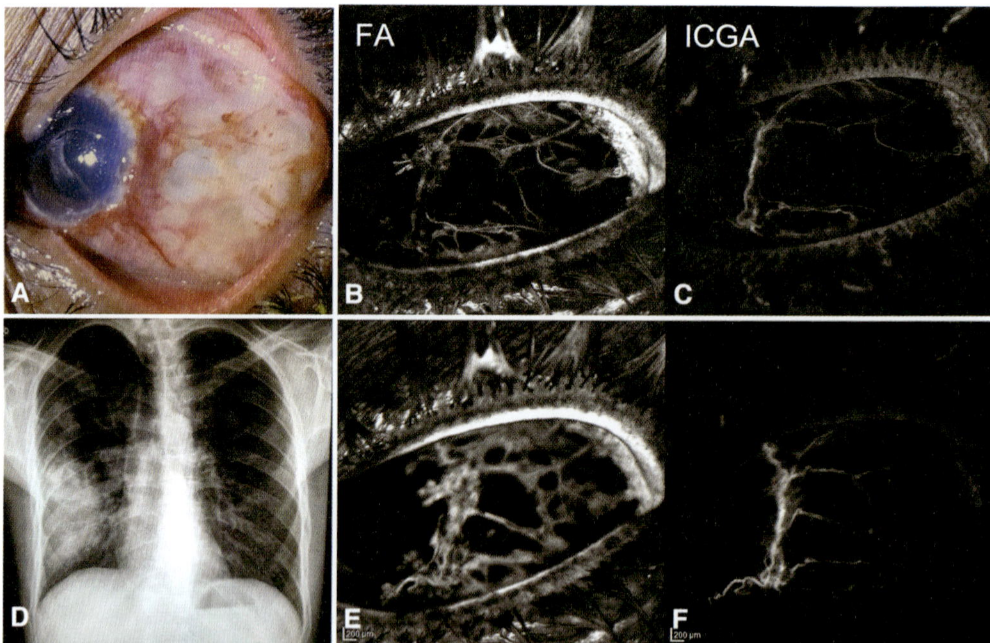

Figure 7-5 Necrotizing scleritis of the granulomatous subtype in a patient with granulomatosis with polyangiitis, with concomitant lung and kidney disease. Infiltration of the sclera and peripheral cornea is seen, with formation of multiple necrotic/avascular plaques **(A)**. Chest radiograph **(D)** shows infiltrates in the right lung (bottom left). Simultaneous fluorescein angiography (FA) **(B, E)** and indocyanine-green angiography (ICGA) **(C, F)** delineate areas of necrosis (with absence of episcleral and of conjunctival vessels) and of predominantly peripheral corneal neovascularization. *(Courtesy of Daniel V. Vasconcelos-Santos, MD, PhD.)*

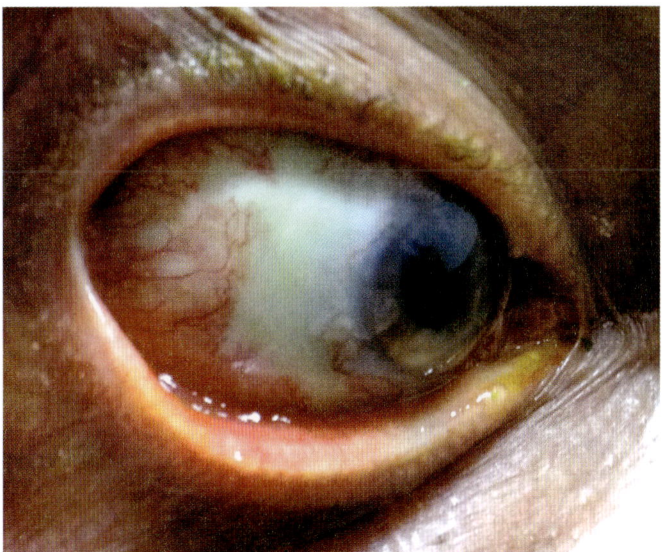

Figure 7-6 Necrotizing scleritis of the vaso-occlusive type, showing a large avascular area adjacent to the limbus. *(Courtesy of Daniel V. Vasconcelos-Santos, MD, PhD.)*

conjunctiva, episclera, and sclera) develop. This granulomatous type is frequently associated with systemic vasculitides, particularly granulomatosis with polyangiitis and polyarteritis nodosa. It is important to note that other subtypes of necrotizing scleritis may also display granulomatous inflammation on histopathology.

The postsurgical type is rare but frequently arises a few months to several years after surgical trauma to the sclera. It may be infectious or noninfectious. Procedures associated with postsurgical scleritis include cataract, strabismus or retinal surgery, trabeculectomy, cryotherapy, and pterygium excision, the last especially with use of mitomycin C or beta radiation. Recalcitrant inflammation, with progressive necrosis of the sclera, develops commonly at the site of the surgical insult (Fig 7-7), or sometimes more distant to the surgical incision. Many of these patients have an underlying autoimmune disease, with scleral surgical injury being the possible trigger for the local inflammatory process. It is important to exclude infection in these cases.

Watson PG, Hazleman BL, McCluskey P, Pavésio CE. *The Sclera and Systemic Disorders.* 3rd ed. London: JP Medical; 2012.

Necrotizing scleritis without (overt) inflammation

Necrotizing scleritis without (overt) inflammation, also called *scleromalacia perforans,* is characterized by lack of significant symptoms and apparent signs of clinical scleral inflammation. On histopathology, however, there is inflammatory cell infiltration in the sclera. The necrotizing granulomatous response leads to progressive (and "silent") destruction of the scleral tissue, which may extend circumferentially, eventually leaving a staphyloma. This entity has been historically misnamed *scleritis without inflammation.* Patients with

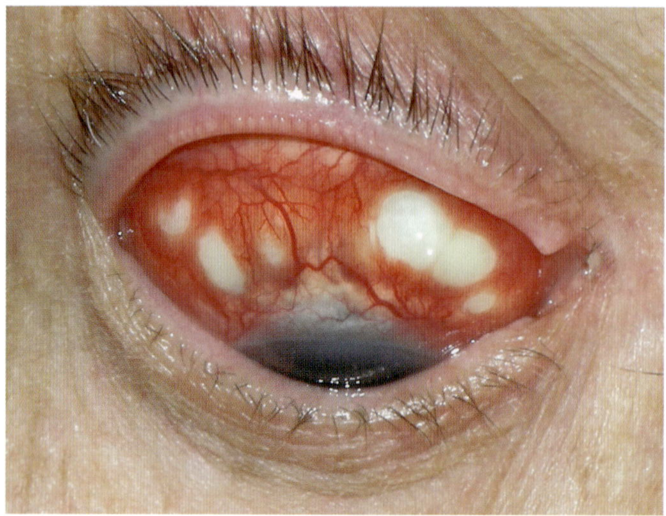

Figure 7-7 Necrotizing scleritis of the postsurgical type (following extracapsular cataract surgery), displaying multiple foci of scleral necrosis. *(Courtesy of Daniel V. Vasconcelos-Santos, MD, PhD.)*

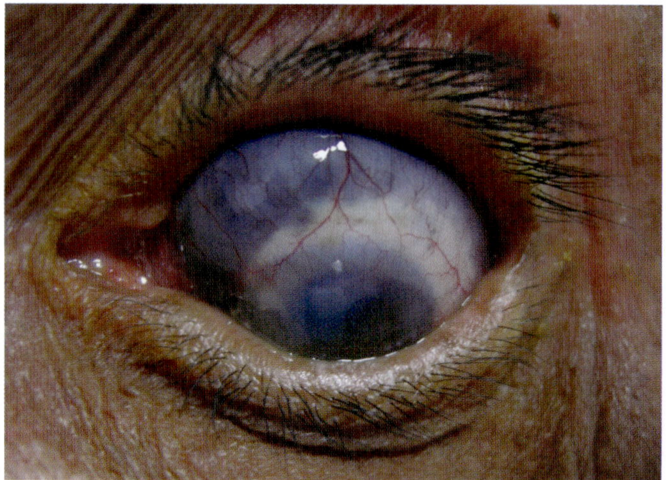

Figure 7-8 Scleromalacia perforans, showing profuse loss of scleral tissue, covered by conjunctiva. No overt inflammatory signs are seen. *(Courtesy of Daniel V. Vasconcelos-Santos, MD, PhD.)*

scleromalacia perforans are often elderly women with long-standing rheumatoid arthritis. They typically present with yellowish or white necrotic scleral plaques involving the sclera and episclera (sequestrum) of both eyes. These plaques are surrounded by mildly dilated episcleral vessels. Associated staphylomata are covered by conjunctiva and a thin translucent layer of fibrous tissue (Fig 7-8). Despite the term "perforans," these lesions do not usually perforate spontaneously.

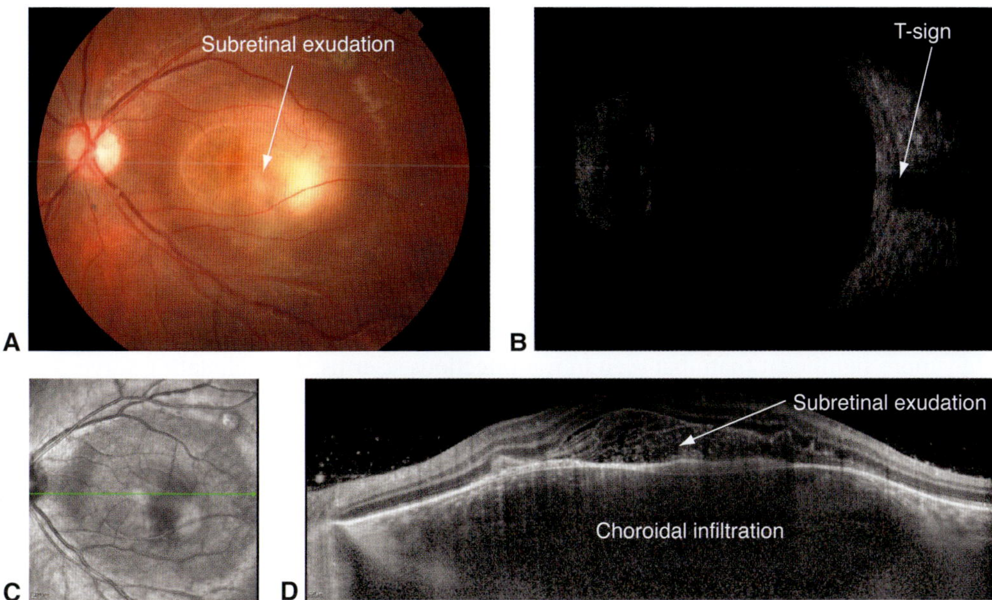

Figure 7-9 Posterior scleritis. **A,** Submacular exudation is seen on fundus photography. **B,** B-scan discloses accumulation of sub-Tenon fluid continuous to the optic nerve shadow (T-sign). **C, D,** Spectral-domain optical coherence tomography shows marked choroidal infiltration leading to serous detachment of the neurosensory retina and of the underlying retinal pigment epithelium. Fibrin deposition can also be seen in the subretinal space. *(Courtesy of Daniel V. Vasconcelos-Santos, MD, PhD.)*

Posterior Scleritis

Posterior scleritis is a sight-threatening entity that is defined by inflammation posterior to the ora serrata. It may be difficult to recognize because of lack of inflammatory signs in the anterior part of the sclera unless it is concomitant to anterior scleritis. The rate of association with inflammatory systemic conditions is comparable to that of anterior scleritis. Patients often report severe deep, boring pain and tenderness to palpation, but in 30%–40% of patients, these symptoms may be mild or absent. Decreased vision is often reported, but also depends on the topography of scleral inflammation and involvement of underlying structures. Possible signs include choroidal detachment and folds, subretinal fluid, and optic disc edema (Fig 7-9). Anterior rotation of the ciliary body pars plicata can displace the iridolenticular diaphragm anteriorly, leading to angle closure and acute elevation of intraocular pressure. Involvement of extraocular muscles (myositis) occasionally leads to diplopia.

McCluskey PJ, Watson PG, Lightman S, Haybittle J, Restori M, Branley M. Posterior scleritis: clinical features, systemic associations, and outcome in a large series of patients. *Ophthalmology.* 1999;106(12):2380–2386.

Infectious Scleritis

A wide variety of agents can infect the sclera, including *Pseudomonas* organisms (most common after pterygium excision), *Actinomyces* and *Nocardia* species, mycobacteria, fungi such as *Fusarium* and *Aspergillus* species, and gram-positive cocci (*Staphylococcus pneumococcus* and *Streptococcus* species). In addition, herpes simplex virus and varicella-zoster virus can cause chronic infectious scleritis. Infectious scleritis can occur after any previous ocular surgery, including pterygium surgery (especially when beta radiation or mitomycin C is used), scleral buckling, cataract surgery, and pars plana vitrectomy. Trauma with a penetrating injury contaminated by soil or vegetable matter may also result in infectious scleritis.

Infectious scleritis can present with pain, redness, and decreased vision, as with noninfectious scleritis. Nodular and necrotizing scleral disease are more common in this setting, and patients may also have intraocular inflammation (sclerouveitis) that is disproportionately more significant than that seen in noninfectious scleritis. A precipitating surgery may be recent or remote (in rare cases, many years before). The sclera appears necrotic, thin, and avascular, with inflammation at the edges (see Fig 7-3), usually at the site of a surgical or traumatic wound. A mucopurulent discharge may be present, depending on the infectious agent.

Raiji VR, Palestine AG, Parver DL. Scleritis and systemic disease association in a community-based referral practice. *Am J Ophthalmol.* 2009;148(6):946–950.

Riono WP, Hidayat AA, Rao NA. Scleritis: a clinicopathologic study of 55 cases. *Ophthalmology.* 1999;106(7):1328–1333.

Watson PG, Hazleman BL, McCluskey P, Pavésio CE. *The Sclera and Systemic Disorders.* 3rd ed. London: JP Medical; 2012.

Diagnosis

Diagnosis of scleritis is based on a detailed clinical history, close inspection, and slit-lamp and fundus examination. Sometimes it may be easier to appreciate scleritis by looking at the eye externally without the slit lamp. Complementary B-scan ultrasonography, fundus angiography, and optical coherence tomography (OCT) can help better delineate scleral involvement. An appropriate laboratory workup is warranted to rule out underlying systemic inflammatory diseases (Table 7-2), which may be very frequent and life-threatening, especially in the setting of necrotizing scleritis. Finally, it is important to consider the possibility of drug-induced scleral inflammation (mainly associated with bisphosphonates).

B-scan ultrasonography is useful for confirming suspicion of posterior scleritis or assessing concomitant posterior scleral involvement. Imaging typically reveals thickening of the sclera, associated with accumulation of fluid in the sub-Tenon space. When adjacent to the optic nerve shadow, this may lead to the classic "T-sign" (see Fig 7-9). Ultrasonography may also be helpful to assess involvement of adjacent structures, including the choroid, ciliary body, retina, extraocular muscles, and orbit. Computed tomography (CT) and magnetic resonance imaging (MRI) can also assist in the assessment of orbital structures in posterior scleritis.

Posterior segment spectral-domain optical coherence tomography (SD-OCT), including enhanced depth imaging (EDI), may also be useful to delineate fundus changes

Table 7-2 Investigations for Noninfectious Inflammatory Conditions Associated With Scleritis

Disease	Potentially Useful Investigations
Rheumatoid arthritis	RF, anti-CCP, ESR/CRP, joint radiographs
Systemic lupus erythematosus	ANA, CBC, urine sediment
Juvenile idiopathic arthritis	ANA, HLA-B27, joint radiographs
Ankylosing spondylitis	HLA-B27, ESR/CRP, lumbosacral radiographs
Reactive arthritis	HLA-B27, ESR/CRP, joint radiographs, cultures (urogenital tract, throat, stool, synovial fluid)
Enteropathic arthritis	HLA-B27, lumbosacral radiographs
Psoriatic arthritis	HLA-B27, ESR/CRP
Granulomatosis with polyangiitis	cANCA (anti-PR3), tissue biopsy, radiographs (chest/sinuses), urine sediment
Polyarteritis nodosa	pANCA (anti-MPO), tissue biopsy, urine sediment
Microscopic polyangiitis	pANCA (anti-MPO)
Relapsing polychondritis	ESR/CRP, cartilage biopsy
Churg-Strauss syndrome	CBC (eosinophilia), pANCA (anti-MPO), tissue biopsy, urine sediment
Leukocytoclastic vasculitis	Anti-HCV, RF, ESR/CRP
Cogan syndrome[a]	Hearing test
Giant cell arteritis	ESR/CRP, CBC, temporal artery biopsy
Takayasu arteritis	Cardiac catheterization
Sarcoidosis	ACE (lysozyme for patients on ACE inhibitors), chest x-ray/CT, tuberculin skin test, tissue biopsy

ACE = angiotensin-converting enzyme; ANA = antinuclear antibodies; ANCA = antineutrophil cytoplasmic antibodies (cANCA = intracytoplasmic staining; pANCA = perinuclear staining); CBC = complete blood count; CCP = cyclic citrullinated peptide; CRP = C-reactive protein; CT = computed tomography; ESR = erythrocyte sedimentation rate; HCV = hepatitis C virus; HLA = human leukocyte antigen; MPO = myeloperoxidase; PR3 = serine proteinase 3; RF = rheumatoid factor.

[a] Refer to BCSC Section 8, *External Disease and Cornea.*

associated with posterior scleritis (see Fig 7-9). Anterior segment SD-OCT may provide noninvasive imaging that documents local changes at the level of the sclera, episclera, Tenon capsule, conjunctiva, cornea, and angle structures, but its clinical utility is unclear at this time. Ultrasound biomicroscopy may be used to image the anterior segment and ciliary body, but this technique is often technically cumbersome in tender and painful eyes with scleritis. In cases of posterior scleritis, fundus fluorescein or indocyanine angiography can identify the extent of disease and may be helpful in differential diagnosis.

In the setting of high suspicion for infectious scleritis, microbiological examination of scleral scrape and even incisional biopsy of the sclera can be very helpful. Biopsy is also valuable in the possibility of neoplastic conditions, such as conjunctival carcinomas and lymphomas. These can masquerade as or even be associated with a variable degree of scleral inflammation. Intraocular tumors, particularly large uveal melanomas, occasionally lead to engorgement of overlying episcleral (so-called *sentinel)* vessels.

Levison AL, Lowder CY, Baynes KM, Kaiser PK, Srivastava SK. Anterior segment spectral domain optical coherence tomography imaging of patients with anterior scleritis. *Int Ophthalmol.* 2016;36(4):499–508.
Nieuwenhuizen J, Watson PG, Emmanouilidis-van der Spek K, Keunen JE, Jager MJ. The value of combining anterior segment fluorescein angiography with indocyanine green angiography in scleral inflammation. *Ophthalmology.* 2003;110(8):1653–1566.
Okhravi N, Odufuwa B, McCluskey P, Lightman S. Scleritis. *Surv Ophthalmol.* 2005;50(4):351–363.
Watson PG, Hazleman BL, McCluskey P, Pavésio CE. *The Sclera and Systemic Disorders.* 3rd ed. London: JP Medical; 2012.

Treatment

Treatment of scleritis depends on the type and extent of scleral inflammation and the results of diagnostic investigations (see Table 7-2). In the presence of an underlying systemic disease, particularly associated with necrotizing scleritis, adequate control of the condition is essential, as it may be a major determinant of mortality. It is also important to manage infectious and neoplastic etiologies accordingly.

Systemic Treatment

Topical therapy is usually not sufficient to treat scleritis; therefore, treatment is systemic. It can range from oral nonsteroidal anti-inflammatory drugs (NSAIDs) to systemic immunomodulatory agents. In individuals with mild-to-moderate noninfectious anterior scleritis, either diffuse or nodular, primary management consists of oral NSAIDs for a few weeks, in the absence of specific contraindications. Caution is advised because of the risk of gastroduodenal ulceration, which may be decreased by concomitant use of histamine-H_2 receptor antagonists or proton-pump inhibitors. It is also important to monitor renal function closely.

Severe noninfectious cases, refractory to NSAIDs or with posterior or necrotizing disease, are managed with systemic corticosteroids, typically with an initial dose of 1 mg/kg/day of prednisone or equivalent, followed by a slow tapering regimen. Careful monitoring for side effects is highly recommended.

When scleral inflammation recurs or is refractory to systemic corticosteroids, especially in necrotizing scleritis, immunomodulatory drugs (mainly antimetabolites, such as methotrexate, mycophenolate mofetil, or azathioprine) are indicated either as corticosteroid-sparing agents or as adjuvants. Biologic immunomodulatory agents, such as tumor necrosis factor inhibitors (eg, infliximab, adalimumab, and rituximab [anti-CD20]), have also been successfully employed for refractory cases.

Intravenous pulse therapy with methylprednisolone (1 g daily for 3 days, followed by high-dose oral prednisone) can be initially used in the setting of severe necrotizing or nonnecrotizing scleritis. Alkylating agents, such as cyclophosphamide, are reserved for severe necrotizing involvement of the sclera and cornea, with impending risk of perforation. They may also be helpful for the control of underlying systemic diseases (eg, granulomatosis with polyangiitis). Scleritis associated with granulomatosis with polyangiitis (formerly called Wegener granulomatosis) and polyarteritis nodosa typically requires more aggressive therapy with rituximab or cyclophosphamide.

Infectious scleritis can be treated with systemic (and topical) antimicrobials and surgical debridement as needed. It is important to differentiate infectious scleritis from noninfectious scleritis, because unopposed corticosteroids or immunosuppressive agents can worsen scleritis in the presence of active infection. Microorganisms may be difficult to eradicate from the sclera, and long-term treatment may be necessary. Scleral patch grafting may be necessary, if there is severe thinning.

Individuals with nonnecrotizing noninfectious scleritis who cannot tolerate systemic therapy or have residual scleral inflammation may be candidates for subconjunctival injection of low-dose subconjunctival triamcinolone (0.5–4 mg). It is important for each case to weigh the risks of cataract and secondary ocular hypertension/glaucoma and, more remotely, of scleral melting and infection against the possible benefits of the injection. Underlying systemic inflammatory diseases should be under control and infectious etiologies must be ruled out before considering local injection of steroids.

Topical corticosteroids can be used to control associated iridocyclitis, present in nearly one-third of individuals with scleritis. This may prevent complications such as anterior/posterior synechiae, uveitic glaucoma, and cataract.

Cao JH, Oray M, Cocho L, Foster CS. Rituximab in the treatment of refractory noninfectious scleritis. *Am J Ophthalmol.* 2016;164:22–28.

Daniel Diaz J, Sobol EK, Gritz DC. Treatment and management of scleral disorders. *Surv Ophthalmol.* 2016;61(6):702–717.

Jabs DA, Mudun A, Dunn JP, Marsh MJ. Episcleritis and scleritis: clinical features and treatment results. *Am J Ophthalmol.* 2000;130(4):469–476.

Sobrin L, Christen W, Foster CS. Mycophenolate mofetil after methotrexate failure or intolerance in treatment of scleritis and uveitis. *Ophthalmology.* 2008;115(8):1416–1421.

Sohn EH, Wang R, Read R, et al. Long-term, multicenter evaluation of subconjunctival injection of triamcinolone for non-necrotizing, noninfectious anterior scleritis. *Ophthalmology.* 2011;118(10):1932–1937.

Surgical Treatment

Surgical treatment can be considered in individuals with severe refractory necrotizing scleritis to reinforce the wall in the setting of an impending perforation or to close a spontaneous or traumatic corneal and/or scleral defect (tectonic grafting). Figure 7-10 shows a postoperative aspect of scleral grafting. Cadaveric donor sclera may be used for grafting, but it can melt. Consequently, some authors have recommended use of autogenous periosteum or donor cornea. In cases of infectious scleritis, scleral debridement can be considered in addition to antibiotics.

Prognosis

The prognosis of scleritis varies upon the severity and extent of involvement of ocular structures and the presence of underlying systemic diseases. Nonnecrotizing noninfectious anterior (diffuse or nodular) scleritis has a good prognosis with treatment, with most eyes

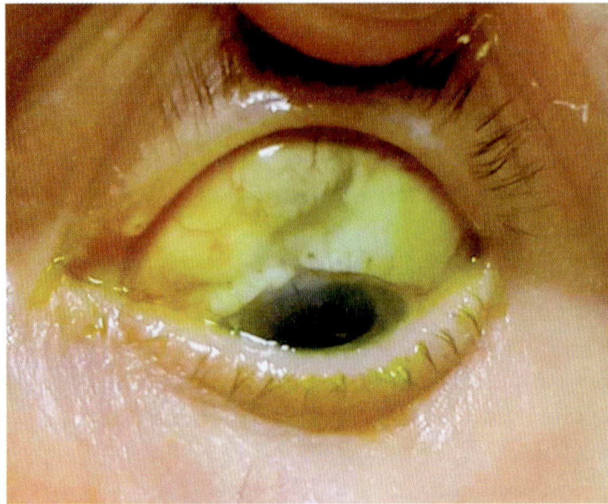

Figure 7-10 Postoperative aspect of scleral grafting. *(Courtesy of Humeyra Karacal, MD.)*

maintaining good visual acuity over time. Patients with posterior scleritis, necrotizing scleritis, or infectious scleritis, however, are at high risk of permanent vision loss. Individuals with necrotizing scleritis are also at risk of higher mortality rates, because of the frequent association with life-threatening vasculitic disorders. Proper and timely management of these disorders is thus very important.

CHAPTER 8

Noninfectious Anterior and Intermediate Uveitis

Highlights

- Noninfectious uveitis can be divided into 4 types: (1) anterior uveitis, (2) intermediate uveitis, (3) posterior uveitis, and (4) panuveitis. This chapter focuses on anterior and intermediate uveitides.
- Anterior uveitis constitutes the majority of all uveitis cases and is often treated with topical corticosteroids.
- The first episode of mild, nongranulomatous, unilateral anterior uveitis may not require further systemic workup.
- Intermediate uveitis can be associated with systemic diseases, including sarcoidosis and multiple sclerosis. Idiopathic intermediate uveitis without associated systemic disease is categorized as pars planitis.
- Ocular inflammatory diseases are either infectious or noninfectious. Noninfectious diseases can be further subdivided into masquerade syndromes and drug-induced, traumatic, and autoimmune ocular inflammatory conditions.

Anterior Uveitis

Anterior uveitis is the most common form of uveitis, accounting for more than 90% of cases in a community-based practice. Incidence in the United States varies by age, from approximately 7 cases per 100,000 person-years in persons aged 14 years and younger up to approximately 220 per 100,000 persons aged 65 years and older.

Because uveitis may occur secondary to inflammation of the cornea and/or sclera, it is important for the physician to evaluate these structures carefully to rule out primary keratitis or scleritis. Inflammation of the sclera and the cornea is covered in depth in BCSC Section 8, *External Disease and Cornea;* see also Chapter 7.

Gritz DC, Wong IG. Incidence and prevalence of uveitis in Northern California; the Northern California Epidemiology of Uveitis Study. *Ophthalmology.* 2004;111(3):491–500.

Reeves SW, Sloan FA, Lee PP, Jaffe GJ. Uveitis in the elderly: epidemiological data from the National Long-term Care Survey Medicare Cohort. *Ophthalmology.* 2006;113(2):307–321.

Acute Nongranulomatous Anterior Uveitis

The classic presentation of acute anterior uveitis is the sudden onset of pain, redness, and photophobia that can be associated with decreased vision. Fine keratic precipitates (KPs) dust the corneal endothelium in most cases. Active disease is characterized by anterior chamber cells and variable flare. Severe cases may show a protein coagulum in the aqueous or, less commonly, a hypopyon (Fig 8-1). Occasionally, a fibrin net forms across the pupillary margin (Fig 8-2), potentially producing a seclusion membrane and iris bombé. Iris vessels may be dilated, and, on rare occasions, a spontaneous hyphema occurs. Cells may also be present in the anterior vitreous. Fundus lesions are not characteristic, although uveitic macular edema and disc edema may be noted. Occasionally, intraocular pressure (IOP) may be elevated because of trabeculitis, blockage of the trabecular meshwork by debris and cells, or pupillary block.

The inflammation usually lasts several days to weeks, up to 3 months. Two patterns may occur. In the first type, the attack is acute and unilateral, with a history of episodes alternating between the 2 eyes; this pattern is typical for HLA-B27–associated anterior uveitis. Either eye may be affected, but recurrence is rarely bilateral. The second pattern is acute and bilateral.

Corticosteroids are the mainstay of treatment to eliminate inflammation, prevent cicatrization, and minimize damage to the uveal structures. Topical corticosteroids are the first line of treatment, and administration every 1–2 hours is often needed. If necessary, periocular or oral corticosteroids may be used for severe episodes. Initial attacks may require all 3 routes of administration, particularly in severe cases.

Ocular morbidity can be reduced by timely diagnosis, aggressive initial therapy, and patient adherence. In cases with a recurrent course, maintenance therapy with low-dose topical corticosteroids may be needed.

Corticosteroid-sparing drugs, such as antimetabolites, and others may be needed for long-term therapy in chronic or frequently recurrent anterior uveitis. Tumor necrosis

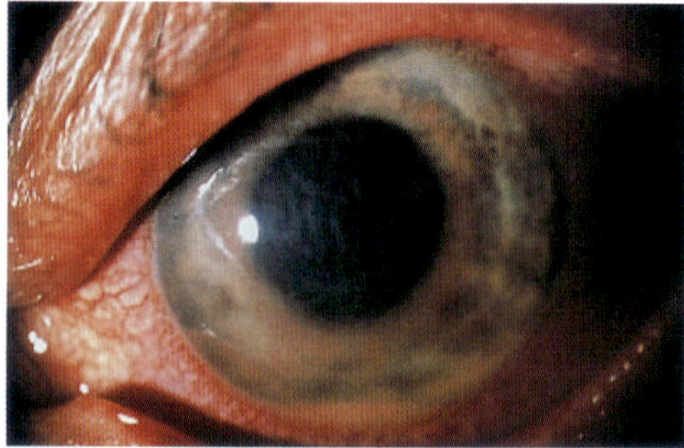

Figure 8-1 Acute HLA-B27–positive anterior uveitis that was accompanied by pain, photophobia, marked injection, fixed pupil, loss of iris detail from corneal edema, and hypopyon. *(Courtesy of David Meisler, MD.)*

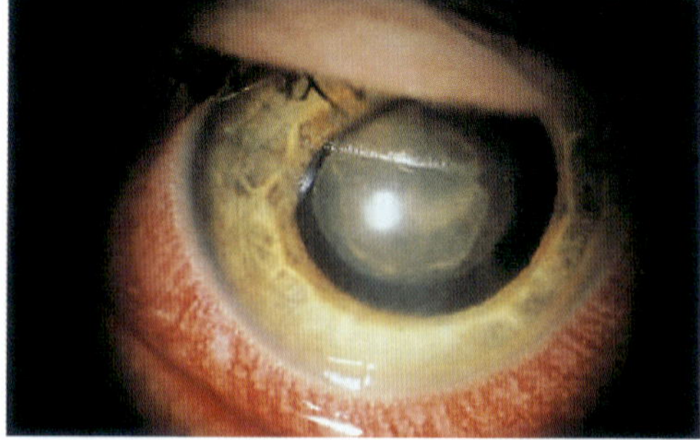

Figure 8-2 Ankylosing spondylitis. Acute unilateral anterior uveitis with severe anterior chamber reaction, central fibrinous exudate contracting anterior to the lens capsule, and posterior synechiae from the 10-o'clock to 12-o'clock position. *(Courtesy of David Meisler, MD.)*

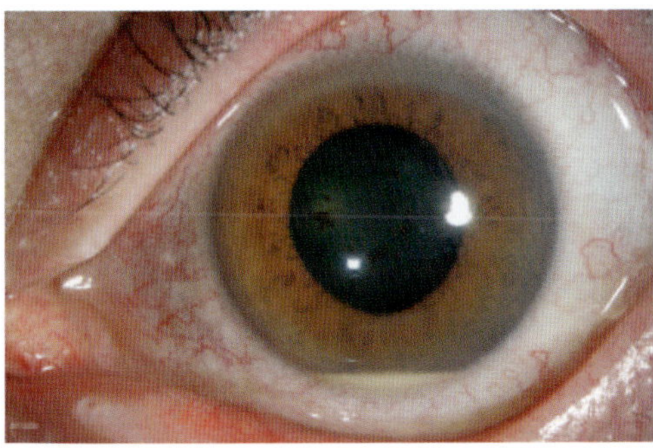

Figure 8-3 Acute nongranulomatous anterior uveitis. Hypopyon and anterior capsular ring of pigment following posterior synechiolysis after intensive treatment with dilating agents. *(Courtesy of H. Nida Sen, MD/National Eye Institute.)*

factor (TNF) inhibitor therapy has been effective in recalcitrant anterior uveitis, particularly in HLA-B27–positive patients. Cycloplegic agents can relieve pain and can break and prevent formation of synechiae. They can be given topically or with conjunctival cotton pledgets soaked in tropicamide, cyclopentolate, or phenylephrine hydrochloride (Fig 8-3).

HLA-B27 is a major histocompatibility complex (MHC) class I antigen present in approximately 8% of the general population in the United States. Approximately 40%–50% of patients with acute anterior uveitis are HLA-B27 positive. Thus, although patients with recurrent anterior nongranulomatous uveitis should be tested for HLA-B27, the presence of HLA-B27 alone does not provide an absolute diagnosis. Further, the precise trigger for acute anterior uveitis in HLA-B27–positive persons remains unclear.

Several autoimmune diseases known collectively as the *seronegative spondyloarthropathies* are strongly associated with both acute anterior uveitis and HLA-B27. Patients with these diseases, by definition, do not test positive for rheumatoid factor. The seronegative spondyloarthropathies include

- ankylosing spondylitis (AS)
- reactive arthritis syndrome
- inflammatory bowel disease
- psoriatic arthritis

These entities are sometimes clinically indistinguishable, and all may be associated with spondylitis and sacroiliitis. Women are more likely than men to experience atypical spondyloarthropathies.

Van Gelder RN. Diagnostic testing in uveitis. *Focal Points: Clinical Modules for Ophthalmologists.* San Francisco: American Academy of Ophthalmology; 2013, module 6.

Wakefield D, Chang JH, Amjadi S, Maconochie Z, Abu El-Asrar A, McCluskey P. What is new HLA-B27 acute anterior uveitis? *Ocul Immunol Inflamm.* 2011;19(2):139–144.

HLA-B27–related diseases

Ankylosing spondylitis AS ranges in severity from asymptomatic to crippling. Symptoms of this disorder include lower back pain and morning stiffness. Up to 90% of patients with AS test positive for HLA-B27, although most HLA-B27–positive individuals do not develop the disease. The chance that an HLA-B27–positive patient will develop spondyloarthritis or eye disease is 1 in 4. Family members may also have AS or anterior uveitis. Often, persons with anterior uveitis lack symptoms of back disease.

The ophthalmologist may be the first physician to suspect AS in an individual patient. Symptoms or family history of back problems together with HLA-B27 positivity suggest the diagnosis. Sacroiliac imaging studies should be obtained when indicated by a suggestive history of morning lower back stiffness that improves with exertion. Patients should be informed of the risk of deformity and referred to a rheumatologist. Pulmonary apical fibrosis and cardiovascular disease (aortic valvular insufficiency) may also develop.

Nonsteroidal anti-inflammatory agents (NSAIDs) are the mainstay of systemic treatment for AS. Sulfasalazine may be used in patients whose joint disease is not controlled with NSAIDs, and it may reduce the frequency of uveitis recurrences. However, TNF inhibitors are gaining favor for second-line treatment in recalcitrant cases given their rapid therapeutic effect and overall efficacy. Ophthalmologists should also recognize that early diagnosis is important because nonpharmacologic interventions such as exercise, physical therapy, and smoking cessation may help slow disease progression.

Braun J, Baraliakos X, Listing J, Sieper J. Decreased incidence of anterior uveitis in patients with ankylosing spondylitis treated with the anti-tumor necrosis factor agents infliximab and etanercept. *Arthritis Rheum.* 2005;52(8):2447–2451.

Monnet D, Breban M, Hudry C, Dougados M, Brézin AP. Ophthalmic findings and frequency of extraocular manifestations in patients with HLA-B27 uveitis: a study of 175 cases. *Ophthalmology.* 2004;111(4):802–809.

Reactive arthritis syndrome Reactive arthritis syndrome, formerly known as *Reiter syndrome,* consists of the classic diagnostic triad of nonspecific urethritis, polyarthritis, and conjunctival inflammation, often accompanied by nongranulomatous anterior uveitis. The HLA-B27 marker is found in approximately 50%–75% of patients. The condition constitutes less than 2% of all spondyloarthropathies and occurs most frequently in young adult men, although 10% of patients are female.

Episodes of diarrhea or dysentery without urethritis can trigger reactive arthritis syndrome. *Ureaplasma urealyticum* as well as *Chlamydia, Shigella, Salmonella,* and *Yersinia* species have all been implicated as triggering infections, although pathogens cannot be isolated from affected joints. Arthritis begins within 30 days of infection in 80% of patients. The knees, ankles, feet, and wrists are affected asymmetrically and in an oligoarticular (4 or fewer joints) distribution. Sacroiliitis is present in as many as 70% of patients.

In addition to the classic triad, 2 other conditions are considered major diagnostic criteria:

- *keratoderma blennorrhagicum:* a scaly, erythematous, irritating disorder of the palms and soles of the feet (Fig 8-4)
- *circinate balanitis:* a persistent, scaly, erythematous, circumferential rash of the distal penis

Extraarticular findings such as nail bed pitting, oral ulcers, conjunctivitis, uveitis, and constitutional symptoms help establish a diagnosis of reactive arthritis syndrome. Most cases resolve after a short episode. Occasionally, the disease becomes chronic. Eye

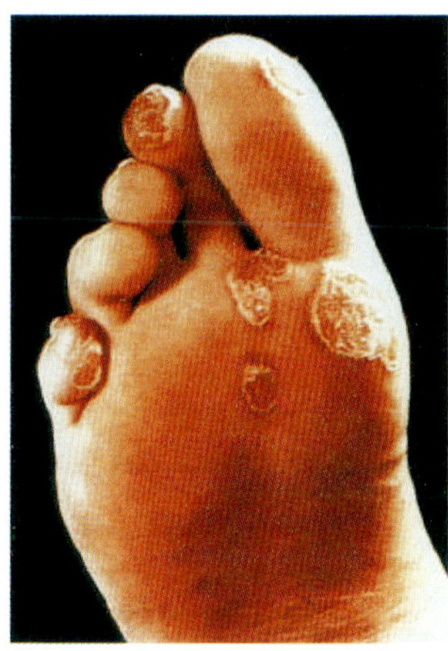

Figure 8-4 Reactive arthritis syndrome with pedal discoid keratoderma blennorrhagicum. *(Courtesy of John D. Sheppard Jr, MD.)*

involvement occurs in approximately 20%. Conjunctivitis is the most common eye finding associated with this disease, and it is usually mucopurulent and papillary. Punctate and subepithelial keratitis may also occur, occasionally leaving permanent corneal scars. Acute nongranulomatous anterior uveitis occurs in up to 10% of patients and may become bilateral and chronic.

Inflammatory bowel disease Ulcerative colitis and Crohn disease (granulomatous ileocolitis) are both associated with acute anterior uveitis. Up to 12% of patients with ulcerative colitis and 2.4% of patients with Crohn disease develop acute anterior uveitis. Occasionally, bowel disease is asymptomatic and follows the onset of uveitis. Twenty percent of patients with inflammatory bowel disease have sacroiliitis; of these, 60% are HLA-B27 positive. Patients with both acute anterior uveitis and inflammatory bowel disease (IBD) are more likely to be HLA-B27 positive and have sacroiliitis. Patients with IBD may also develop sclerouveitis, but these individuals are more commonly HLA-B27 negative, have symptoms resembling rheumatoid arthritis, and usually do not develop sacroiliitis. HLA-B27–negative IBD patients may also be more likely to develop intermediate uveitis.

Psoriatic arthritis The diagnosis of psoriatic arthritis is made according to findings of typical cutaneous changes (Fig 8-5), terminal phalangeal joint inflammation (Fig 8-6), and ungual involvement. Twenty percent of patients may have sacroiliitis, and IBD occurs more frequently than would be expected by chance. Up to 25% of patients develop anterior uveitis, which tends to be insidious and bilateral; it is also more likely to be chronic than is the uveitis associated with other spondyloarthropathies. Risk is particularly high in psoriatic spondylitis patients. Uveitis may be more severe in HLA-B27–positive patients. Treatment consists of cycloplegic and mydriatic agents and corticosteroids, which are usually given topically. In severe cases, periocular or systemic corticosteroids may be required, and chronic cases may need immunomodulatory therapy (IMT).

Anterior uveitis in patients with psoriasis without arthritis has distinct clinical features. The mean age of onset is older than in idiopathic or HLA-B27–associated uveitis and may be bilateral and of longer duration. Posterior segment involvement can be present.

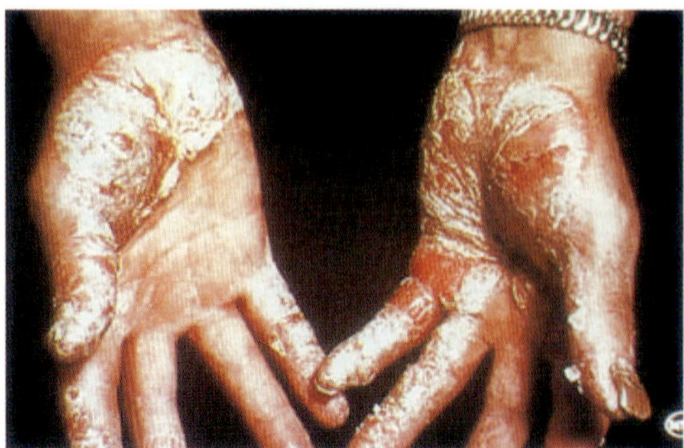

Figure 8-5 Psoriatic arthritis with classic erythematous, hyperkeratotic rash. *(Courtesy of John D. Sheppard Jr, MD.)*

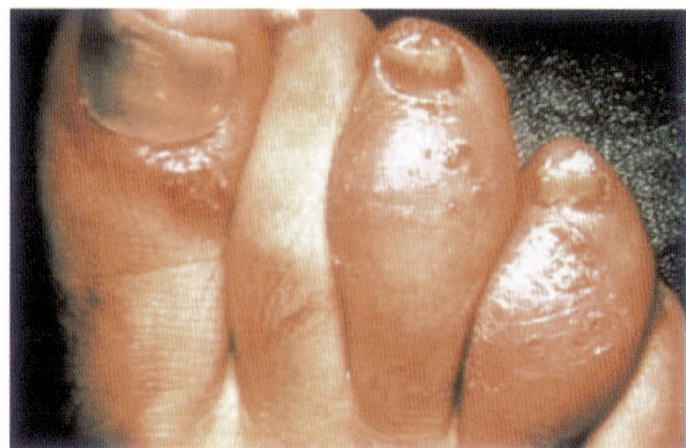

Figure 8-6 Psoriatic arthritis with "sausage" digits resulting from tissue swelling and distal interphalangeal joint inflammation. *(Courtesy of John D. Sheppard Jr, MD.)*

de Azevedo Fraga NA, Paim de Oliveira MF, Follador I, de Oliveira Rocha B, Rêgo VR. Psoriasis and uveitis: a literature review. *An Bras Dermatol.* 2012;87(6):877–883.

Egeberg A, Khalid U, Gislason GH, Mallbris L, Skov L, Hansen PR. Association of psoriatic disease with uveitis: a Danish nationwide cohort study. *JAMA Dermatol.* 2015;151(11):1200–1205.

Sampaio-Barros PD, Pereira IA, Hernández-Cuevas C, et al; RESPONDIA Group. An analysis of 372 patients with anterior uveitis in a large Ibero-American cohort of spondyloarthritis: the RESPONDIA Group. *Clin Exp Rheumatol.* 2013;(4):484–489.

Tubulointerstitial nephritis and uveitis syndrome

Tubulointerstitial nephritis and uveitis (TINU) syndrome occurs predominantly in adolescent girls and women up to their early 30s; the mean age of onset is 21 years. Uveitis is typically a bilateral, nongranulomatous, anterior uveitis. Ocular symptoms and findings are more severe in patients with recurrent disease, with development of fibrin, posterior synechiae, larger KPs, and, rarely, hypopyon. Posterior segment involvement is rare but may include vitritis, multifocal chorioretinal lesions, and retinal vascular leakage as well as optic nerve and macular edema (Fig 8-7).

Patients may present with ophthalmic findings before systemic symptoms and tubulointerstitial nephritis develop. More commonly, however, patients present with systemic symptoms before the development of uveitis. The following criteria are required for a clinical diagnosis of TINU syndrome:

- abnormal serum creatinine level or decreased creatinine clearance
- abnormal urinalysis findings, with increased β2-microglobulin level, proteinuria, presence of eosinophils, pyuria or hematuria, urinary white cell casts, and normoglycemic glycosuria
- associated systemic illness, consisting of fever, weight loss, anorexia, fatigue, arthralgias, and myalgias; there may also be abnormal liver function, eosinophilia, and an elevated erythrocyte sedimentation rate

The etiology remains unclear. Seroreactivity against retinal and renal antigens has been demonstrated. The syndrome has been reported to be strongly associated with

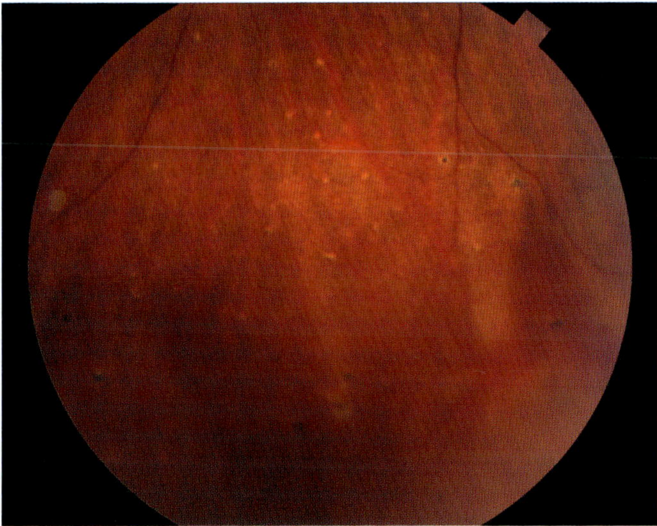

Figure 8-7 Tubulointerstitial nephritis–associated uveitis with chorioretinal scars in peripheral retina. *(Courtesy of Debra A. Goldstein, MD.)*

HLA-DRB1*0102. The predominance of activated CD4+ (helper) T lymphocytes in the kidney interstitium suggests a role for cellular immunity. Renal biopsies have shown severe interstitial fibrosis. TINU syndrome is very responsive to treatment with high-dose oral corticosteroids. Some patients with a prolonged course may require IMT.

Ali A, Rosenbaum JT. TINU (tubulointerstitial nephritis uveitis) can be associated with chorioretinal scars. *Ocul Immunol Inflamm.* 2014;22(3):213–217.

Mackensen F, Billing H. Tubulointerstitial nephritis and uveitis syndrome. *Curr Opin Ophthalmol.* 2009;20(6):525–531.

Mandeville JT, Levinson RD, Holland GN. The tubulointerstitial nephritis and uveitis syndrome. *Surv Ophthalmol.* 2001;46(3):195–208.

Glaucomatocyclitic crisis

Glaucomatocyclitic crisis, also known as *Posner-Schlossman syndrome (PSS),* usually manifests as a recurrent unilateral, mild, acute nongranulomatous anterior uveitis. Symptoms are vague: discomfort, blurred vision, and halos. Signs include markedly elevated IOP, corneal edema, KPs, low-grade cell and flare, and a slightly dilated pupil. Episodes last from several hours to several days, and recurrences are common over many years. Historically treatment has been topical corticosteroids and antiglaucoma medications, including, if necessary, systemic carbonic anhydrase inhibitors. Recent studies suggest cytomegalovirus (CMV) as a possible cause of PSS, with distinct genotypes of CMV being associated with PSS and anterior uveitis as opposed to retinitis. Corneal endotheliitis, linear KPs, and male preponderance are more common among CMV-associated PSS. An anterior chamber tap can be done to confirm the diagnosis of CMV by polymerase chain reaction testing. There may be a possible role for antiviral therapy in such cases.

Chee SP, Jap A. Presumed Fuchs heterochromic iridocyclitis and Posner-Schlossman syndrome: comparison of cytomegalovirus-positive and negative eyes. *Am J Ophthalmol.* 2008;146(6):883–889.

Oka N, Suzuki T, Inoue T, Kobayashi T, Ohashi Y. Polymorphisms in cytomegalovirus genotype in immunocompetent patients with corneal endotheliitis or iridocyclitis. *J Med Virol.* 2015;87(8):1441–1445.

Lens-associated uveitis

An immune reaction to lens material may result in ocular inflammatory disease. This reaction may follow disruption of the lens capsule (traumatic or surgical), termed *phacoantigenic uveitis,* or leakage of lens protein through the intact lens capsule in mature or hypermature cataracts, termed *phacolytic uveitis* (Figs 8-8, 8-9). The exact mechanism of lens-induced uveitis, although unknown, is thought to represent an immune reaction to lens proteins. Experimental animal studies suggest that altered tolerance to lens protein leads to the inflammation, which usually has an abrupt onset but occasionally occurs insidiously. Patients previously sensitized to lens protein (eg, after cataract extraction in the fellow eye) can experience inflammation within 24 hours after capsular rupture.

Phacoantigenic uveitis Phacoantigenic uveitis was previously termed *phacoanaphylactic uveitis.* This nomenclature is incorrect because anaphylaxis involves immunoglobulin

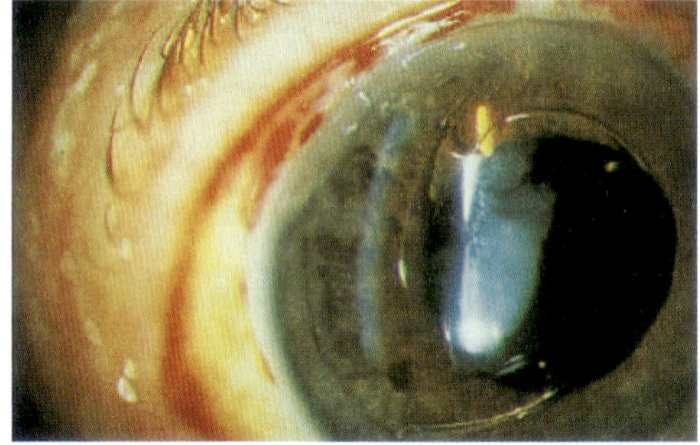

Figure 8-8 Low-grade postoperative uveitis in this patient could be secondary to retained lens cortex or to the anterior chamber intraocular lens. *(Courtesy of John D. Sheppard Jr, MD.)*

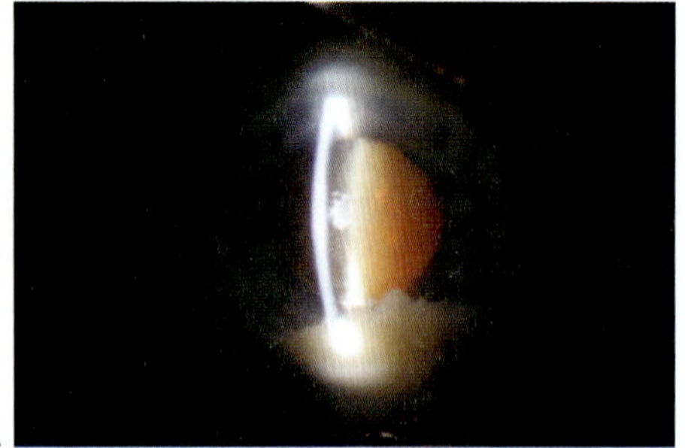

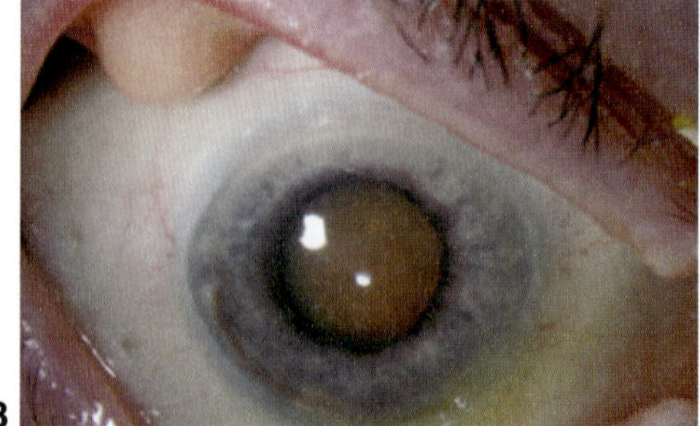

Figure 8-9 Phacolytic uveitis. **A,** Phacolytic uveitis with glaucoma, corneal edema, granulomatous anterior uveitis, and pseudohypopyon in a patient with hypermature cataract. **B,** Resolution of anterior chamber inflammation with intense topical corticosteroid use; treatment eventually necessitated cataract surgery. *(Courtesy of H. Nida Sen, MD/National Eye Institute.)*

E (IgE), mast cells, and basophils, none of which are present in the more appropriately termed phacoantigenic uveitis. Clinically, patients exhibit an anterior uveitis that may be granulomatous or nongranulomatous. Small or large KPs are usually present. Anterior chamber reaction varies from mild (eg, postoperative inflammation involving a small amount of retained cortex) to severe (eg, traumatic lens capsule disruption); hypopyon may be present. Posterior synechiae are common, and IOP is often elevated. Inflammation in the anterior vitreous cavity is common, but fundus lesions do not occur.

Histologically, a zonal granulomatous inflammation is centered at the site of lens injury. Neutrophils are present around the lens material with surrounding lymphocytes, plasma cells, epithelioid cells, and occasional giant cells.

Treatment consists of topical and, in severe cases, systemic corticosteroids, as well as cycloplegic and mydriatic agents. Surgical removal of all lens material is usually curative. When small amounts of lens material remain, corticosteroid therapy alone may be sufficient to allow resorption of the inciting material. It is important to differentiate some of these entities from postoperative endophthalmitis.

Phacolytic uveitis Phacolytic uveitis (or *phacolytic glaucoma,* as it is frequently referred to) involves an acute increase in IOP caused by clogging of the trabecular meshwork by macrophages engorged with lens proteins leaking through the intact capsule of a hypermature cataract. The diagnosis is suggested by the presence of elevated IOP, refractile bodies in the aqueous (representing lipid-laden macrophages), and a lack of KPs and synechiae. Therapy includes pressure reduction, often through use of osmotic agents and topical medications, followed quickly by cataract extraction. An aqueous tap may reveal swollen macrophages.

Kalogeropoulos CD, Malamou-Mitsi VD, Asproudis I, Psilas K. The contribution of aqueous humor cytology in the differential diagnosis of anterior uvea inflammations. *Ocul Immunol Inflamm.* 2004;12(3):215–225.

Postoperative inflammation: infectious endophthalmitis

Infectious endophthalmitis must be included in the differential diagnosis of postoperative inflammation and hypopyon. Infection with low-virulence organisms such as *Propionibacterium acnes* and *Staphylococcus epidermidis* as well as fungal species can cause delayed or late-onset endophthalmitis after cataract surgery. Infectious endophthalmitis is discussed in more detail in Chapter 12.

Postoperative inflammation: intraocular lens–associated uveitis

Intraocular lens (IOL)–associated uveitis ranges from mild inflammation to the uveitis-glaucoma-hyphema (UGH) syndrome. Surgical manipulation results in breakdown of the blood–aqueous barrier, leading to vulnerability in the early postoperative period. IOL implantation can activate complement cascades and promote neutrophil chemotaxis. This leads to cellular deposits on the IOL, synechiae formation, capsular opacification, and anterior capsule phimosis. Retained lens material from extracapsular cataract extraction can exacerbate the usual transient postoperative inflammation. Rarely, iris chafing caused by the edges or loops of IOLs on either the anterior or the posterior surface of the iris can result in mechanical irritation and inflammation. The motion of

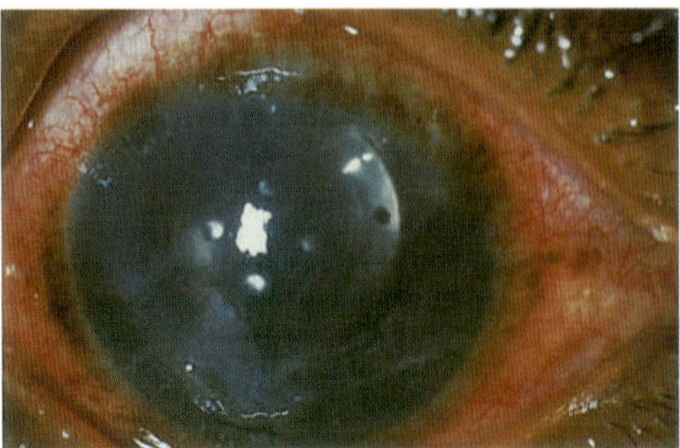

Figure 8-10 Pseudophakic bullous keratopathy and chronic anterior uveitis caused by an iris-fixated anterior chamber intraocular lens, with corneal touch, iris stromal erosion, and chronic recalcitrant uveitic macular edema. *(Courtesy of John D. Sheppard Jr, MD.)*

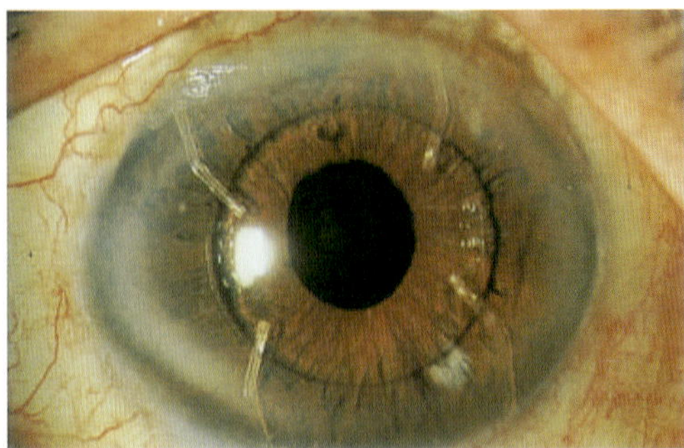

Figure 8-11 Fixed-haptic anterior chamber intraocular lens associated with peripheral and superior corneal edema, chronic low-grade anterior uveitis, peripheral anterior synechiae, globe tenderness, and intermittent microhyphema. *(Courtesy of John D. Sheppard Jr, MD.)*

an iris-supported IOL or anterior chamber IOL (ACIOL) can cause intermittent corneal touch and lead to corneal endothelial damage or decompensation, low-grade anterior uveitis, peripheral anterior synechiae, recalcitrant glaucoma, and macular edema (Figs 8-10, 8-11). These lenses should be removed and exchanged when penetrating keratoplasty is performed.

Irritation of the iris root by an intraocular implant can cause UGH syndrome. Flexible ACIOLs are less likely than older rigid ACIOLs to cause UGH syndrome. Because ACIOL use is rare, UGH syndrome is encountered most commonly with sulcus placement of a single-piece hydrophobic acrylic IOL (something that should never be intentionally done). The syndrome can occur even with the appropriate placement of a 3-piece IOL in the sulcus. Ultrasound biomicroscopy or anterior segment optical coherence tomography (OCT) can be helpful in evaluating lens position in cases of chronic pseudophakic uveitis. Many cases can be managed with topical corticosteroids only, although some may require IOL explantation or repositioning. UGH syndrome and chronic uveitis are also discussed in BCSC Section 11, *Lens and Cataract.*

In general, the more biocompatible the IOL material, the less likely it is to incite an inflammatory response. Irregular or damaged IOL surfaces as well as polypropylene haptics have been associated with enhanced bacterial and leukocyte binding and should be avoided in patients with uveitis. In general, acrylic IOLs appear to have excellent biocompatibility, with low rates of cellular deposits and capsular opacification. Persistent postoperative anterior uveitis (postsurgical uveitis) is very rare and occur more commonly in eyes experiencing intraoperative complications. Foldable implant materials have also been found to be well tolerated in many patients with uveitis.

One of the most important factors in the success of cataract surgery is aggressive control of intraocular inflammation in the perioperative period. For further discussion and illustrations, see Chapter 14 and BCSC Section 11, *Lens and Cataract.*

Ozdal PC, Mansour M, Deschênes J. Ultrasound biomicroscopy of pseudophakic eyes with chronic postoperative inflammation. *J Cataract Refract Surg.* 2003;29(6):1185–1191.

Patel C, Kim SJ, Chomsky A, Saboori M. Incidence and risk factors for chronic uveitis following cataract surgery. *Ocul Immunol Inflamm.* 2013;21(2):130–134.

Roesel M, Heinz C, Heimes B, Koch JM, Heiligenhaus A. Uveal and capsular biocompatibility of two foldable acrylic intraocular lenses in patients with endogenous uveitis—a prospective randomized study. *Graefes Arch Clin Exp Ophthalmol.* 2008;246(11):1609–1615.

Taravati P, Lam DL, Leveque T, Van Gelder RN. Postcataract surgical inflammation. *Curr Opin Ophthalmol.* 2012;23(1):12–18.

Drug-induced uveitis

Some drugs are associated with the development of intraocular inflammation. These include rifabutin (an antibiotic used in the treatment of *Mycobacterium avium-intracellulare* infection), systemic fluoroquinolones (especially moxifloxacin, which may induce iris depigmentation and uveitis), bisphosphonates, sulfonamides, diethylcarbamazine (an antifilarial drug), and oral contraceptives. Paradoxically, certain TNF inhibitors (eg, etanercept, adalimumab) have also been associated with new-onset uveitis, psoriasis-like rash (Fig 8-12), and

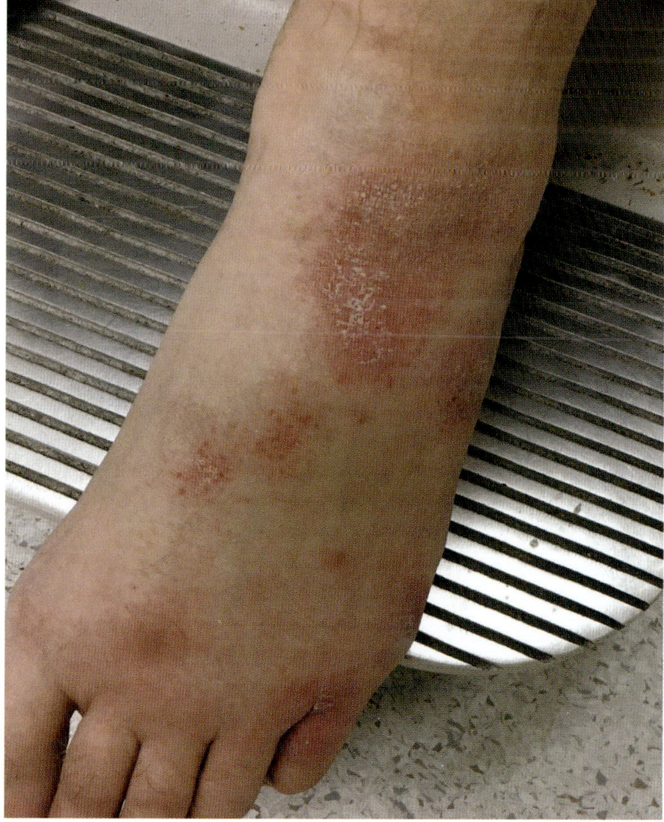

Figure 8-12 Adalimumab-induced, psoriasis-like rash on dorsal surface of left foot of a young patient with chronic pars planitis. The rash resolved upon discontinuation of the drug.

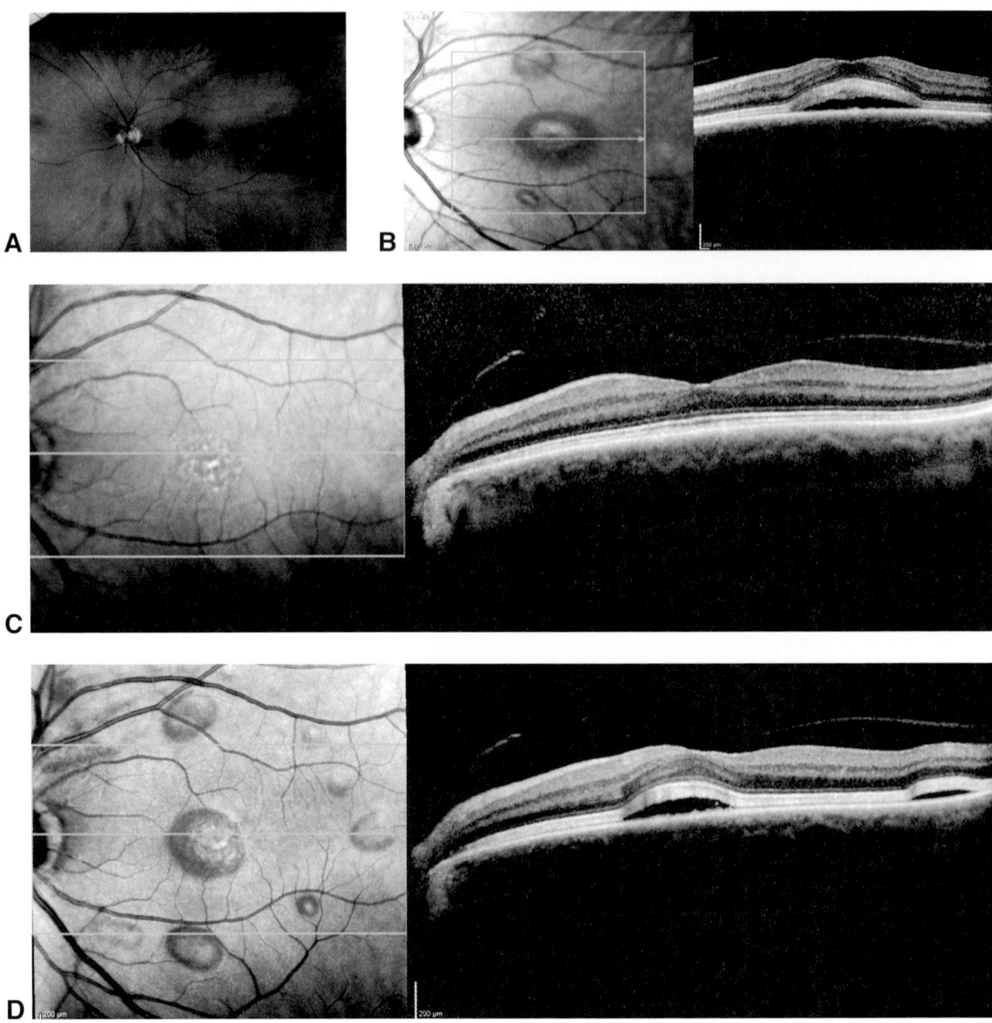

Figure 8-13 Immune checkpoint inhibitor (nivolumab)–induced Vogt-Koyanagi-Harada–like syndrome in a patient with metastatic melanoma. **A, B,** Subretinal fluid noted on optical coherence tomography, despite relatively unremarkable fundus findings. **C,** Fluid resolved with periocular corticosteroids with residual retinal pigment epithelium changes noted on infrared *(left)*. **D,** There was recurrence when the next cycle of anticancer treatment was started. *(Courtesy of Bryn M. Burkholder, MD, and H. Nida Sen, MD.)*

a systemic sarcoid-like syndrome. Vaccines such as BCG vaccine and influenza vaccines, as well as the purified protein derivative used in the tuberculin skin test, have also been implicated in the development of uveitis. Intravesical BCG vaccine (sometimes used in the treatment of bladder cancer) can result in uveitis that may be immune-mediated or infectious. More recently, a spectrum of intraocular inflammation—ranging from mild anterior uveitis to retinal vasculitis, choroiditis, and Vogt-Koyanagi-Harada (VKH) syndrome–like panuveitis—has been associated with cancer immunotherapy, particularly with immune checkpoint inhibitors (Fig 8-13).

Numerous topical antiglaucoma medications have been associated with uveitis. These include metipranolol (a nonselective beta-blocking drug used in the treatment of glaucoma), acetylcholinesterase inhibitors, prostaglandin $F_{2\alpha}$ analogues, and brimonidine (α_2-adrenergic agonist). While prostaglandin analogues have been suggested to induce or worsen macular edema, evidence is anecdotal, and these glaucoma drops are generally used in uveitis patients when other topicals are not sufficient to lower IOP. Drugs that are injected directly into the eye have also been associated with uveitis. These medications include antibiotics, urokinase (a plasminogen activator), cidofovir (a cytosine analogue effective against CMV) and vascular endothelial growth factor (VEGF) inhibitors. Treatment generally involves topical corticosteroids and cycloplegic drugs, if necessary. Recalcitrant cases may require cessation or tapering of the offending medication.

Conrady CD, Larochelle M, Pecen P, Palestine A, Shakoor A, Singh A. Checkpoint inhibitor-induced uveitis: a case series. *Graefes Arch Clin Exp Ophthalmol.* 2018;256(1):187–191.

Cunningham ET Jr, Pasadhika S, Suhler EB, Zierhut M. Drug-induced inflammation in patients on TNF-α inhibitors. *Ocul Immunol Inflamm.* 2012;20(1):2–5.

Horsley MB, Chen TC. The use of prostaglandin analogs in the uveitic patient. *Semin Ophthalmol.* 2011;26(4–5):285–289.

Moorthy RS, London NJ, Garg SJ, Cunningham ET Jr. Drug-induced uveitis. *Curr Opin Ophthalmol.* 2013;24(6):589–597.

Chronic Anterior Uveitis

Inflammation of the anterior segment that is persistent and relapses less than 3 months after discontinuation of therapy is termed *chronic anterior uveitis;* it may persist for years. This type of inflammation usually starts insidiously, with variable amounts of redness, discomfort, and photophobia. Some patients have no symptoms. The disease can be unilateral or bilateral, and the amount of inflammatory activity is variable. Uveitic macular edema, cataract progression, and secondary glaucoma are common.

Juvenile idiopathic arthritis

Juvenile idiopathic arthritis (JIA; formerly referred to as *juvenile chronic arthritis* and *juvenile rheumatoid arthritis*), is the most common systemic disorder associated with anterior uveitis in the pediatric age group. It is characterized by arthritis beginning before age 16 years and lasting for at least 6 weeks.

Ocular involvement JIA can be classified into 5 types according to medical history and other presenting factors according to International League of Associations of Rheumatology (ILAR) guidelines:

- *Systemic onset (Still disease).* This type, usually observed in children under age 5 years, accounts for approximately 10%–15% of all cases of JIA. It is characterized by fever, rash, lymphadenopathy, and hepatosplenomegaly. Joint involvement may be minimal or absent initially. Ocular involvement is rare.
- *Polyarticular onset.* Patients with this type show involvement of more than 4 joints in the first 6 months of the disease; it represents 40% of JIA cases overall but only

about 10% of cases of JIA-associated anterior uveitis. Patients who are positive for rheumatoid factor may not develop uveitis.
- *Oligoarticular onset.* This type, previously also known as *pauciarticular onset,* constitutes 40%–50% of all cases of JIA and includes 80%–90% of patients with JIA-associated uveitis. Four or fewer joints may be involved during the first 6 months of disease, and patients may have no joint symptoms. Girls under age 5 years and positive for antinuclear antibody (ANA) are at increased risk of developing chronic anterior uveitis; 25%–35% of these patients will develop uveitis, most in the first 4 years.

Other subgroups of JIA include enthesitis-related arthritis (ERA) and psoriatic arthritis (or psoriatic JIA). ERA accounts for 10%–20% of cases of JIA. Enthesitis, axial disease, and HLA-B27 positivity are common. The uveitis in these patients is more likely to be acute and recurrent, with pain, redness, and photophobia.

The average age of onset of uveitis in patients with JIA is 6 years. Uveitis generally develops within 5–7 years of the onset of joint disease but may occur as long as 28 years after the development of arthritis. There is usually little or no correlation between severity or timing of ocular and joint inflammation. Risk factors for the development of chronic uveitis in patients with JIA include female sex, oligoarticular onset, and the presence of circulating ANA. Most patients test negative for rheumatoid factor. HLA-DRB1*11 and *13 may be associated with increased risk of uveitis among JIA patients.

The eye is frequently white. Symptoms may include mild to moderate pain, photophobia, and blurring, although some patients are asymptomatic. Often, the eye disease is found incidentally during a routine screening or physical examination. The signs of inflammation include fine KPs, band keratopathy, flare and cells, posterior synechiae, and cataract (Fig 8-14). Patients in whom JIA is suspected should undergo ANA testing and be evaluated by a pediatric rheumatologist because the joint disease may be minimal or absent at the time the uveitis is diagnosed. The differential diagnosis includes TINU, Fuchs uveitis syndrome, sarcoidosis, Blau disease, Behçet disease, the seronegative spondyloarthropathies, herpetic uveitis, and Lyme disease.

Prognosis Because of the frequently asymptomatic nature of the uveitis, profound silent ocular damage can occur, and long-term prognosis often depends on the extent of structural complications at the time of first diagnosis. Complications are frequent and often severe; they include band keratopathy, cataract, glaucoma, macular edema, chronic hypotony, and phthisis. Children with JIA, especially those who are ANA positive or have oligoarticular disease, should undergo regular slit-lamp examinations. Table 8-1 outlines the recommended schedule for screening patients with JIA for development of uveitis, as developed by the American Academy of Pediatrics.

Treatment The American College of Rheumatology and the Arthritis Foundation expert panels developed evidence-based recommendations for the screening, monitoring, and treatment of JIA-associated anterior uveitis. Patients with inactive uveitis (or <1 AC cells) should be monitored every 3 months, unless tapering or discontinuing treatment. Patients should be seen at least 1 month after each change in topical medication, and within 2 months of changing systemic treatment. Initial treatment consists of topical corticosteroids. More

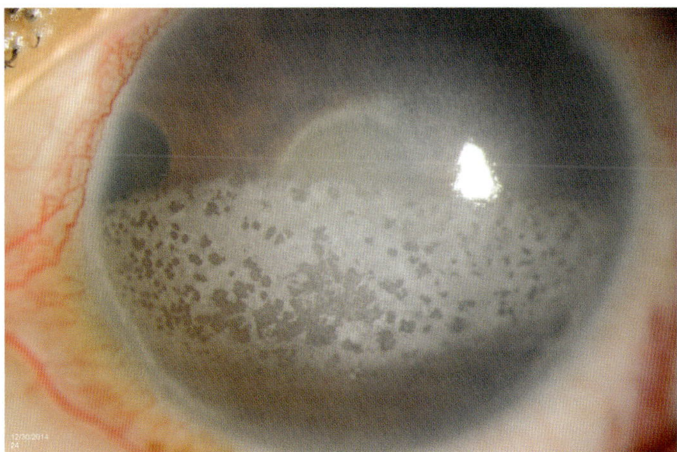

Figure 8-14 JIA with complicated chronic calcific band keratopathy, cataract, and glaucoma in a patient with peripheral iridectomy superonasally. *(Courtesy of H. Nida Sen, MD/National Eye Institute.)*

Table 8-1 Frequency of Ophthalmologic Examination in Patients With JIA

Type	ANA	Age at Onset, y	Duration of Disease, y	Risk Category	Eye Examination Frequency, mo
Oligoarthritis or polyarthritis	+	≤6	≤4	High	3
	+	≤6	>4	Moderate	6
	+	≤6	>7	Low	12
	+	>6	≤4	Moderate	6
	+	>6	>4	Low	12
	–	≤6	≤4	Moderate	6
	–	≤6	>4	Low	12
	–	>6	NA	Low	12
Systemic disease (fever, rash)	NA	NA	NA	Low	12

ANA = antinuclear antibodies; JIA = juvenile idiopathic arthritis; NA = not applicable.
Recommendations for follow-up continue through childhood and adolescence.

Reprinted with permission from Cassidy J, Kivlin J, Lindsley C, Nocton J; Section on Rheumatology; Section on Ophthalmology. Ophthalmologic examinations in children with juvenile rheumatoid arthritis. *Pediatrics.* 2006;117(5):1844.

severe cases may require use of systemic corticosteroids or IMT. The goal is to eliminate active inflammation (anterior chamber cells) and prevent new complications. Short-acting mydriatic drugs may be useful in patients with chronic flare to keep the pupil mobile and to prevent posterior synechiae formation. Use of systemic NSAIDs may permit a lower dose of corticosteroids.

Because of the chronic nature of the inflammation, corticosteroid-induced complications are common. Long-term use of systemic corticosteroids in children may lead to growth retardation from premature closure of the epiphyses. Also, prolonged use of topical corticosteroids leads to cataracts and glaucoma. Because long-term use of topical corticosteroids at doses ≥3 times daily can increase the risk of cataract formation, systemic IMT should be considered for such cases. Topical corticosteroids should be tapered as soon as inflammation is controlled on systemic therapy. There is also evidence that even low-grade inflammation, if present for a prolonged period, can result in unacceptable ocular morbidity and loss of vision. For these reasons, many children are treated with methotrexate. Numerous studies have shown that this treatment regimen can effectively control the uveitis, is generally well tolerated, and can spare patients the complications of long-term corticosteroid use. In addition, several studies have demonstrated a benefit from TNF inhibitors and other biologic agents.

Treatment of cataracts in patients with JIA remains a challenge, and the use of IOLs remains controversial. Children who are left aphakic may develop amblyopia. Cataract surgery in patients with JIA-associated anterior uveitis has a high complication rate due to the difficulty in controlling the more aggressive inflammatory response present in these children. Lensectomy and vitrectomy via the pars plana have been advocated.

There have been reports, however, of more successful cataract surgery with IOL implants in patients with JIA. These reports highlight the importance of well-controlled uveitis through systemic IMT and the use of perioperative corticosteroids.

The following considerations are useful when selecting patients with JIA for cataract surgery with IOL implants:

- Patients' intraocular inflammation must be well controlled with systemic IMT for at least 3 months before surgery and must not require frequent instillation of topical corticosteroids.
- Only acrylic lenses should be implanted.
- Patients must be monitored frequently after cataract surgery to watch for any inflammation, and inflammation that occurs must be aggressively treated.
- IMT must be used preoperatively and postoperatively, not just perioperatively.
- Because long-term results are not available, patients must be strongly advised about the need for careful, regular, lifelong follow-up to detect late complications that may lead to loss of the eye.
- The ophthalmologist must have a low threshold for IOL explantation in patients who have persistent postoperative inflammation and recurrent cyclitic membranes.

Patients with band keratopathy should be treated (eg, using chelation with sodium ethylenediaminetetraacetic acid [EDTA]) and allowed to heal well before cataract surgery is attempted. See also Chapter 14 and BCSC Section 6, *Pediatric Ophthalmology and Strabismus,* Chapter 24.

Glaucoma should be treated with medical therapy initially, although surgical intervention is often necessary in severe cases. Standard filtering procedures are usually unsuccessful, and the use of antifibrotic drugs or aqueous drainage devices is usually required for successful control of the glaucoma.

Angeles-Han S, Yeh S. Prevention and management of cataracts in children with juvenile idiopathic arthritis–associated uveitis. *Curr Rheumatol Rep.* 2012;14(2):142–149.

Clarke SL, Sen ES, Ramanan AV. Juvenile idiopathic arthritis-associated uveitis. *Pediatr Rheumatol Online J.* 2016;14(1):27.

Grajewski RS, Zurek-Imhoff B, Roesel M, Heinz C, Heiligenhaus A. Favourable outcome after cataract surgery with IOL implantation in uveitis associated with juvenile idiopathic arthritis. *Acta Ophthalmol.* 2012;90(7):657–662.

Gregory AC 2nd, Kempen JH, Daniel E, Kaçmaz RO, et al; Systemic Immunosuppressive Therapy for Eye Diseases Cohort Study Research Group. Risk factors for loss of visual acuity among patients with uveitis associated with juvenile idiopathic arthritis: the Systemic Immunosuppressive Therapy for Eye Diseases Study. *Ophthalmology.* 2013;120(1):186–192.

Mehta PJ, Alexander JL, Sen HN. Pediatric uveitis: new and future treatments. *Curr Opin Ophthalmol.* 2013;24(5):453–462.

Simonini G, Taddio A, Cattalini M, et al. Superior efficacy of adalimumab in treating childhood refractory chronic uveitis when used as first biologic modifier drug: adalimumab as starting anti-TNF-α therapy in childhood chronic uveitis. *Pediatr Rheumatol Online J.* 2013;11(1):16.

Thorne JE, Woreta FA, Dunn JP, Jabs DA. Risk of cataract development among children with juvenile idiopathic arthritis–related uveitis treated with topical corticosteroids. *Ophthalmology.* 2010;117(7):1436–1441.

Zannin ME, Birolo C, Gerloni VM, et al. Safety and efficacy of infliximab and adalimumab for refractory uveitis in juvenile idiopathic arthritis: 1-year followup data from the Italian Registry. *J Rheumatol.* 2013;40(1):74–79.

Fuchs uveitis syndrome

Fuchs uveitis syndrome (sometimes called *Fuchs heterochromic iridocyclitis* or *Fuchs heterochromic uveitis)* constitutes 2%–3% of patients referred to uveitis clinics. This condition is usually unilateral, and symptoms vary from none to mild blurring and discomfort. Signs include

- diffuse iris stromal atrophy with variable pigment epithelial layer atrophy (Fig 8-15)
- small, white, stellate KPs scattered diffusely over the entire endothelium (Fig 8-16)
- iris nodules
- cells in the anterior chamber as well as in the anterior vitreous
- late staining of the optic nerve on fluorescein angiography
- glaucoma and cataracts, which occur frequently

In addition, synechiae, chorioretinal scars, and retinal periphlebitis are rare or absent and macular edema is seldom present.

The diagnosis is made according to the distribution of KPs, presence of heterochromia, lack of synechiae, and lack of symptoms. Heterochromia may be subtle in a brown-eyed patient, and the clinician must look carefully for signs of iris stromal atrophy. Often, the inflammation is discovered during a routine examination, such as when a unilateral cataract develops. Usually, but not invariably, a lighter-colored iris indicates the involved eye. In blue-eyed persons, however, the affected eye may become darker as the stromal atrophy progresses and the darker iris pigment epithelium shows through.

Fuchs uveitis syndrome is now known to be associated with viral infections such as rubella and CMV. Association with ocular toxoplasmosis has also been reported.

Patients generally do well with cataract surgery, and IOLs can usually be implanted successfully. However, some patients experience substantial visual disability because of extensive vitreous opacification. Pars plana vitrectomy should be carefully considered in such instances. Glaucoma control can be difficult. Abnormal vessels bridging the angle

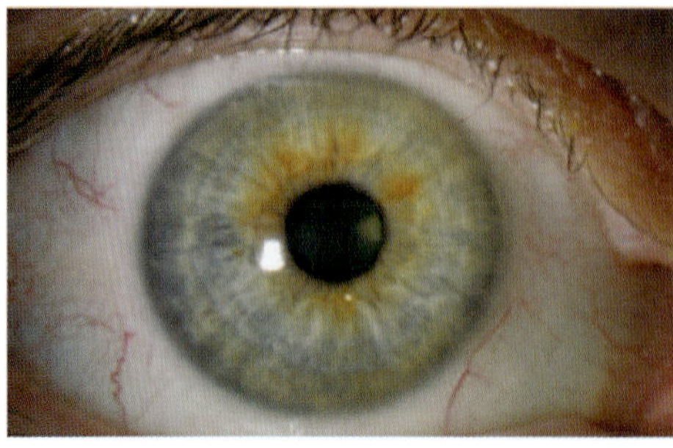

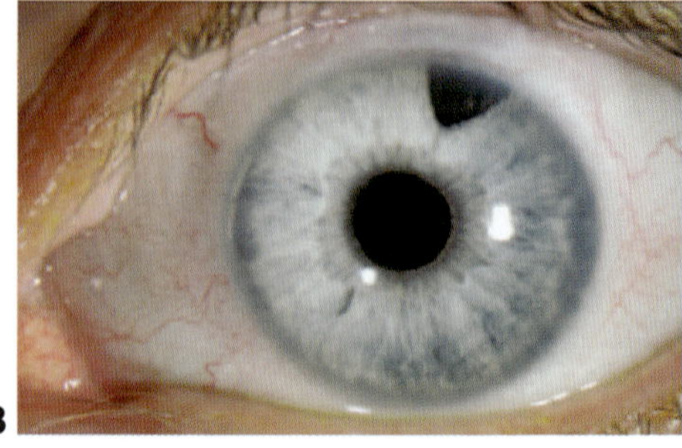

Figure 8-15 Heterochromia in Fuchs uveitis syndrome. **A,** Right (unaffected) eye. **B,** Left (affected) eye in the same patient. Note the lighter iris color and stromal atrophy ("moth-eaten appearance") in the affected eye, which underwent surgical iridectomy at the same time as cataract surgery. *(Courtesy of H. Nida Sen, MD/National Eye Institute.)*

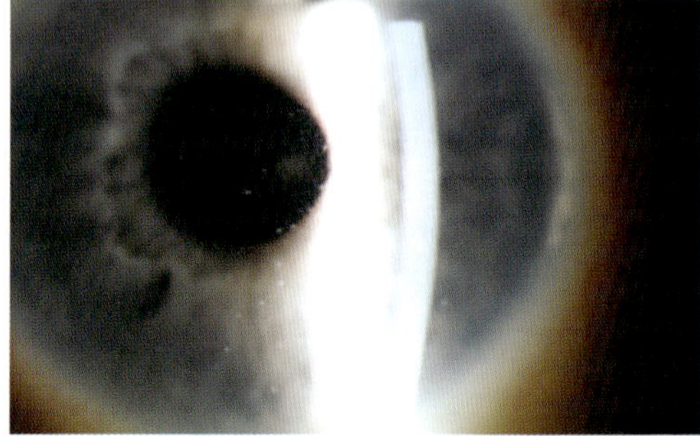

Figure 8-16 Diffusely distributed stellate keratic precipitates in a patient with Fuchs uveitis syndrome. *(Courtesy of H. Nida Sen, MD/National Eye Institute.)*

can be seen on gonioscopy. These vessels may bleed during surgery, resulting in postoperative hyphema.

Few cases require therapy for inflammation. The prognosis is good in most cases, even when the inflammation persists for decades. Because topical corticosteroids can lessen the inflammation but typically do not resolve it, aggressive treatment to eradicate the cellular reaction is not indicated. Cycloplegia is seldom necessary. See BCSC Section 10, *Glaucoma,* for further discussion of Fuchs heterochromic uveitis (Fuchs uveitis syndrome).

Accorinti M, Spinucci G, Pirraglia MP, Bruschi S, Pesci FR, Iannetti L. Fuchs' heterochromic iridocyclitis in an Italian tertiary referral centre: epidemiology, clinical features, and prognosis. *J Ophthalmol.* 2016;2016:1458624.

Birnbaum AD, Tessler HH, Schultz KL, et al. Epidemiologic relationship between Fuchs heterochromic iridocyclitis and the United States rubella vaccination program. *Am J Ophthalmol.* 2007;144(3):424–428.

de Groot-Mijnes JD, de Visser L, Rothova A, Schuller M, van Loon AM, Weersink AJ. Rubella virus is associated with Fuchs heterochromic iridocyclitis. *Am J Ophthalmol.* 2006;141(1):212–214.

Undifferentiated anterior uveitis

Inability to positively identify a diagnosis, as is the case in many patients with chronic anterior uveitis, does not preclude treatment with topical steroids and/or cycloplegics, other steroids, or systemic steroid-sparing agents, assuming infectious causes have been ruled out. In some cases initially labeled idiopathic, repeat diagnostic testing at a later date as the clinical picture evolves may reveal an underlying systemic condition.

Intermediate Uveitis

The Standardization of Uveitis Nomenclature (SUN) Working Group defines *intermediate uveitis* as the subset in which the predominant site of inflammation is in the vitreous; this subset accounts for up to 15% of all cases of uveitis. Intermediate uveitis is characterized by ocular inflammation concentrated in the vitreous and the vitreous base overlying the ciliary body and peripheral retina–pars plana complex. Inflammatory cells may aggregate in the vitreous ("snowballs"), where some coalesce. In some patients, inflammatory exudative accumulation on the inferior pars plana ("snowbanking") seems to correlate with a more severe disease process. There may be associated peripheral retinal phlebitis. Anterior chamber reaction of varying severity may also occur.

Intermediate uveitis can be associated with various conditions, including sarcoidosis, multiple sclerosis (MS), Lyme disease, peripheral toxocariasis, syphilis, tuberculosis, primary Sjögren syndrome, and infection with human T-cell lymphotropic virus type 1 (HTLV-1).

Pars Planitis

The term *pars planitis* refers to the subset of intermediate uveitis that is idiopathic with no associated infection or systemic disease. It is the most common form of intermediate uveitis, constituting approximately 85%–90% of cases. Previously also known as *chronic cyclitis* and *peripheral uveitis,* the condition most commonly affects persons aged 5–40 years. It has a bimodal distribution, concentrating in younger (5–15 years) and older (20–40 years) groups. No overall sex predilection is apparent. The pathogenesis of pars planitis is not well understood.

Clinical characteristics

Approximately 80% of cases of pars planitis are bilateral, which can often be asymmetric in severity. In children, the initial presentation may consist of significant anterior chamber inflammation accompanied by redness, photophobia, and discomfort. The onset in teenagers and young adults may be more insidious, with the presenting complaint generally being floaters. Ocular manifestations include anterior chamber inflammatory cells, vitreous cells, snowballs (Fig 8-17), and pars plana exudates. Inferior peripheral retinal phlebitis with retinal venous sheathing is common. With long-standing inflammation, macular edema often develops; this condition becomes chronic and refractory in approximately 10% of patients and is the major cause of vision loss. Ischemia from retinal phlebitis, combined with angiogenic stimuli from intraocular inflammation, can lead to neovascularization along the inferior snowbank in up to 10% of cases. These neovascular complexes can result in vitreous hemorrhages, more common in children than adults; they also may contract, leading to peripheral tractional and rhegmatogenous retinal detachments. In rare cases, the complexes evolve into secondary peripheral retinal vasoproliferative tumors—vascular masses

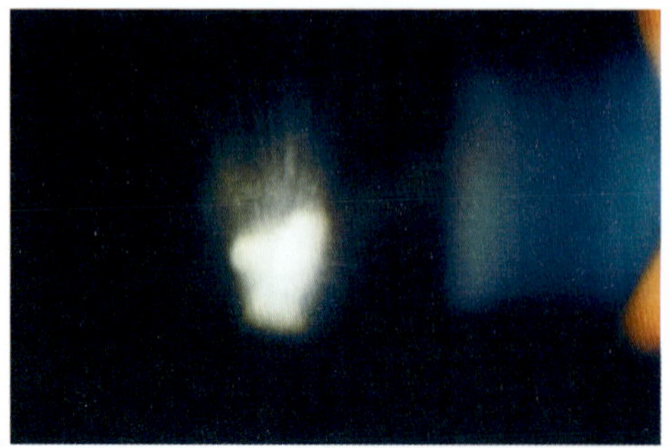

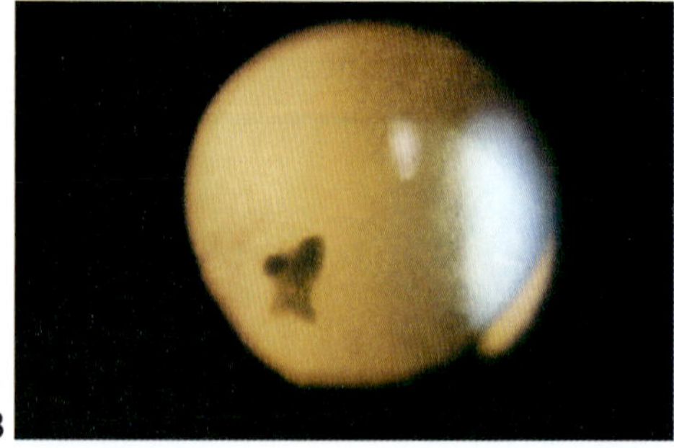

Figure 8-17 Pars planitis. **A,** Vitreous "snowball" opacity in the anterior, inferior retrolental vitreous. **B,** Same vitreous snowball opacity shown in retroillumination, revealing its location with respect to the lens as well as evidence of vitreous cellularity. *(Courtesy of Ramana S. Moorthy, MD/National Eye Institute.)*

with exudative retinopathy and minimally dilated vessels—years after the initial diagnosis. Rhegmatogenous retinal detachments are rare but localized peripheral detachments (serous or tractional) that can occur in 4%–10% of patients with pars planitis. With chronicity, posterior synechiae and band keratopathy may also develop. Other possible causes of loss of vision include cataracts, epiretinal membrane, and vitreous opacification.

Differential diagnosis

The differential diagnosis of intermediate uveitis includes syphilis, tuberculosis, Lyme uveitis, sarcoidosis, intermediate uveitis associated with MS, and toxocariasis. Syphilis should be checked in all uveitis patients, including those with intermediate uveitis. Measurement of Lyme antibody titers may be useful in regions where the disease is endemic, especially in patients with a history of tick bite or cutaneous and articular disease. Anterior and intermediate uveitis may occur in up to 20% of patients with MS. Sarcoidosis-associated uveitis presents as an intermediate disease in 7% of cases. A peripheral granuloma such as that seen in toxocariasis can mimic the unilateral pars plana snowbank in a child and should be ruled out. Serologic testing can be helpful in these cases.

Vitritis without other ocular findings can be suggestive of primary central nervous system (CNS) lymphoma. These patients are generally much older at presentation than patients with pars planitis, usually in their fifth or sixth decade of life or older.

Ancillary tests and histologic findings

The diagnosis of intermediate uveitis is made according to classic clinical findings. Laboratory workup to evaluate for other causes of intermediate uveitis, including sarcoidosis, Lyme disease in high-risk cases, and syphilis, is important. Measurement of serum angiotensin-converting enzyme (ACE) and Lyme antibody titers, chest imaging, and syphilis testing should be considered. Fluorescein angiography (FA) may show diffuse peripheral venous leakage, disc leakage, and macular edema. Ultrasound biomicroscopy may be used in the case of a small pupil or dense cataract to demonstrate peripheral exudates or membranes over the pars plana.

Histologic examination of eyes with pars planitis shows vitreous condensation and cellular infiltration in the vitreous base. The inflammatory cells consist mostly of macrophages,

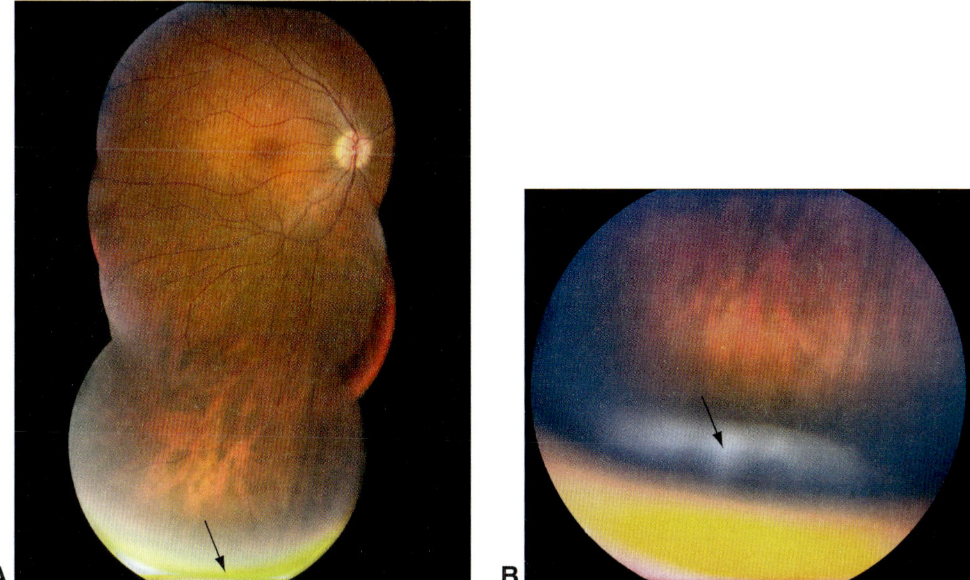

Figure 8-18 Fundus examination of a patient with undifferentiated intermediate uveitis (pars planitis). **A, B,** Note pars plana membrane inferiorly *(arrows)*. *(Courtesy of H. Nida Sen, MD/National Eye Institute.)*

lymphocytes, and a few plasma cells. Pars planitis is also characterized by peripheral lymphocytic cuffing of venules and a loose fibrovascular membrane over the pars plana (Fig 8-18).

Prognosis

The clinical course of pars planitis may be divided into 3 types. Approximately 10% of cases have a self-limiting, benign course; 30% have a smoldering course with remissions and exacerbations; and 60% have a prolonged course without exacerbations. Pars planitis can remain active for many years. In some cases, the disease "burns out" after a few years. If macular edema is treated until resolution and kept from returning by adequate control of inflammation, the long-term visual prognosis can be good, with nearly 75% of patients maintaining visual acuity of 20/40 or better after 10 years.

Treatment

Therapy should be directed toward treating the underlying cause of the inflammation, and infectious etiologies should be ruled out prior to initiating therapy. If an underlying condition is not identified, as in pars planitis, or if therapy of an associated condition consists of nonspecific control of inflammation, as in sarcoidosis, anti-inflammatory therapy should be implemented.

Corticosteroids, oral or periocular, usually constitute the first line of therapy. Periocular depot corticosteroid injections of triamcinolone or methylprednisolone may be given via the posterior sub-Tenon (see Chapter 6) or orbital floor route. These can be repeated as frequently as every 3–4 weeks. In most cases, the inflammation responds and the macular edema improves; however, some cases prove recalcitrant and macular edema may recur. Patients, especially those with a history of glaucoma, must be carefully monitored for corticosteroid-induced IOP elevation. Other complications of periocular corticosteroids include aponeurotic ptosis, fat prolapse, enophthalmos, and, in rare instances, globe perforation. Cataract formation can occur with any form of corticosteroid therapy.

Intravitreal corticosteroid injections may be an alternative to periocular injections in refractory cases. These injections carry risks of sustained IOP elevation and glaucoma and very small risks of retinal detachment, vitreous hemorrhage, and endophthalmitis. Injections should be administered away from areas of snowbanking and areas with peripheral retinal pathology.

Other forms of local steroid injections, such as dexamethasone intravitreal implants, can also be considered. Local treatment with corticosteroid injections is a particularly appealing approach in unilateral cases.

Systemic corticosteroid therapy may also be used, especially in severe or bilateral cases. Patients may be treated with an initial dosage of 1 mg/kg/day, with gradual tapering every 1–2 weeks to dosages of less than 10 mg/day after 8 weeks of treatment.

As with all autoimmune uveitis, if corticosteroid therapy fails or long-term use of high doses of corticosteroids is needed to control the inflammation, immunomodulatory treatment is indicated. Systemic immunomodulatory drugs such as antimetabolites, T-cell inhibitors, biologic agents, and alkylating drugs can be considered. Several reports from the Systemic Immunosuppressive Therapy for Eye Diseases (SITE) cohort study indicated that cyclosporine, azathioprine, and mycophenolate mofetil were effective in achieving sustained control of inflammation in 70%–80% of patients with intermediate uveitis. The TNF inhibitor adalimumab is approved by the United States Food and Drug Administration for the treatment of uveitis, including intermediate uveitis. Because TNF inhibitors can exacerbate MS, it is important to consider an extensive workup for MS, including magnetic resonance imaging of the brain, before initiating this therapy. See Chapter 6 for more detailed information on IMT in uveitis.

Alternative therapies for pars planitis include peripheral ablation of the pars plana snowbank with cryotherapy and/or indirect laser photocoagulation to the peripheral retina. Cryotherapy is rarely used because of concerns about further inducing inflammation. Laser photocoagulation can be used in cases of retinal ischemia and neovascularization to prevent vitreous hemorrhage; it does not seem to increase the risk of rhegmatogenous retinal detachment. Intravitreal anti-VEGF treatment can also be used for retinal or choroidal neovascularization in pars planitis in otherwise quiet eyes.

Pars plana vitrectomy, with or without laser photocoagulation, can also be helpful in treating complications of pars planitis or in cases recalcitrant to IMT. In such cases, a perioperative increase in systemic immunosuppression and/or corticosteroids should be considered. Pars plana vitrectomy may be necessary to treat severe vision loss caused by vitreous hemorrhage or traction, retinal detachment, or epiretinal membrane. It can also be considered for cases with significant vitreous opacities despite adequate IMT. In cases involving epiretinal membrane or vitreomacular traction, separation of the posterior hyaloid membrane during vitrectomy may have a beneficial effect in reducing macular edema. Potential complications include retinal detachment, endophthalmitis, and cataract formation.

Complications

Complications of pars planitis include cataract, glaucoma, macular edema, retinal neovascularization, vitreous hemorrhage, retinoschisis, and tractional or rhegmatogenous retinal detachment. Cataracts occur in up to 60% of cases. Cataract surgery with IOL implantation may be complicated by smoldering low-grade inflammation; recurring opacification of the posterior capsule despite capsulotomy; recurrent retrolental membranes; and chronic macular edema, even in cases in which there is no active cellular inflammation. Combining pars plana vitrectomy with cataract extraction and IOL implantation may reduce the risk of these complications. Glaucoma—both angle-closure and open-angle—occurs in approximately 10% of patients with pars planitis. Macular edema may occur in 50% of patients with intermediate uveitis and is a hallmark of pars planitis. Neovascularization of the retina, disc, and peripheral snowbank has been reported. Occasionally, vitreous hemorrhage is the presenting sign of pars planitis, especially in children; it can be treated effectively with pars plana vitrectomy. Tractional and rhegmatogenous retinal detachments can occur in up to 10% of patients and may require scleral buckling, sometimes combined with vitrectomy. Risk factors for rhegmatogenous retinal detachment include severe inflammation, use of cryotherapy at the time of a vitrectomy, and neovascularization of the pars plana snowbank.

Donaldson MJ, Pulido JS, Herman DC, Diehl N, Hodge D. Pars planitis: a 20-year study of incidence, clinical features, and outcomes. *Am J Ophthalmol.* 2007;144(6):812–817.

Lauer AK, Smith JR, Robertson JE, Rosenbaum JT. Vitreous hemorrhage is a common complication of pediatric pars planitis. *Ophthalmology.* 2002;109(1):95–98.

Leder HA, Jabs DA, Galor A, Dunn JP, Thorne JE. Periocular triamcinolone acetonide injections for cystoid macular edema complicating noninfectious uveitis. *Am J Ophthalmol.* 2011;152(3):441–448.

Mackensen F, Jakob E, Springer C, et al. Interferon versus methotrexate in intermediate uveitis with macular edema: results of a randomized controlled clinical trial. *Am J Ophthalmol.* 2013;156(3):478–486.

Pato E, Muñoz-Fernández S, Francisco F, et al; Uveitis Working Group from Spanish Society of Rheumatology. Systematic review on the effectiveness of immunosuppressants and biological therapies in the treatment of autoimmune posterior uveitis. *Semin Arthritis Rheum.* 2011;40(4):314–323.

Shin YU, Shin JY, Ma DJ, Cho H, Yu HG. Preoperative inflammatory control and surgical outcome of vitrectomy in intermediate uveitis. *J Ophthalmol.* 2017;2017:5946240.

Multiple Sclerosis

Uveitis is 10 times more common in MS patients than in the general population. The frequency of uveitis in patients with MS is reported to be as high as 30%, and the onset of uveitis may precede the diagnosis of MS in up to 25% of patients and by 5–10 years. MS usually affects White women 20–50 years of age, and intermediate uveitis is the most common manifestation of MS-associated uveitis. Up to 95% of cases are bilateral. Up to 15% of patients with pars planitis may eventually develop MS. Intermediate uveitis appears to be of milder severity in MS than in idiopathic cases. Macular edema is less common. Most patients develop mild vitritis with periphlebitis. Periphlebitis in MS is not clearly related to optic neuritis, systemic exacerbations, or disease severity.

The immunopathogenesis of MS is not well understood but appears to involve humoral, cellular, and immunogenetic components directed against myelin. HLA-DR15 appears to be associated with the combination of MS and uveitis. Immunocytologic studies have shown some cross-reactivity between myelin-associated glycoprotein and Müller cells.

Treatment of MS with interferon may have a beneficial effect on intermediate uveitis and associated macular edema. More recently, daclizumab, an interleukin-2 receptor blocking antibody, was approved for the treatment of MS and may be helpful in controlling uveitis. Fingolimod therapy for MS, on the other hand, can lead to macular edema. As biologic therapies for uveitis become more common, it is particularly important to consider the possibility of MS in any patient who presents with intermediate uveitis or pars planitis, as TNF inhibitors have been associated with exacerbations of MS.

Becker MD, Heiligenhaus A, Hudde T, et al. Interferon as a treatment for uveitis associated with multiple sclerosis. *Br J Ophthalmol.* 2005;89(10):1254–1257.

Bielekova B. Daclizumab therapy for multiple sclerosis. *Neurotherapeutics.* 2013;10(1):55–67.

Chen L, Gordon LK. Ocular manifestations of multiple sclerosis. *Curr Opin Ophthalmol.* 2005;16(5):315–320.

Zein G, Berta A, Foster CS. Multiple sclerosis–associated uveitis. *Ocul Immunol Inflamm.* 2004;12(2):137–142.

CHAPTER 9

Posterior Uveitis and Panuveitis

Highlights

- Posterior uveitis is inflammation that involves primarily the retina and/or choroid.
- Panuveitis is inflammation that involves all anatomical components of the eye—anterior chamber, vitreous, retina, and/or choroid.
- Posterior uveitis and panuveitis may be associated with systemic infection or autoimmune disease, which can be diagnosed by history and physical examination, review of systems, and focused workup.
- Initial treatment of noninfectious posterior uveitis and panuveitis typically involves systemic and/or local corticosteroids. Systemic immunomodulatory therapy may be beneficial for patients who are intolerant of corticosteroids, require high doses of corticosteroids to control their disease, or require long-term treatment.

Posterior Uveitis

Posterior uveitis is defined by the Standardization of Uveitis Nomenclature classification system as intraocular inflammation that involves primarily the retina and/or choroid. Inflammatory cells may be observed diffusely throughout the vitreous cavity, adjacent to foci of active inflammation, or on the posterior vitreous face. The presence of posterior segment structural complications—such as macular edema, peripheral retinal vasculitis, optic disc edema, and retinal or choroidal neovascularization—is not considered when determining whether a patient has posterior uveitis. For instance, the presence of macular edema as part of HLA-B27–associated anterior uveitis does not mean that the patient also has posterior uveitis. Noninfectious syndromes with primarily posterior segment involvement are included in this section; diagnoses routinely producing both anterior and posterior segment involvement are addressed in the Panuveitis section later in the chapter.

Collagen Vascular Diseases

Systemic lupus erythematosus

Systemic lupus erythematosus (SLE) is a multisystem connective tissue disorder that affects primarily women of childbearing age, with higher incidence rates among African American and Hispanic persons in the United States. The pathogenesis of SLE is incompletely understood. It is thought to be an autoimmune disorder characterized by

B-lymphocyte hyperactivity, polyclonal B-lymphocyte activation, hypergammaglobulinemia, autoantibody formation, and T-lymphocyte autoreactivity with immune complex deposition, leading to end-organ damage. Autoantibodies associated with SLE include antinuclear antibodies (ANA), antibodies to both single- and double-stranded DNA (anti-ssDNA and anti-dsDNA), antibodies to cytoplasmic components (anti-Sm, anti-Ro, and anti-La), and antiphospholipid antibodies.

D'Cruz DP, Khamashta MA, Hughes GR. Systemic lupus erythematosus. *Lancet.* 2007;369(9561):587–596.

Manifestations The systemic manifestations of SLE include acute cutaneous diseases in approximately 70%–80% of patients (malar rash, discoid lupus, photosensitivity, and mucosal lesions), arthritis in 80%–85%, renal disease in 50%–75%, Raynaud phenomenon in 30%–50%, and neurologic involvement in 35%. Cardiac, pulmonary, hepatic, and hematologic abnormalities can also occur. The diagnosis is clinical and based on criteria established by the American College of Rheumatology.

Ocular manifestations occur in 50% of patients with SLE and include cutaneous lesions on the eyelids (discoid lupus erythematosus), secondary Sjögren syndrome, scleritis, cranial nerve palsies, optic neuropathy, retinal and choroidal vasculopathy, and, in rare cases, uveitis.

Lupus retinopathy, the most well-recognized posterior segment manifestation, is considered an important marker of systemic disease activity. Prevalence ranges from 3% among patients with mild disease to 29% among those with more active disease. Its clinical spectrum varies and is characterized by the following signs:

- *Cotton-wool spots with or without intraretinal hemorrhages.* These lesions can be seen without concurrent hypertension and are thought to be due to the underlying microangiopathy of the disease (Fig 9-1).
- *Severe retinal vascular occlusive disease (arterial and venous thrombosis).* Retinal vascular occlusion results in retinal nonperfusion and ischemia, secondary retinal neovascularization, and vitreous hemorrhage (Fig 9-2). More severe retinal vascular occlusive disease in SLE appears to be associated with central nervous system (CNS) lupus and the presence of antiphospholipid antibodies. Retinal vascular thrombosis is thought to be related to a hypercoagulable state induced by autoantibodies, rather than to an inflammatory retinal vasculitis. See BCSC Section 1, *Update on General Medicine,* for a discussion of antiphospholipid antibodies.
- *Lupus choroidopathy.* This entity is characterized by an immune-mediated choroidal vasculopathy, causing serous elevations of the retina and/or retinal pigment epithelium (RPE), as well as choroidal infarction and choroidal neovascularization (CNV). It almost always occurs in patients with known, and usually severe, systemic vascular disease, due to either hypertension from lupus nephritis or systemic vasculitis (Fig 9-3). SLE-induced hypertension and nephritis may also result in arteriolar narrowing, retinal hemorrhage, and disc edema.

American College of Rheumatology. 1997 update of the 1982 American College of Rheumatology revised criteria for classification of systemic lupus erythematosus. Available at https://bit.ly/2pYkcqJ. Accessed November 16, 2020.

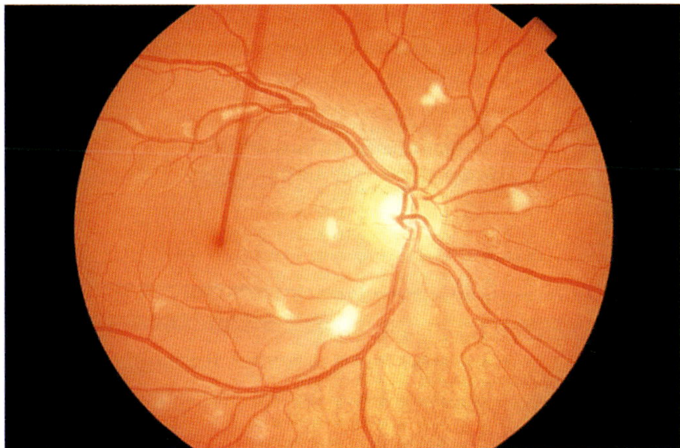

Figure 9-1 Systemic lupus erythematosus fundus photograph showing multiple cotton-wool spots. *(Courtesy of E. Mitchel Opremcak, MD.)*

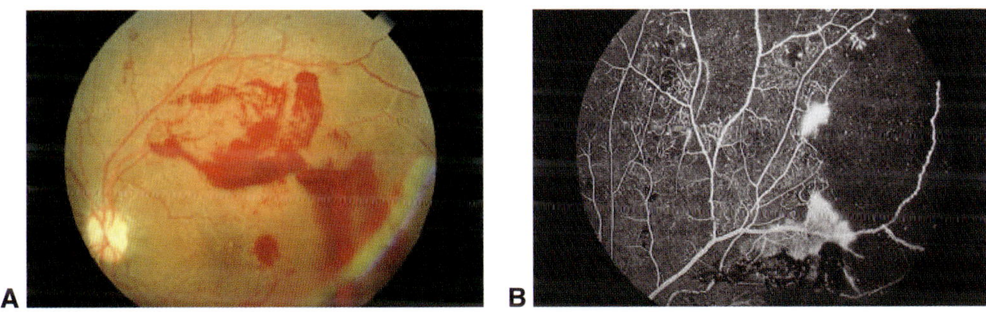

Figure 9-2 Systemic lupus erythematosus (SLE). **A,** Fundus photograph showing ischemic retinal vasculitis and neovascularization in a patient with SLE. **B,** Fluorescein angiogram of the same patient, showing capillary nonperfusion. *(Courtesy of E. Mitchel Opremcak, MD.)*

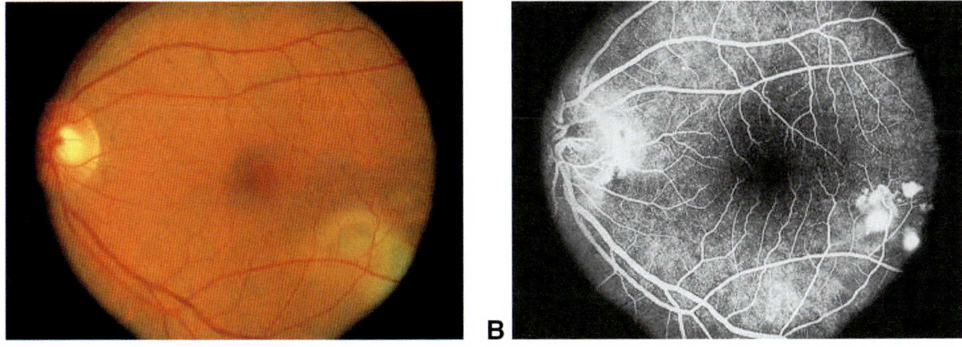

Figure 9-3 Systemic lupus erythematosus (SLE). **A,** Fundus photograph of multifocal choroiditis in a patient with SLE. **B,** Fluorescein angiogram showing multifocal areas of hyperfluorescence. *(Courtesy of E. Mitchel Opremcak, MD.)*

Jabs DA, Fine SL, Hochberg MC, Newman SA, Heiner GG, Stevens MB. Severe retinal vaso-occlusive disease in systemic lupus erythematosus. *Arch Ophthalmol.* 1986;104(4):558–563.
Nguyen QD, Uy HS, Akpek EK, Harper SL, Zacks DN, Foster CS. Choroidopathy of systemic lupus erythematosus. *Lupus.* 2000;9(4):288–298.
Palejwala NV, Walia HS, Yeh S. Ocular manifestations of systemic lupus erythematosus: a review of the literature. *Autoimmune Dis.* 2012;2012:290898.

Limits to ANA testing Uveitis is not commonly associated with SLE. However, ANA testing is often done in patients with uveitis who have no systemic or ocular findings to suggest SLE. Under those circumstances, the test has a very high false-positive rate; ANA testing should be limited to use in patients with signs or symptoms suggestive of SLE or who have juvenile idiopathic arthritis (JIA), for whom the test can help determine the level of risk for uveitis.

Treatment The treatment of ophthalmic disease in SLE is directed toward control of the underlying systemic disease, which may involve corticosteroids and IMT (immunomodulatory therapy), including hydroxychloroquine. Patients with severe vaso-occlusive disease or antiphospholipid antibodies may benefit from antiplatelet therapy or systemic anticoagulation. Ischemic complications, including proliferative retinopathy and vitreous hemorrhage, are managed with panretinal photocoagulation, intravitreal anti-vascular endothelial growth factor (VEGF) injections, and, in some cases, vitrectomy.

Some patients with SLE may remain on glucocorticoids for extended periods and thus need monitoring for cataracts and glaucoma. In addition, patients taking hydroxychloroquine should be informed about the ophthalmic risks and the need for regular ophthalmic examinations to screen for retinal toxicity. For further information, see BCSC Section 12, *Retina and Vitreous.*

Marmor MF, Kellner U, Lai TY, Melles RB, Mieler WF; American Academy of Ophthalmology. Recommendations on screening for chloroquine and hydroxychloroquine retinopathy (2016 revision). *Ophthalmology.* 2016;123(6):1386–1394.

Polyarteritis nodosa

Polyarteritis nodosa (PAN) is an uncommon systemic vasculitis characterized by subacute or chronic, focal, necrotizing inflammation of medium-sized and small arteries. The disease presents in patients between the ages of 40 and 60 years and affects men 3 times more frequently than women; the annual incidence rate is approximately 0.7 per 100,000 individuals. Although there are no racial or geographic predisposing factors, 10% of patients test positive for hepatitis B surface antigen, implicating hepatitis B as an etiologic agent. Indeed, the demonstration of circulating immune complexes composed of hepatitis B antigen and antibodies to hepatitis B in vessel walls during the early stages of the disease strongly implicates immune-complex–mediated mechanisms in the pathogenesis of PAN.

Manifestations PAN most commonly affects skin, nerves, kidneys, and gastrointestinal tract. Fatigue, fever, weight loss, and arthralgia are present in up to 75% of patients. Vasculitis-induced peripheral neuropathies are also common, as are skin manifestations, which include subcutaneous nodules, purpura, livedo reticularis, and Raynaud phenomenon. Renal involvement often manifests as secondary hypertension and affects approximately one-third of patients. Gastrointestinal disease with small-bowel ischemia and infarction occurs less frequently but may lead to serious complications. Other systemic manifestations include coronary arteritis, pericarditis, and hematologic abnormalities. CNS disease associated with PAN is rare. The American College of Rheumatology has developed specific criteria for the diagnosis of PAN.

Ocular involvement is present in up to 20% of patients with PAN and arises because of the underlying vascular disease. Posterior pole manifestations include hypertensive retinopathy, characterized by macular star formation, cotton-wool spots, intraretinal hemorrhages, retinal artery occlusions, and choroidal infarcts. Patients may have a retinal vasculitis (Fig 9-4) or a vasculitis involving the posterior ciliary arteries and choroidal vessels, with resultant exudative retinal detachments. Elschnig spots—focal areas of choroidal hyperpigmentation surrounded by hypopigmentation—may be observed in the posterior pole because of lobular choroidal ischemia and infarcts (see BCSC Section 12, *Retina and Vitreous*). Neuro-ophthalmic manifestations include cranial nerve palsies, amaurosis fugax, homonymous hemianopia, Horner syndrome, and optic atrophy. Scleral inflammatory disease of all types, including necrotizing and posterior scleritis, has been reported. Peripheral ulcerative keratitis (PUK), typically accompanied by scleritis, may be the presenting manifestation of PAN.

American College of Rheumatology. 1990 criteria for the classification of polyarteritis nodosa. Available at https://bit.ly/2xtKZxU. Accessed November 16, 2020.

Perez VL, Chavala SH, Ahmed M, et al. Ocular manifestations and concepts of systemic vasculitides. *Surv Ophthalmol.* 2004;49(4):399–418.

Rothschild PR, Pagnoux C, Seror R, Brézin AP, Delair E, Guillevin L. Ophthalmologic manifestations of systemic necrotizing vasculitides at diagnosis: a retrospective study of 1286 patients and review of the literature. *Semin Arthritis Rheum.* 2013;42(5):507–514.

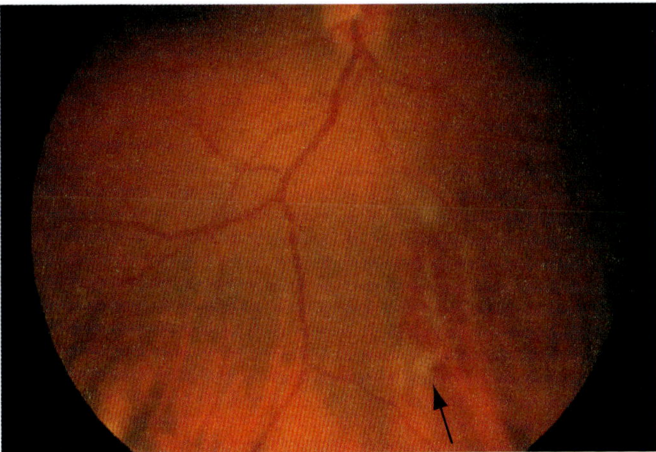

Figure 9-4 Polyarteritis nodosa. Fundus photograph indicating retinal vasculitis associated with vascular sheathing *(arrow)* and intraretinal hemorrhage. *(Courtesy of E. Mitchel Opremcak, MD.)*

Treatment and prognosis Unlike granulomatosis with polyangiitis (GPA; previously known as *Wegener granulomatosis*), polyarteritis nodosa is not associated with antineutrophil cytoplasmic antibodies (ANCA). The 5-year mortality rate of untreated PAN is 90%. Although systemic corticosteroid use may reduce this rate to 50%, combination therapy with IMT, such as cyclophosphamide, improves 5-year survival to 80% and may induce long-term remission of the disease. It is therefore important to consider PAN in the differential diagnosis of retinal vasculitis presenting in patients in whom an underlying necrotizing vasculitis is suspected; appropriate diagnosis and management can be life-saving. Tissue biopsy confirms the diagnosis.

Gayraud M, Guillevin L, le Toumelin P, et al; French Vasculitis Study Group. Long-term followup of polyarteritis nodosa, microscopic polyangiitis, and Churg-Strauss syndrome: analysis of four prospective trials including 278 patients. *Arthritis Rheum.* 2001;44(3):666–675.

Granulomatosis with polyangiitis

Granulomatosis with polyangiitis is a multisystem autoimmune disorder characterized by the classic triad of necrotizing granulomatous vasculitis of the upper and lower respiratory tract, focal segmental glomerulonephritis, and necrotizing vasculitis of small arteries and veins. Involvement of the paranasal sinuses is the most characteristic clinical feature of this disorder, followed by pulmonary and renal disease. Renal involvement may or may not be evident at presentation, but its early detection is important, as glomerulonephritis develops in up to 85% of patients during the course of the disease and carries significant mortality if left untreated. A limited form of this disease has been described, consisting of granulomatous inflammation involving the respiratory tract without overt involvement of the kidneys.

Another entity believed to belong to the GPA spectrum is microscopic polyangiitis (MPA). Patients with MPA may have clinical features similar to those of GPA but lack granulomatous changes on biopsy. Patients with MPA are also more likely to have ANCA directed at myeloperoxidase (MPO; discussed further shortly). There is some controversy in the rheumatologic literature about differentiating the 2 entities; however, ophthalmic involvement is much less common in MPA.

Manifestations Patients with GPA may present with sinusitis associated with bloody nasal discharge, pulmonary symptomatology, and arthritis. Dermatologic involvement is present in approximately one-half of patients, with purpura involving the lower extremities occurring most frequently; less common are ulcers and subcutaneous nodules. Nervous system involvement may occur in approximately one-third of patients. Mononeuritis multiplex is the most common, but cranial neuropathies, seizures, stroke syndromes, and cerebral vasculitis may also occur.

Ocular or orbital involvement is found in 15% of patients at presentation and in up to 50% of patients during the course of the disease. Orbital involvement is usually secondary to contiguous extension of the granulomatous inflammatory process from the paranasal sinuses into the orbit. Orbital cellulitis and dacryocystitis may arise from the involved and secondarily infected nasal mucosa. Orbital pseudotumor, distinct from the sinus

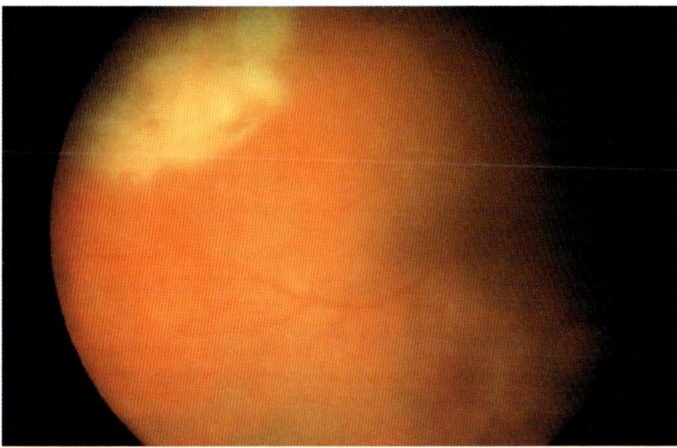

Figure 9-5 Granulomatosis with polyangiitis. Fundus photograph of retinitis. The appearance of the retinitis may be similar to that of a viral retinitis. *(Courtesy of E. Mitchel Opremcak, MD.)*

inflammation, may also occur. Scleritis of any type, particularly diffuse anterior or necrotizing disease, with or without peripheral ulcerative keratitis, affects up to 40% of patients. Posterior scleritis has been reported.

Approximately 10% of patients with GPA and ocular involvement have been reported to have an associated nonspecific, unilateral or bilateral anterior, intermediate, or posterior uveitis, with varying degrees of vitritis. Retinal involvement is relatively uncommon, occurring in up to 10% of patients. Retinal vascular manifestations range from relatively benign cotton-wool spots, with or without associated intraretinal hemorrhages, to more severe vaso-occlusive disease, including branch or central retinal artery or vein occlusion. Retinitis has been reported in up to 20% of patients; those with accompanying retinal vasculitis may develop retinal neovascularization, vitreous hemorrhage, and neovascular glaucoma (Fig 9-5). Orbital involvement can lead to compressive ischemic optic neuropathy. Vision loss in GPA may occur in up to 40% of patients, especially among those with long-standing or inadequately treated disease.

Kubal AA, Perez VL. Ocular manifestations of ANCA-associated vasculitis. *Rheum Dis Clin North Am*. 2010;36(3):573–586.

Pakrou N, Selva D, Leibovitch I. Wegener's granulomatosis: ophthalmic manifestations and management. *Semin Arthritis Rheum*. 2006;35(5):284–292.

Diagnosis Tissue biopsy establishes the histologic diagnosis; chest radiograph may disclose nodular, diffuse, or cavitary lesions; and laboratory evaluation may reveal proteinuria or hematuria, elevated erythrocyte sedimentation rate (ESR) and C-reactive protein levels, as well as the presence of ANCA. ANCA are antibodies directed against cytoplasmic azurophilic granules of neutrophils and monocytes that are specific markers for a group of related systemic vasculitides, including GPA, MPA, eosinophilic GPA (Churg-Strauss syndrome), renal-limited vasculitis, and pauci-immunoglomerulonephritis. Two main classes of ANCA have been described according to their immunofluorescence staining patterns:

- The cytoplasmic, or c-ANCA, pattern is both sensitive to and specific for GPA and is present in up to 95% of patients; proteinase 3 is the most common target antigen (referred to as PR3-ANCA).
- The perinuclear, or p-ANCA, pattern is associated with MPA, renal-limited vasculitis, and pauci-immunoglomerulonephritis.

Myeloperoxidase is the most common antigenic target (MPO-ANCA). Standardized testing for ANCA should include both immunofluorescence testing for c- and p-ANCA and specific antibody testing for PR3-ANCA and MPO-ANCA; the latter 2 are most specific.

Treatment Appropriate treatment of GPA mandates combination therapy with oral corticosteroids and IMT, such as rituximab and cyclophosphamide. Without therapy, the 1-year mortality rate is 80%. However, 93% of patients treated with cyclophosphamide and corticosteroids successfully achieve remission with resolution of eye disease. The ophthalmologist's role in recognizing GPA-associated eye disease can be critical, since timely diagnosis and treatment are essential in reducing not only ocular morbidity but also patient mortality.

Susac Syndrome

Susac syndrome (also known as *SICRET syndrome,* for *s*mall *i*nfarctions of *c*ochlear, *r*etinal, and *e*ncephalic *t*issue) is a rare entity, initially reported in 1979 by Susac and colleagues. The clinically observed triad consists of encephalopathy, hearing loss, and branch retinal artery occlusions (BRAO). The syndrome occurs mostly in young women but has been noted in patients aged 16–58 years.

Manifestations

The differential diagnosis at presentation includes multiple sclerosis, herpetic encephalitis, acute disseminated encephalomyelitis, and Behçet disease; however, ocular findings are highly specific and may aid in diagnosis. Ophthalmoscopy shows diffuse or localized narrowing of retinal arteries with a "boxcar" segmentation of the blood column at

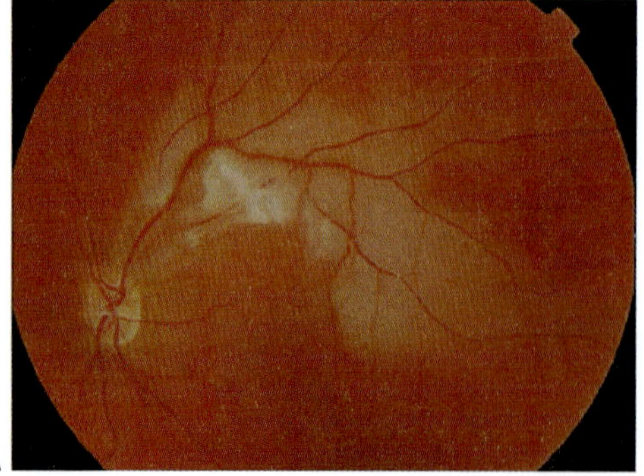

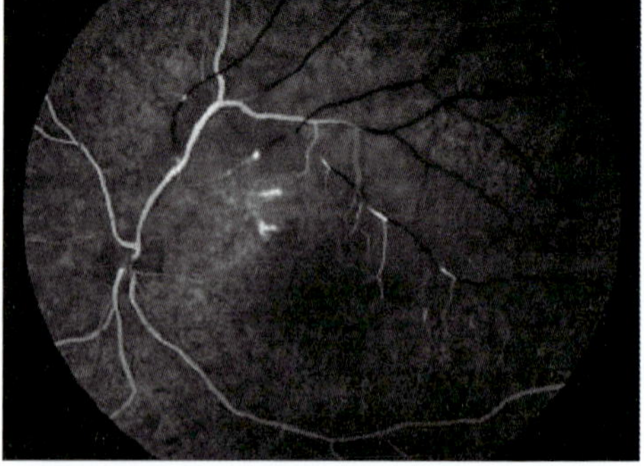

Figure 9-6 Susac syndrome. **A,** Color fundus photograph revealing an area of intraretinal whitening corresponding to a superotemporal branch artery occlusion in the left eye. **B,** Fluorescein angiogram showing a superotemporal branch artery occlusion with multiple areas of segmental staining well away from sites of bifurcation. *(Courtesy of Albert T. Vitale, MD.)*

the level of peripheral retinal arteries (Fig 9-6A). Vitreous haze or cells are absent. Angiography demonstrates focal nonperfused retinal arterioles with hyperfluorescent walls (Fig 9-6B). There is usually no evidence of embolic material or inflammatory reactions around the vessels. Magnetic resonance imaging (MRI) is another useful diagnostic tool and shows multifocal supratentorial white matter lesions; the corpus callosum may be involved. Audiometry should be performed in any patient being evaluated for this entity; sensorineural hearing loss is a common finding.

Dörr J, Krautwald S, Wildemann B, et al. Characteristics of Susac syndrome: a review of all reported cases. *Nat Rev Neurol.* 2013;9(6):307–316.

Treatment Treatment remains controversial and includes high-dose intravenous corticosteroids, anticoagulants, and IMT, such as intravenous immunoglobulin and mycophenolate mofetil. The course of Susac syndrome is not always self-limiting, and isolated retinal arteriolar involvement may occur as a very late manifestation.

Inflammatory Chorioretinopathies of Unknown Etiology

The inflammatory chorioretinopathies, or white dot syndromes, are a heterogeneous group of inflammatory disorders with overlapping clinical features that share the presence of discrete, multiple, well-circumscribed, yellow-white lesions at the level of the retina, outer retina, RPE, choriocapillaris, and/or choroid during some phase of their course. The white dot syndromes consist of the predominantly noninfectious ocular syndromes listed in Table 9-1.

Their differential diagnosis includes systemic and ocular infectious entities such as syphilis, diffuse unilateral subacute neuroretinitis (DUSN), and ocular histoplasmosis syndrome (OHS), as well as noninfectious entities such as sarcoidosis, sympathetic ophthalmia, Vogt-Koyanagi-Harada (VKH) syndrome, and intraocular lymphoma. Common presenting symptoms include photopsias, blurred vision, nyctalopia, floaters, and visual field loss contiguous with the blind spot. In many cases, a prodromal viral syndrome can be identified. Bilateral involvement, albeit asymmetrically (with the exception of multiple evanescent white dot syndrome [MEWDS]), is the rule. Excepting patients with birdshot chorioretinopathy or serpiginous choroiditis, most individuals are younger than 50 years of age. A female predominance is observed in patients with MEWDS, birdshot chorioretinopathy, multifocal choroiditis and panuveitis, punctate inner choroiditis (PIC), subretinal fibrosis and uveitis syndrome, and acute zonal occult outer retinopathy.

The etiology of the white dot syndromes is unknown. Some investigators have postulated an infectious cause; others have suggested an autoimmune/inflammatory pathogenesis arising in individuals with common non–disease-specific genetics, triggered by some exogenous agent. An increased prevalence of systemic autoimmune disease, both in patients with white dot syndromes and in their first- and second-degree relatives, suggests that inflammatory chorioretinopathies may occur in families with inherited immune dysregulation that predisposes to autoimmunity. It is also unclear whether the white dot syndromes represent a clinical spectrum of a single disease entity or are discrete diseases.

Table 9-1 Inflammatory Chorioretinopathies

	Birdshot Chorioretinopathy	APMPPE	Serpiginous Choroiditis	MCP	PIC	SFU	MEWDS	ARPE	AZOOR
Age, years	30–70	20–50	20–60	10–70	20–40	10–35	10–50	15–40	15–65
Sex	F>M	M=F	M=F	F (3:1)	F (90%)	F (>95%)	F (3:1)	M=F	F (3:1)
Laterality	Bilateral	Bilateral	Bilateral, asymmetric	Bilateral	Bilateral	Bilateral, asymmetric	Unilateral	Unilateral (75%)	Bilateral (76%)
Systemic associations	80%–98% HLA-A29	Viral prodrome, cerebro-vasculitis, CSF abnormalities	Rule out TB-associated disease	None	None	None	Viral prodrome (50%)	None	Systemic autoimmune disease (28%)
Onset	Insidious	Acute	Variable	Insidious	Acute	Insidious	Acute	Acute	Insidious
Course	Chronic, recurrent	Self-limited	Chronic, recurrent	Chronic, recurrent	Self-limited	Chronic, recurrent	Self-limited	Self-limited	Chronic, recurrent (31%)
Symptoms	Blurred vision, floaters, photopsias, disturbed night and color vision	Blurred vision, scotomata, photopsias	Blurred vision, scotomata	Blurred vision, floaters, photopsias, meta-morphopsia, scotomata	Paracentral scotomata, photopsias, metamor-phopsia	Blurred vision,	Blurred vision, scotomata, photopsias	Central metamor-phopsia, scotomata	Photopsias, scotomata
Examination	Vitritis; ovoid, creamy, white-yellow, postequatorial lesions, 50–1500 μm, do not pigment	Multifocal, flat, gray-white lesions, 1–2 disc areas, outer retina/RPE with evolving pigmentation	Geographic, yellow-gray, peripapillary, macular chorioretinal lesions with centrifugal extension; activity at leading peripheral edge with RPE/chorio-capillaris atrophy in its wake	Myopia, anterior uveitis (50%), vitritis (100%), active white-yellow chorioreti-nal lesions, 50–200 μm, evolving to punched-out scars	Myopia, vitritis absent, white-yellow chorio-retinal lesions, 100-200 μm, may develop pigment	Moderate vitritis, 50–500 μm yellow-white lesions posterior pole to midperiphery, RPE, hypertrophy, atrophy, large stellate zones of subretinal fibrosis	Myopia; mild anterior uveitis; vitritis; small white-orange, evanescent, perifoveal dots, 100–200 μm, outer retina/RPE; macular granularity	Small, hyper-pigmented lesions with yellow halo, 100–200 μm, mild/no vitritis	Initially normal to subtle RPE changes, late pigment migration, focal perivenous sheathing

Structural complications	Retinal vasculitis, disc edema, ME, CNVM (6%)	Disc edema, pigment alterations	CNVM (25%), RPE mottling, scarring, loss of choriocapillaris	Optic disc edema, peripapillary pigment changes, ME (14%–44%), CNVM (33%)	CNVM (17%–40%), serous detachment over confluent lesions	Neurosensory retinal detachment, ME, CNVM	Disc edema, venous sheathing	None	RPE mottling, occasional ME
Fluorescein angiography	Early hypofluorescence vs silence, subtle late stain; leakage from disc, vessels, ME; delayed retinal circulation time	Acute lesions: early blockage, late staining; late window defects	Early hypofluorescence, late staining/leak of active border, leakage in presence of CNVM	Early blockage, late staining of lesions, leakage from ME, CNVM	Early blockage or hyperfluorescence, variable late leakage/staining of acute lesions, leakage in presence of ME, CNVM	Multiple areas of alternating hypo- and hyperfluorescence; early, late staining	Early punctate hyperfluorescence, wreath-like configuration, late staining of lesions, optic nerve	Early hypercyanescence with surrounding halo of hyperfluorescence and late staining	In acute stage, normal with increased retinal circulation time; in late stage, diffuse hyperfluorescence, RPE atrophy
Indocyanine green angiography	Corresponding hypocyanescent lesions more numerous than on exam, FA	Hypocyanescent spots corresponding to those seen on exam, FA	Early hypocyanescence, late staining, more widespread extent than seen on exam, FA	Multiple hypocyanescent lesions, confluence around optic nerve, more numerous than on exam, FA	Multiple hypocyanescent, peripapillary, posterior pole lesions, corresponding to those seen on exam, FA	Hypocyanescent lesions in 1 report	Multiple hypocyanescent spots, more numerous than on exam, FA	Early- and midphase patchy macular hypercyanescence; late hypercyanescent halo in the macula	Hypocyanescence in atrophic areas with late leakage in subacute areas
Fundus autofluorescence	Hypoautofluorescent spots more numerous than clinically apparent lesions; placoid macular hypoautofluorescence	Hyperautofluorescent areas correspond to FA blockage; hypoautofluorescent areas correspond to areas of staining; FAF findings lag FA findings	Hyperautofluorescent active lesions; hypofluorescent regressed lesions	Acute lesions variably hyper- to hypoautofluorescent; may be more numerous with FAF than clinically	Similar to MCP	NI	Hyperautofluorescent spots corresponding to lesions on clinical exam	Normal or hypoautofluorescent spots corresponding to lesions on clinical exam	Lesions may have central hypoautofluorescence with peripheral hyperautofluorescence

(Continued)

Table 9-1 *(continued)*

	Birdshot Chorioretinopathy	APMPPE	Serpiginous Choroiditis	MCP	PIC	SFU	MEWDS	ARPE	AZOOR
Optical coherence tomography	Macular edema; loss of inner/outer segment line (ellipsoid zone); suprachoroidal fluid	Outer retinal hyper-reflectivity with intra- and subretinal fluid	Outer retinal hyper-reflectivity in active lesions; retinal and RPE atrophy in regressed lesions	Sub-RPE deposits with overlying outer retinal disruption	Similar to MCP	Variable retinal edema; subretinal fluid and subretinal fibrosis	Abnormal reflectivity of the inner/outer segment line	Transient disruption of the inner/outer segment line (ellipsoid zone) and of the RPE inner band	Loss of the inner/outer segment line (ellipsoid zone)
Electrophysiology, visual fields	ERG: abnormal rod and cone responses; diminished b-wave	EOG: variably abnormal	ERG: normal	ERG: abnormal, extinguished responses	ERG: normal; VF: enlargement of blind spot (41%)	ERG and EOG markedly attenuated	ERG: diminished a-wave, early receptor potentials (reversible); VF: enlarged blind spot, paracentral scotomata	ERG: normal; EOG: abnormal	ERG, mfERG: abnormal; VF: temporal, superior defects, enlarged blind spot
Visual prognosis	Guarded without treatment	Good	Guarded	Guarded	Good in absence of CNVM	Guarded	Excellent	Excellent	Guarded
Treatment	Systemic or local cortico-steroids, IMT	Observation; systemic cortico-steroids with CNS involvement	Systemic or local cortico-steroids, IMT. Anti-VEGF agents with or without laser for CNVM	Systemic or local cortico-steroids, IMT. Anti-VEGF agents with or without laser for CNVM	Observation; systemic or local cortico-steroids. Anti-VEGF agents with or without laser for CNVM	Corticosteroids for CME; IMT of equivocal efficacy long term	Observation	None	Corticosteroids, IMT, antivirals of equivocal efficacy

APMPPE = acute posterior multifocal placoid pigment epitheliopathy; ARPE = acute retinal pigment epitheliitis; AZOOR = acute zonal occult outer retinopathy; CNVM = choroidal neovascular membrane; CNS = central nervous system; EOG = electro-oculogram; ERG = electroretinogram; FA = fluorescein angiography; FAF = fundus autofluorescence; IMT = immunomodulatory therapy; MCP = multifocal choroiditis and panuveitis syndrome; ME = macular edema; MEWDS = multiple evanescent white dot syndrome; mfERG = multifocal electroretinogram; NI = no information; PIC = punctate inner choroiditis; RPE = retinal pigment epithelium; SFU = subretinal fibrosis and uveitis syndrome; TB = tuberculosis; VEGF = vascular endothelial growth factor; VF = visual fields.

Although they share common features, the white dot syndromes can be differentiated by their variable lesion morphology and evolution, distinct natural histories, and appearance with multimodal imaging. This differentiation has important implications with respect to disease-specific treatments and visual prognosis.

Abu-Yaghi NE, Hartono SP, Hodge DO, Pulido JS, Bakri SJ. White dot syndromes: a 20-year study of incidence, clinical features, and outcomes. *Ocul Immunol Inflamm.* 2011;19(6):426–430.

Gass JD. Are acute zonal occult outer retinopathy and the white spot syndromes (AZOOR complex) specific autoimmune diseases? *Am J Ophthalmol.* 2003;135(3):380–381.

Jampol LM, Becker KG. White spot syndromes of the retina: a hypothesis based on the common genetic hypothesis of autoimmune/inflammatory disease. *Am J Ophthalmol.* 2003;135(3):376–379.

Pearlman RB, Golchet PR, Feldmann MG, et al. Increased prevalence of autoimmunity in patients with white spot syndromes and their family members. *Arch Ophthalmol.* 2009;127(7):869–874.

Quillen DA, Davis JB, Gottlieb JL, et al. The white dot syndromes. *Am J Ophthalmol.* 2004;137(3):538–550.

Birdshot chorioretinopathy

Birdshot chorioretinopathy (also known as *birdshot uveitis, birdshot retinochoroidopathy,* and *vitiliginous chorioretinitis*) is an uncommon disease presenting predominantly in White women of northern European descent past the fourth decade of life. Although no consistent systemic disease association has been identified, birdshot chorioretinopathy is highly correlated with the HLA-A29 gene, with a sensitivity of 96% and a specificity of 93%. The presence of the haplotype confers considerably increased relative risk (224-fold) for the development of this disease. HLA-A29 is confirmatory rather than diagnostic, as 7% of the general population carries this haplotype, and in the absence of characteristic clinical features, an alternative diagnosis should be considered.

Manifestations Presenting symptoms include blurred vision, floaters, nyctalopia, and disturbance of color vision. Visual complaints may be out of proportion to the measured Snellen visual acuity, reflecting the diffuse retinal dysfunction that occurs in this disease. Patients may also report unusual peripheral visual phenomena, such as pinwheels, sparkles, or flickering lights, and these symptoms may be indicators of subtle disease activity. Anterior segment inflammation may be minimal or absent; however, varying degrees of vitritis are commonly noted.

Funduscopy reveals characteristic multifocal, hypopigmented, ovoid, cream-colored lesions (50–1500 μm) at the level of the choroid and RPE in the postequatorial fundus. Typically, these lesions show a nasal and radial distribution, emanating from the optic nerve, and frequently they follow the underlying choroidal vessels (Fig 9-7). The lesions do not become pigmented over time and are best appreciated by indirect ophthalmoscopy, although they may not be readily apparent at presentation. Retinal vasculitis, uveitic macular edema, and optic nerve head inflammation are important components of active disease. Late complications include optic atrophy, epiretinal membrane (ERM) formation, and, rarely, CNV.

Fluorescein angiography (FA) findings are variable, depending on duration of disease and clinical activity. Although early birdshot chorioretinopathy lesions may show initial

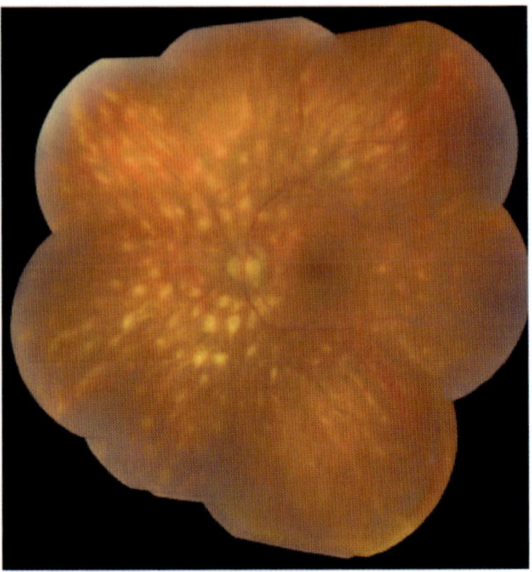

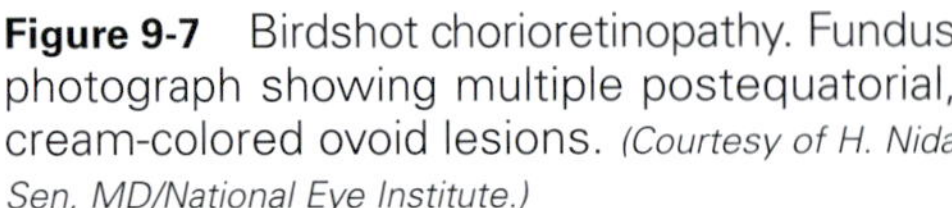

Figure 9-7 Birdshot chorioretinopathy. Fundus photograph showing multiple postequatorial, cream-colored ovoid lesions. *(Courtesy of H. Nida Sen, MD/National Eye Institute.)*

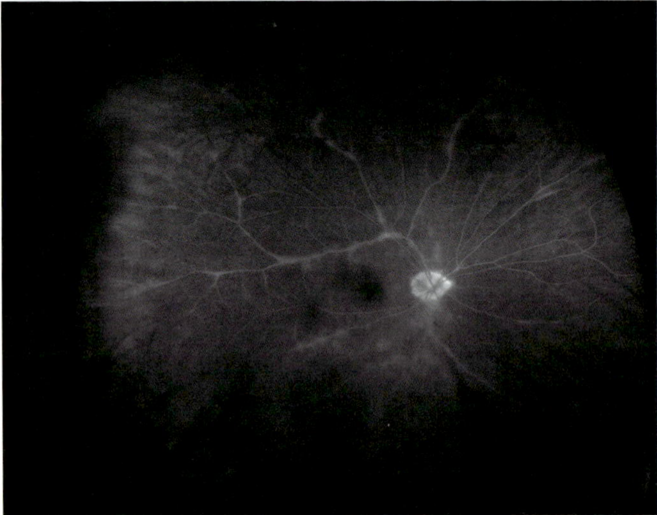

Figure 9-8 Birdshot chorioretinopathy. Fluorescein angiogram showing diffuse retinal phlebitis. *(Courtesy of Bryn M. Burkholder, MD.)*

hypofluorescence with subtle late staining, in general, FA is more useful in identifying more subtle indices of active inflammation, such as retinal vasculitis, macular edema, and optic nerve head leakage (Fig 9-8). Indocyanine green (ICG) angiography discloses multiple hypocyanescent spots, which are typically more numerous than those apparent on clinical examination or FA (Fig 9-9).

Fundus autofluorescence (FAF) imaging reveals hypoautofluorescence in areas of RPE atrophy that are more numerous and not uniformly correspondent with lesions on examination, suggesting that the choroid and RPE may be affected independently (Fig 9-10).

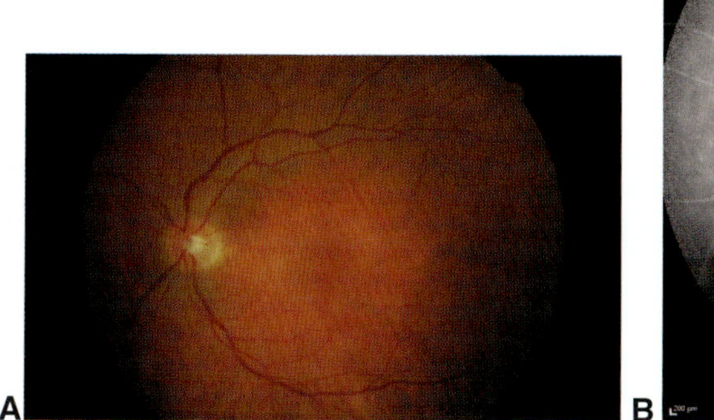

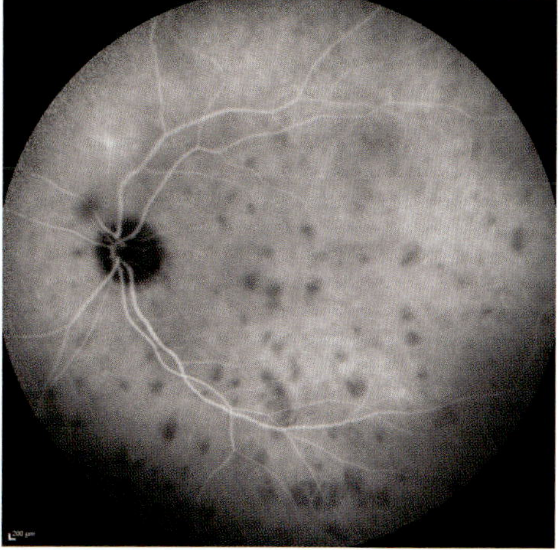

Figure 9-9 Birdshot chorioretinopathy. **A,** Fundus photograph showing very subtle, yellow choroidal spots. **B,** On indocyanine green angiogram, these spots are much more visible as hypocyanescent spots. *(Courtesy of Bryn M. Burkholder, MD.)*

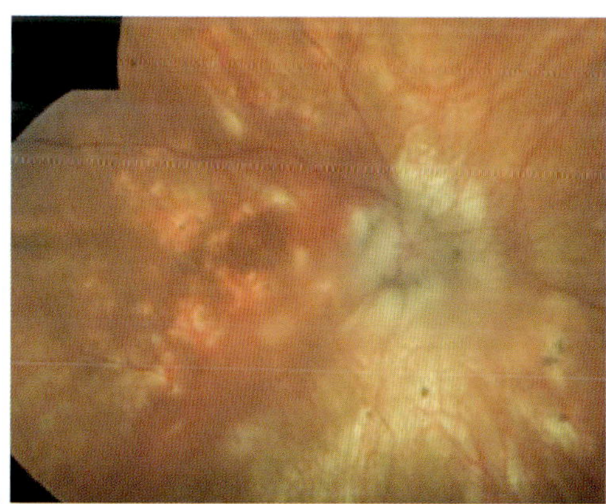

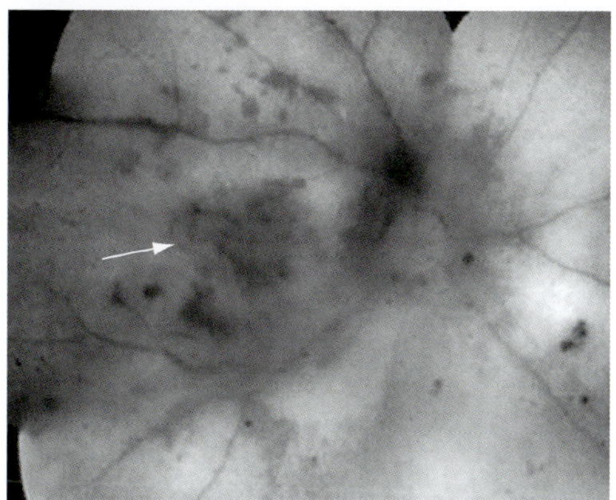

Figure 9-10 Birdshot chorioretinopathy. **A,** Color fundus photograph showing multifocal hypopigmented spots within the macula and outside the arcades. **B,** Autofluorescence image showing placoid hypoautofluorescence in the central macula *(arrow)*. *(Reprinted with permission from Koizumi H, Pozzoni MC, Spaide RF. Fundus autofluorescence in birdshot chorioretinopathy.* Ophthalmology. *2008:115[5]: e15–20.)*

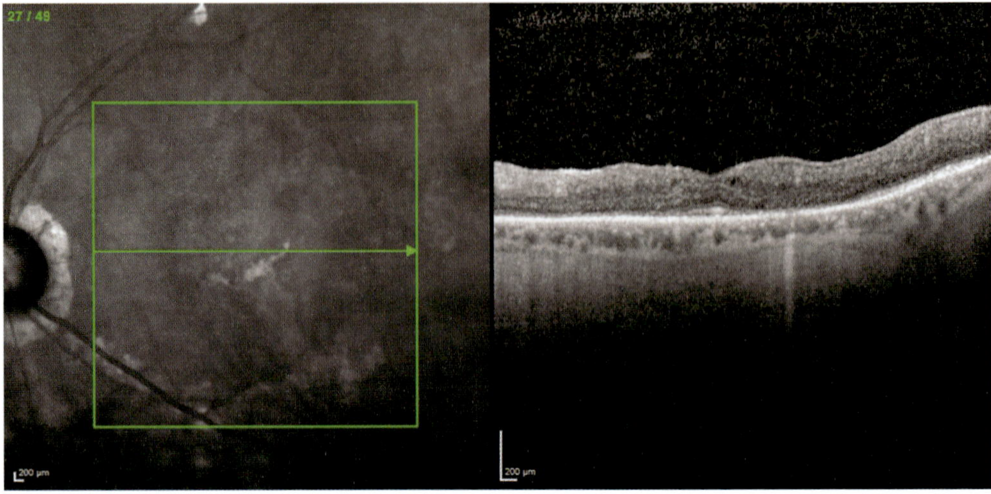

Figure 9-11 Birdshot chorioretinopathy. Optical coherence tomography scan demonstrating mild macular edema, retinal atrophy, and patchy loss of photoreceptors. *(Courtesy of Bryn M. Burkholder, MD.)*

Macular hypoautofluorescence has been associated with vision loss and disease severity. Optical coherence tomography (OCT) may show macular edema or demonstrate patchy or diffuse loss of photoreceptors (inner/outer segment line or ellipsoid zone) and macular atrophy, especially with long-standing disease (Fig 9-11). Enhanced-depth OCT imaging may be useful to evaluate choroidal thickening early in the disease course and thinning in advanced disease.

Böni C, Thorne JE, Spaide RF, et al. Choroidal findings in eyes with birdshot chorioretinitis using enhanced-depth optical coherence tomography. *Invest Ophthalmol Vis Sci.* 2016;57(9):591–599.

Piffer AL, Boissonnot M, Gobert F, et al. Relevance of wide-field autofluorescence imaging in birdshot retinochoroidopathy: descriptive analysis of 76 eyes. *Acta Ophthalmol.* 2014;92(6):e463–469.

Differential diagnosis Important differential diagnostic considerations include pars planitis, VKH syndrome, sympathetic ophthalmia, OHS, intraocular lymphoma, and especially sarcoidosis, which may present with chorioretinal lesions of similar morphology and distribution as those present in birdshot chorioretinopathy.

Disease course Birdshot chorioretinopathy can be insidious, and simply monitoring visual acuity and clinical examination findings is insufficient to protect patients from vision loss. Progressive worsening of the visual field and abnormal electroretinogram (ERG) results are commonly found with extended follow-up. This suggests a more diffuse retinal dysfunction not fully explained by the presence of uveitic macular edema or other structural abnormality. For this reason, full-field ERGs (with attention to the 30-Hz flicker implicit time and scotopic b-wave amplitudes) and Goldmann and automated visual field

(30-2 with attention to the mean deviation) testing are more useful parameters for monitoring disease course and response to therapy than are changes in funduscopic examination or visual acuity.

A small subset of patients with birdshot chorioretinopathy may have self-limited disease and do well without treatment. However, there is no way to determine which patients will have disease progression, so close monitoring with the testing modalities discussed earlier is critical. Studies have shown that early and aggressive control of inflammation in this disease results in better visual outcomes.

Gordon LK, Monnet D, Holland GN, Brézin AP, Yu F, Levinson RD. Longitudinal cohort study of patients with birdshot chorioretinopathy. IV. Visual field results at baseline. *Am J Ophthalmol.* 2007;144(6):829–837.

Holder GE, Robson AG, Pavesio C, Graham EM. Electrophysiological characterisation and monitoring in the management of birdshot chorioretinopathy. *Br J Ophthalmol.* 2005;89(6):709–718.

Thorne JE, Jabs DA, Peters GB, Hair D, Dunn JP, Kempen JH. Birdshot retinochoroidopathy: ocular complications and visual impairment. *Am J Ophthalmol.* 2005;140(1):45–51.

Treatment Treatment consists of the initial administration of systemic and/or local corticosteroids, with early introduction of corticosteroid-sparing IMT. Birdshot chorioretinopathy is typically incompletely responsive to corticosteroid monotherapy. Extended IMT is anticipated in most patients, given the chronic nature of the disease. Treatment with IMT may include cyclosporine, mycophenolate mofetil, azathioprine, methotrexate, and tumor necrosis factor α (TNF-α) inhibitors. This approach is effective in reducing intraocular inflammation, inflammatory recurrences, and the risk of developing uveitic macular edema, as well as in preserving visual acuity and visual field. Periocular or intravitreal corticosteroid injections are useful as adjunctive therapy in managing macular edema and inflammatory recurrences. The intravitreal fluocinolone acetonide implant is an option for patients who cannot tolerate systemic therapy, or in whom systemic therapy is insufficient, although multiple implants may be necessary to maintain inflammation control over time.

Kiss S, Ahmed M, Letko E, Foster CS. Long-term follow-up of patients with birdshot retinochoroidopathy treated with corticosteroid-sparing systemic immunomodulatory therapy. *Ophthalmology.* 2005;112(6):1066–1071.

Menezo V, Taylor SR. Birdshot uveitis: current and emerging treatment options. *Clin Ophthalmol.* 2014;8:73–81.

Tomkins-Netzer O, Taylor SR, Lightman S. Long-term clinical and anatomic outcome of birdshot chorioretinopathy. *JAMA Ophthalmol.* 2014;132(1):57–62.

Acute posterior multifocal placoid pigment epitheliopathy

Acute posterior multifocal placoid pigment epitheliopathy (APMPPE) is an uncommon condition presenting in otherwise healthy young adults, affecting men and women equally. It may be associated with an influenza-like illness (50%) and may have a genetic predisposition, given the association of HLA-B7 and HLA-DR2 with this entity.

Several noninfectious systemic conditions have been reported in connection with APMPPE, including erythema nodosum, GPA, PAN, cerebral vasculitis, scleritis and episcleritis, sarcoidosis, and ulcerative colitis. Infectious etiologies, including group A streptococcus, adenovirus type 5, tuberculosis, Lyme disease, and mumps virus have also been associated with APMPPE, as has hepatitis B vaccination. It has been postulated that APMPPE is an immune-driven vasculitis. Of greatest concern is the rare but potentially life-threatening association of APMPPE with cerebral vasculitis. Patients presenting with symptoms suggestive of CNS disease should undergo urgent neurologic evaluation.

Manifestations Patients typically present with a sudden onset of unilateral vision loss associated with central and paracentral scotomata; the fellow eye becomes involved within days to weeks. Photopsias may precede loss of vision. There is minimal or no anterior segment inflammation; vitritis may be present but is usually mild. Funduscopic examination demonstrates multiple large, flat, yellow-white placoid lesions at the level of the RPE. The lesions vary in size from 1 to 2 disc areas and are scattered throughout the posterior pole (Fig 9-12). New peripheral lesions may appear in a linear or radial array over the next few weeks. Papillitis may be observed, but macular edema is uncommon. Atypical findings include retinal vasculitis, retinal vascular occlusive disease, retinal neovascularization, and exudative retinal detachment. The lesions resolve over a period of 2–6 weeks, leaving a permanent, well-defined alteration in the RPE, consisting of alternating areas of depigmentation and pigment clumping. Rapid evolution of the pigmentary changes, often over days, is a typical feature of the disease.

Diagnosis The diagnosis of APMPPE is based on the characteristic clinical presentation and FA findings during the acute phase of the disease: early hypofluorescent lesions (Fig 9-13A) corresponding to, but typically more numerous than, those apparent on funduscopy and late hyperfluorescent staining (Fig 9-13B). Subacute lesions may show increased central hyperfluorescence with late staining; with resolution, transmission defects are typically observed.

Indocyanine green angiography reveals choroidal hypocyanescence with hypervisualization of the underlying choroidal vessels in both the acute and inactive stages of the disease; these lesions become smaller in the inactive stages (Fig 9-14). Choroidal perfusion

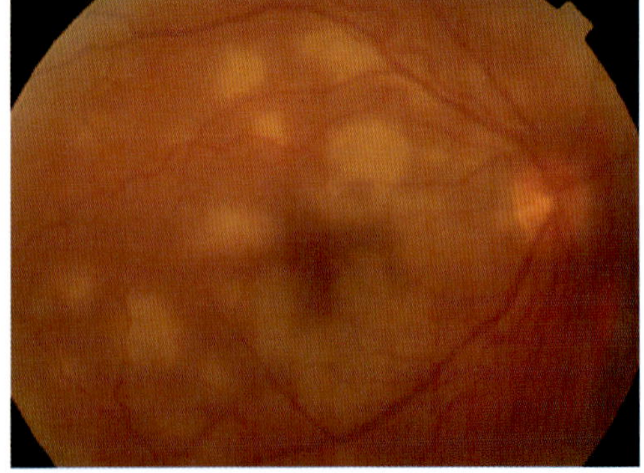

Figure 9-12 Acute posterior multifocal placoid pigment epitheliopathy. Fundus photograph showing multifocal, placoid lesions in the macula. *(Courtesy of Albert T. Vitale, MD.)*

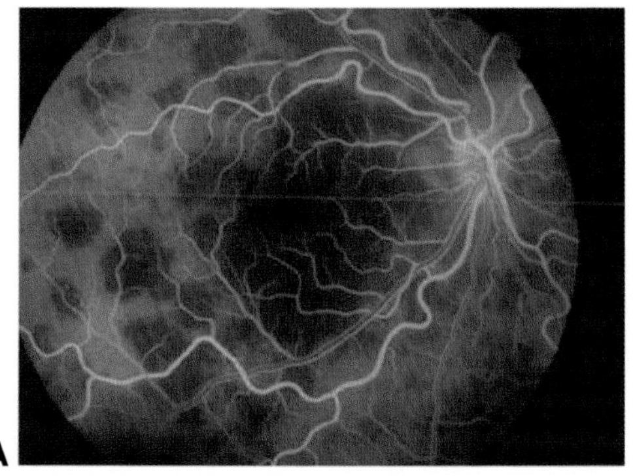

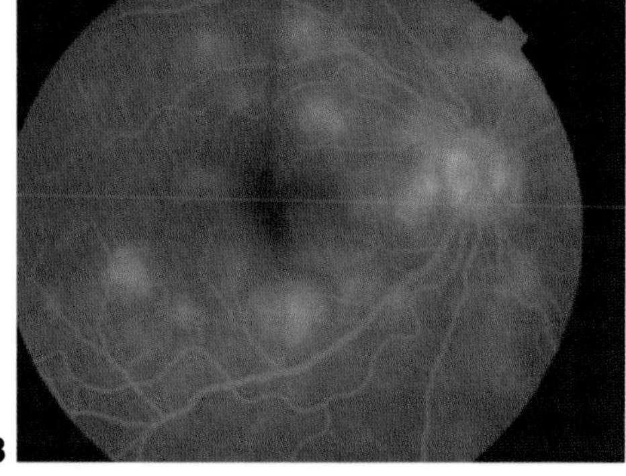

Figure 9-13 Fluorescein angiography image from a patient with acute posterior multifocal placoid pigment epitheliopathy. **A,** Early blockage of choroidal circulation. **B,** Late-phase staining. *(Courtesy of Albert T. Vitale, MD.)*

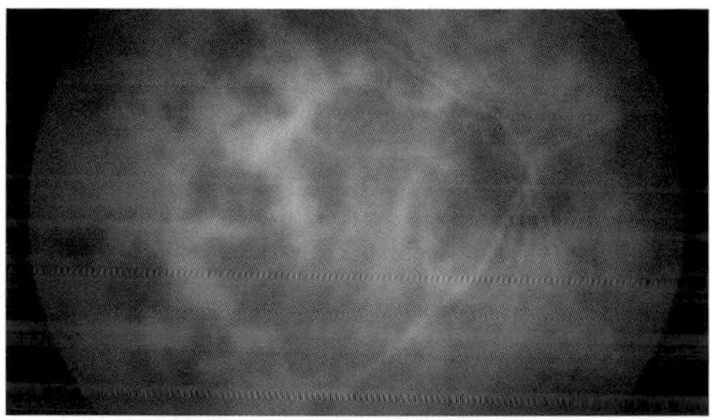

Figure 9-14 Indocyanine green angiography image from a patient with acute posterior multifocal placoid pigment epitheliopathy showing multiple midphase hypocyanescent spots. *(Courtesy of Albert T. Vitale, MD.)*

abnormalities revealed early on FA and ICG angiography are more numerous than the overlying placoid lesions.

Abnormalities noted on FAF imaging lag the clinical appearance of these lesions and are fewer in number. Typically, lesions are initially hyperautofluorescent and may evolve into areas of hypoautofluorescence over time (Fig 9-15). RPE alterations observed during recovery appear well after the choroid is affected.

It remains controversial whether the lesions of APMPPE are due primarily to involvement of the RPE or represent choroidal/choriocapillary perfusion abnormalities with secondary involvement of the RPE and photoreceptors; however, taken together, the FA, ICG, and FAF imaging findings suggest a primary choroidal process. OCT of acute lesions demonstrates hyperreflectivity of the outer retinal layers; subretinal or intraretinal fluid may also be present (Fig 9-16). As the lesions resolve, outer retinal and photoreceptor loss may be observed.

An important differential diagnostic consideration—in addition to choroidal metastasis, viral retinitis, sarcoidosis, VKH syndrome, and pneumocystis choroiditis—is serpiginous choroiditis. APMPPE is an acute, usually nonrecurring disease, whereas serpiginous choroiditis is insidious and progressive.

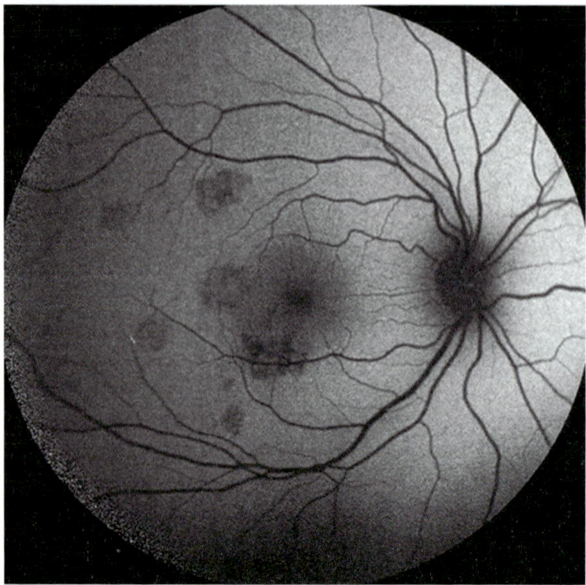

Figure 9-15 Acute posterior multifocal placoid pigment epitheliopathy. Fundus autofluorescence image showing scattered, hypoautofluorescent inactive lesions. *(Courtesy of Bryn M. Burkholder, MD.)*

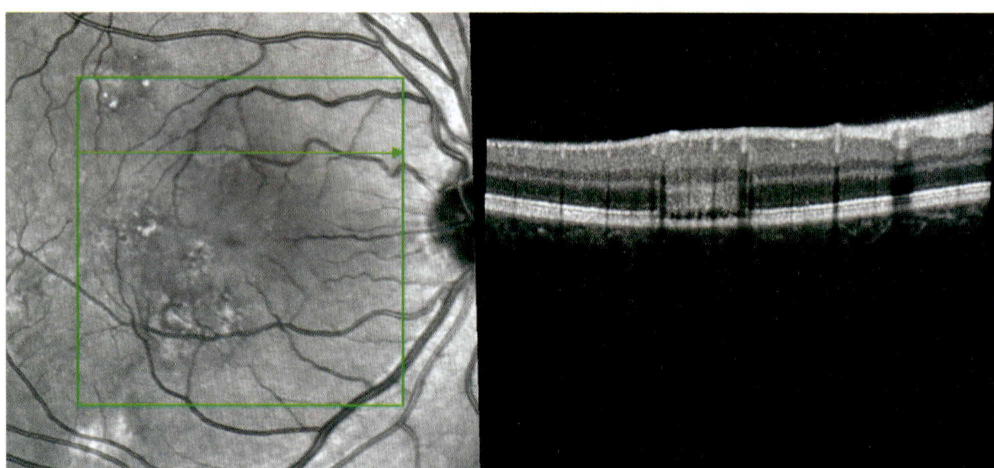

Figure 9-16 Acute posterior multifocal placoid pigment epitheliopathy. Optical coherence tomography image through an active lesion *(arrows)*, demonstrating hyperreflectivity of the outer retina and retinal pigment epithelium, a sliver of subretinal fluid, and focal disruption of the photoreceptor layer. *(Courtesy of Bryn M. Burkholder, MD.)*

Steiner S, Goldstein DA. Imaging in the diagnosis and management of APMPPE. *Int Ophthalmol Clin.* 2012;52(4):211–219.

Prognosis In most patients with APMPPE, visual acuity returns to 20/40 or better within 6 months, although 20% are left with residual visual dysfunction. Risk factors for loss of vision include foveal involvement at presentation, older age at presentation, unilateral disease, a longer interval between initial and fellow eye involvement, and recurrence. No convincing data suggest that treatment with systemic corticosteroids is beneficial in altering the visual outcome, although some authorities advocate such treatment in patients presenting with extensive macular involvement in an effort to limit subsequent RPE derangement of the foveal center. Systemic corticosteroids are also indicated in individuals with an associated CNS vasculitis.

Fiore T, Iaccheri B, Androudi S, et al. Acute posterior multifocal placoid pigment epitheliopathy: outcome and visual prognosis. *Retina*. 2009;29(7):994–1001.

Kaplan HJ. Acute posterior multifocal placoid pigment epitheliopathy and "ampiginous choroiditis" [AAO annual meeting video]. American Academy of Ophthalmology; 2012. https://www.aao.org/annual-meeting-video/apmppe-ampiginous-choroiditis-how-should-these-be-. Accessed November 16, 2020.

Relentless placoid chorioretinitis An uncommon variant termed *relentless placoid chorioretinitis* or *ampiginous choroiditis* has features of both serpiginous choroiditis and APMPPE. Men or women between the second and sixth decades of life present with floaters, photopsias, paracentral scotomata, and decreased vision, as well as variable degrees of anterior segment inflammation and vitritis. The acute retinal lesions are similar to those of APMPPE or serpiginous choroiditis, both clinically and angiographically, but the clinical course is atypical for both entities. Patients have numerous posterior and peripheral lesions predating or occurring simultaneously with macular involvement (Fig 9-17). Acute lesions heal over a period of weeks, with resultant chorioretinal atrophy. Older pigmented areas are observed together with new, active, white placoid lesions that are not necessarily extensions of previous areas of activity. Prolonged periods of disease activity occur, with the appearance of numerous (>50) multifocal lesions scattered throughout the fundus. Relapses are common, and new lesions may appear and progress for up to 2 years after the initial presentation. FA demonstrates early hypofluorescence and late staining of these lesions. Although macular involvement can result in vision loss, metamorphopsia, or scotomata, visual acuity is preserved in most patients upon healing of the lesions.

The precise roles of systemic steroids, antiviral drugs, and IMT in the treatment of relentless placoid chorioretinitis are incompletely understood. Systemic corticosteroids

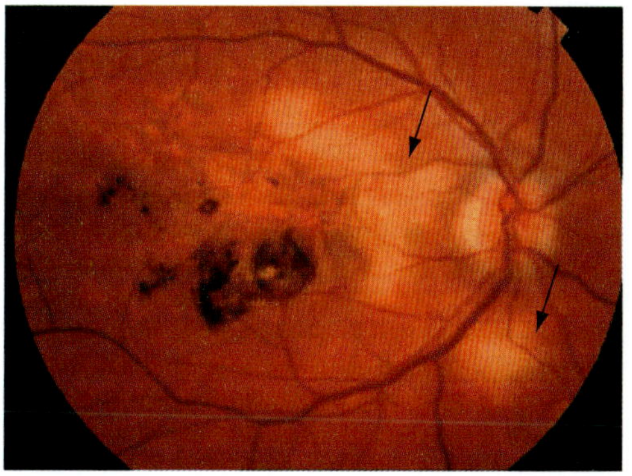

Figure 9-17 Relentless placoid chorioretinitis. Fundus photograph showing retinal pigment epithelial hyperpigmentation and atrophy in the central macula in areas of previous inflammation, with new, yellow-white foci of active disease temporal and inferior to the optic nerve *(arrows)*. *(Courtesy of Albert T. Vitale, MD.)*

are commonly employed, but the disease may recur despite their use. It is important to rule out the presence of tuberculosis-associated serpiginous-like choroiditis.

Jones BE, Jampol LM, Yannuzzi LA, et al. Relentless placoid chorioretinitis: a new entity or an unusual variant of serpiginous chorioretinitis? *Arch Ophthalmol.* 2000;118(7):931–938.

Pagliarini S, Piguet B, Ffytche TJ, Bird AC. Foveal involvement and lack of visual recovery in APMPPE associated with uncommon features. *Eye (Lond).* 1995;9(Pt. 1):42–47.

Serpiginous choroiditis

Serpiginous choroiditis, also known as *geographic* or *helicoid choroidopathy,* is an uncommon, chronic, progressive inflammatory condition affecting adult men and women equally in the second to seventh decades of life. Its etiology is unknown, but it is thought to represent an immune-mediated occlusive vasculitis. With the exception of tuberculosis, which can cause a serpiginous-like choroidopathy, no other infectious organisms have been definitively implicated in this disease. Serpiginous choroiditis has been reported to occur in patients with Crohn disease, sarcoidosis, and PAN, but no consistent systemic disease associations have been identified.

Manifestations Patients present with painless, paracentral scotomata and decreased vision, with minimal vitreous involvement and a quiet anterior chamber. Although patients may present with unilateral symptoms, funduscopy usually reveals asymmetric bilateral scarring. Active areas appear as gray-white lesions at the level of the RPE that project in a pseudopodial or geographic manner from the optic nerve in the posterior fundus (Fig 9-18). Far less

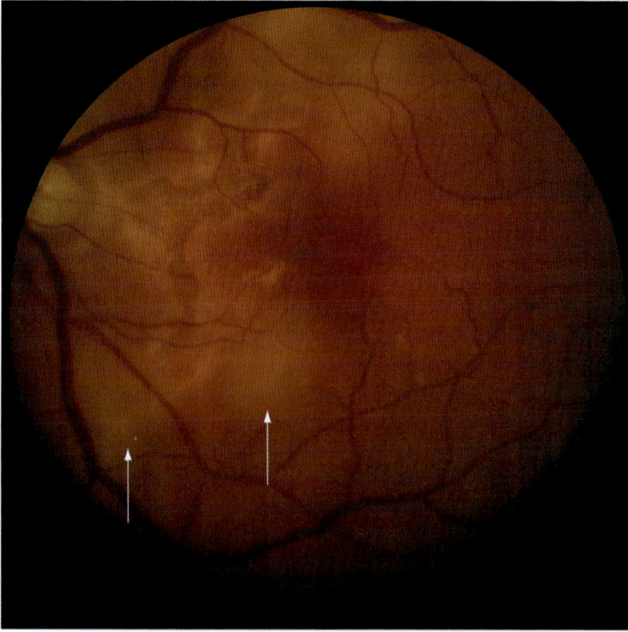

Figure 9-18 Serpiginous choroiditis. Fundus photograph with area of active inflammation inferiorly *(arrows). (Courtesy of Bryn M. Burkholder, MD.)*

commonly, macular or peripheral lesions may present without peripapillary involvement. Disease activity is typically confined to the leading edge of the advancing lesion and may be associated with shallow subretinal fluid. Occasionally, vascular sheathing has been reported along with RPE detachment and neovascularization of the disc. Late findings include atrophy of the choriocapillaris, RPE, and retina, with extensive RPE hyperpigmentation and subretinal fibrosis. CNV may occur at the border of an old scar in up to 25% of patients.

Disease course The disease course is marked by progressive centrifugal extension, with marked asymmetry between the 2 eyes. New lesions and recurrent attacks are typical; up to 38% of affected eyes deteriorate to a visual acuity of 20/200 or worse. Fluorescein angiography may show blockage of the choroidal flush in the early phase and staining of the active edge of the lesion in the later stage of the angiogram (Fig 9-19). In contrast, early hyperfluorescence with late leakage is indicative of the presence of CNV. Indocyanine green angiography reveals hypocyanescence throughout all phases of both acute and old lesions. It may reveal more extensive involvement than FA or clinical examination and may be useful in distinguishing active new serpiginous lesions, which are hypofluorescent, from CNV, which may appear as localized areas of hyperfluorescence during the middle to late phases.

Fundus autofluorescence imaging may be an exquisitely sensitive modality for detecting damage to the RPE and monitoring the clinical course of serpiginous choroiditis. Characteristic hypoautofluorescence corresponds closely to areas of regressed disease activity, and hyperfluorescence highlights areas of active disease (Fig 9-20A). OCT can show increased outer retinal reflectivity and disruption and thickening of the underlying choroid in active disease (Fig 9-20B), and atrophic changes in the retina and RPE in quiescent areas.

Bansal R, Gupta A, Gupta V. Imaging in the diagnosis and management of serpiginous choroiditis. *Int Ophthalmol Clin*. 2012;52(4):229–236.

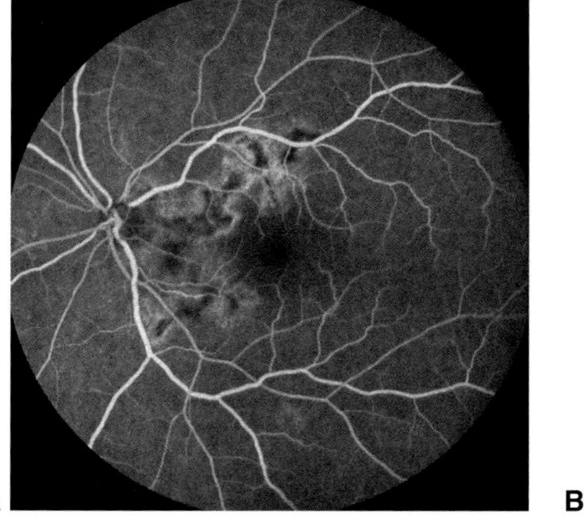

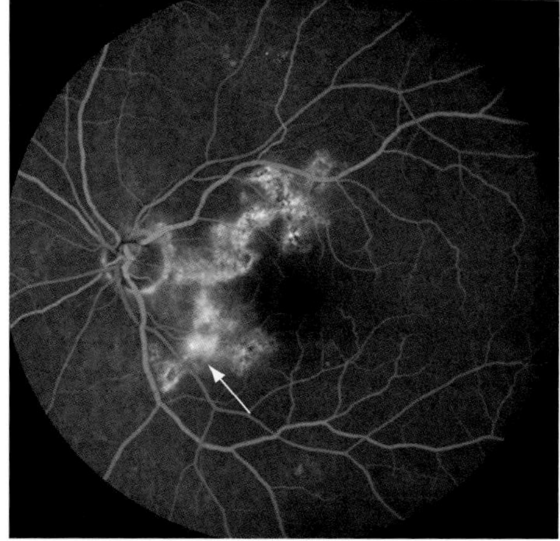

Figure 9-19 Serpiginous choroiditis. Fluorescein angiograms. **A,** Early blocked fluorescence. **B,** Late staining and leakage at the active border of the lesion *(arrow)*. *(Courtesy of Bryn M. Burkholder, MD.)*

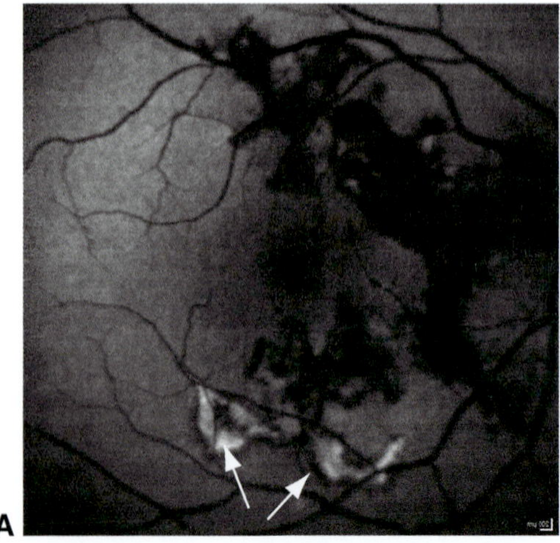

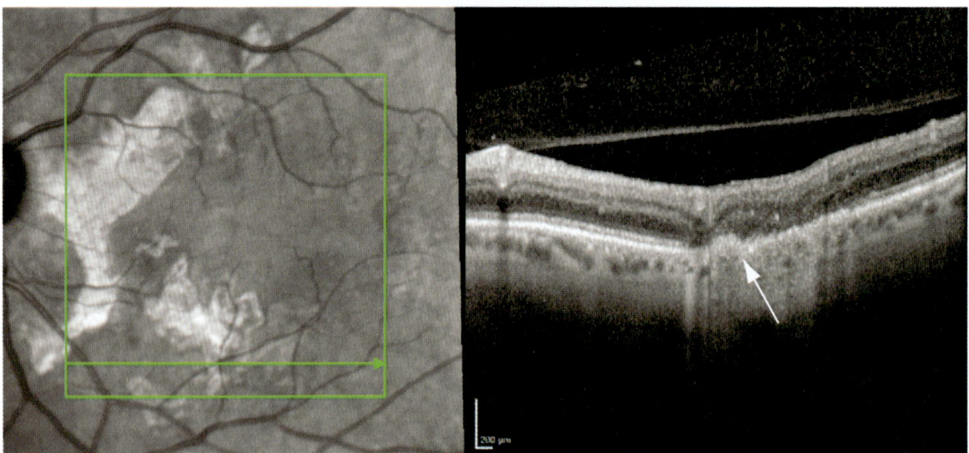

Figure 9-20 Serpiginous choroiditis. **A,** Fundus autofluorescence image showing a hypoautofluorescent area of active inflammation *(arrows)*. **B,** Optical coherence tomography scan through this area demonstrates outer retinal disruption and hyperreflectivity *(arrow)*. *(Courtesy of Bryn M. Burkholder, MD.)*

Treatment Given the small number of patients with serpiginous choroiditis, no consensus has evolved regarding the optimal treatment regimen or its efficacy. Treatments include the following:

- Systemic, periocular, and intravitreal corticosteroids may be used in the treatment of active lesions, particularly lesions threatening the fovea.
- The addition of systemic IMT at the outset has been suggested, as corticosteroids alone are typically insufficient, and patients require prolonged anti-inflammatory therapy.
- Combination therapy with an antimetabolite and a T-cell inhibitor may be effective.

- Cytotoxic therapy with cyclophosphamide or chlorambucil has been shown to induce long, drug-free remissions.
- Intravitreal steroid implants, including the fluocinolone acetonide and dexamethasone implants, may be used in patients intolerant of systemic therapy.
- Intravitreal anti-VEGF drugs, focal laser photocoagulation, and photodynamic therapy are important adjuvant therapies for the treatment of associated CNV.

It is important to distinguish presumed immune-mediated serpiginous choroiditis from infectious entities that can simulate the disease. Although herpetic and syphilitic choroiditis can occasionally mimic serpiginous choroiditis, much more commonly, *Mycobacterium tuberculosis* can cause inflammation in a pattern that simulates typical serpiginous choroiditis. Tuberculosis (TB)-associated disease has been called *multifocal serpiginoid choroiditis* or *serpiginous-like choroiditis* (see Chapter 13).

Patients with serpiginous-like choroiditis tend to be from countries where TB is endemic or have been exposed to active pulmonary TB. In such cases, results of tuberculin skin testing and the interferon-gamma release assay are usually positive for TB, although the chest x-ray often appears normal. The ocular involvement in TB-related serpiginous-like choroiditis is mostly unilateral, with serpiginoid lesions involving the posterior pole, midperiphery, and periphery but usually sparing the juxtapapillary area until late in the disease. The lesions tend to appear and progress in multiple areas rather than to spread out centrifugally as they do in serpiginous choroiditis. Patients with serpiginous-like choroiditis exhibit a more prominent inflammatory cellular reaction in the vitreous than do patients with serpiginous choroiditis. The disease usually responds to anti-TB treatment, although complete control may take months and corticosteroids may also be needed to control inflammation. (See Chapter 9 for a full discussion of TB-associated uveitis.)

Akpek EK, Jabs DA, Tessler HH, Joondeph BC, Foster CS. Successful treatment of serpiginous choroiditis with alkylating agents. *Ophthalmology.* 2002;109(8):1506–1513.

Bansal R, Gupta A, Gupta V, Dogra MR, Sharma A, Bambery P. Tubercular serpiginous-like choroiditis presenting as multifocal serpiginoid choroiditis. *Ophthalmology.* 2012;119(11):2334–2342.

Christmas NJ, Oh KT, Oh DM, Folk JC. Long-term follow-up of patients with serpiginous choroiditis. *Retina.* 2002;22(5):550–556.

Nazari Khanamiri H, Rao NA. Serpiginous choroiditis and infectious multifocal serpiginoid choroiditis. *Surv Ophthalmol.*2013;58(3):203–232.

Rao NA. Serpiginous choroiditis: autoimmune, herpes, or tuberculosis. [American Academy of Ophthalmology Annual Meeting Video Program.] San Francisco: American Academy of Ophthalmology; 2012. Available at www.aao.org/annual-meeting-video/serpiginous-choroiditis-autoimmune-herpes-tubercul. Accessed November 16, 2020.

Multifocal choroiditis and panuveitis

Multifocal choroiditis and panuveitis (MCP), PIC, and the subretinal fibrosis and uveitis syndrome represent a subset of the white dot syndromes. Some authorities regard them as discrete entities, whereas others view them as a single disease with a variable severity continuum. When the disorders are considered a continuum, the term *multifocal choroiditis* may be used to describe all the entities, and the presence of fibrosis or panuveitis is then described separately. For this discussion, the traditional nomenclature is used to discuss the three related diseases as discrete entities.

Essex RW, Wong J, Jampol LM, Dowler J, Bird AC. Idiopathic multifocal choroiditis: a comment on present and past nomenclature. *Retina*. 2013;33(1):1–4.

Manifestations MCP is an idiopathic inflammatory disorder affecting the choroid, retina, and vitreous. It presents asymmetrically, most often in young women with myopia. Symptoms include floaters, photopsias, enlargement of the physiologic blind spot, and decreased vision. The ophthalmoscopic hallmarks include the presence of multiple old, atrophic lesions that appear as punched-out, white-yellow dots (50–200 μm) in a peripapillary, midperipheral, and anterior equatorial distribution (Fig 9-21).

Acute lesions have a creamier, opaque appearance and develop more discrete borders over time. Varying degrees of anterior segment inflammation and vitritis are uniformly present, which differentiate this condition from OHS or PIC. The lesions are smaller than those present in birdshot chorioretinopathy or APMPPE, are larger than those found in PIC, and evolve into atrophic scars with varying degrees of hyperpigmentation. New lesions may appear, and peripheral chorioretinal streaks and peripapillary pigment changes similar to those present in OHS have been observed. Subretinal fibrosis with RPE clumping is much more common in MCP than in OHS. Structural complications noted at presentation may include cataract, uveitis macular edema, ERM, and CNV and are frequent causes of visual impairment.

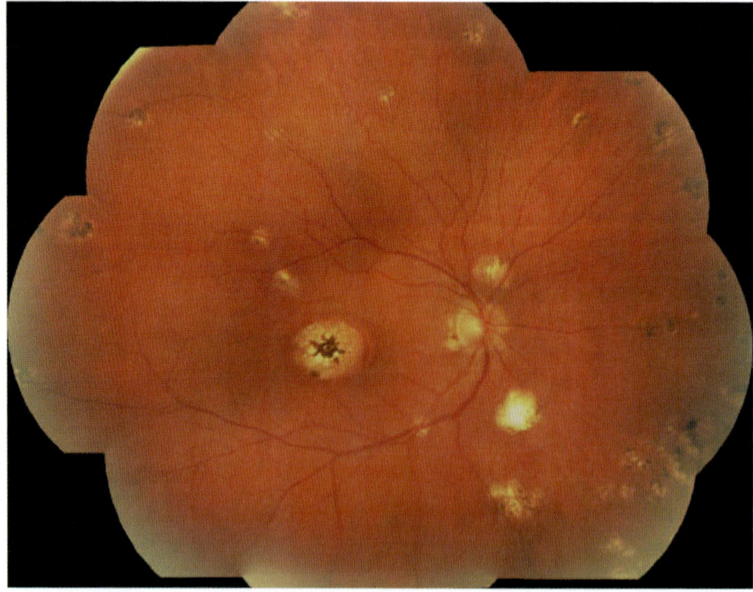

Figure 9-21 Multifocal choroiditis and panuveitis. Fundus photograph. *(Courtesy of Ramana S. Moorthy, MD.)*

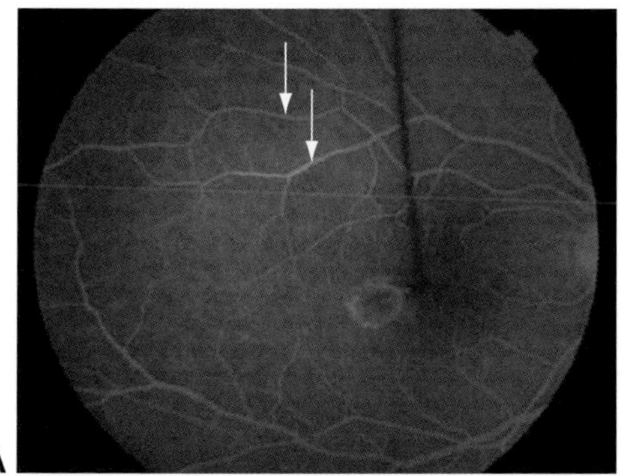

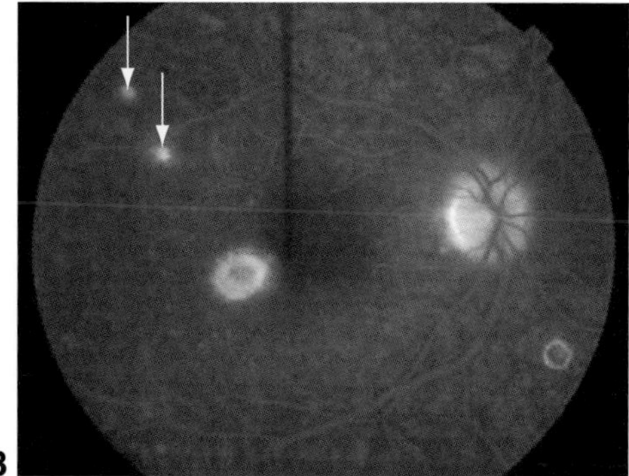

Figure 9-22 Multifocal choroiditis and panuveitis. Fluorescein angiograms. **A,** Early blocked fluorescence *(arrows)*. **B,** Late staining of lesions *(arrows)*. *(Courtesy of Ramana S. Moorthy, MD.)*

Fluorescein angiography shows early hypofluorescence with late staining of acute active lesions, whereas atrophic lesions produce transmission defects (early hyperfluorescence that fades in the late phases of the angiogram). Early hyperfluorescence and late leakage are observed in the presence of macular edema and CNV (Fig 9-22).

As in birdshot chorioretinopathy, ICG angiography reveals multiple midphase hypocyanescent lesions compatible with active choroiditis that are more numerous than those apparent on clinical examination or FA; they are frequently clustered around the optic nerve. This finding may correlate with an enlarged blind spot on visual field testing. The hypofluorescent spots may fade with resolution of the intraocular inflammation.

The most common findings on FAF imaging are punctate hypoautofluorescent spots (≥125 μm) corresponding to multiple areas of chorioretinal atrophy; however, smaller (<125 μm) spots numbering in the hundreds may be seen in the macular and peripapillary regions that are not visible on fundus examination. Some of these lesions will later develop into clinically evident chorioretinal scars (Fig 9-23). Active MCP lesions display hyperautofluorescence that disappears with minimal RPE disruption following anti-inflammatory treatment. Fundus autofluorescence findings in MCP suggest that patients have more widespread involvement of the RPE than indicated by other imaging modalities; therefore, FAF may be useful in monitoring response to treatment.

Optical coherence tomography may show drusenlike material beneath the RPE at the site of visible spots that can be associated with more widespread disruption of the overlying outer retina (Fig 9-24). There is also choroidal hyperreflectivity beneath these deposits.

The herpes simplex and Epstein-Barr viruses have been implicated in this disease process; however, a viral etiology has not been proven. Pathologic specimens obtained from eyes with MCP have shown variable findings, ranging from large numbers of B lymphocytes in the choroid to a predominance of T lymphocytes, suggesting that different immune mechanisms may produce a similar clinical picture, and that an initial viral infection may trigger an autoimmune process.

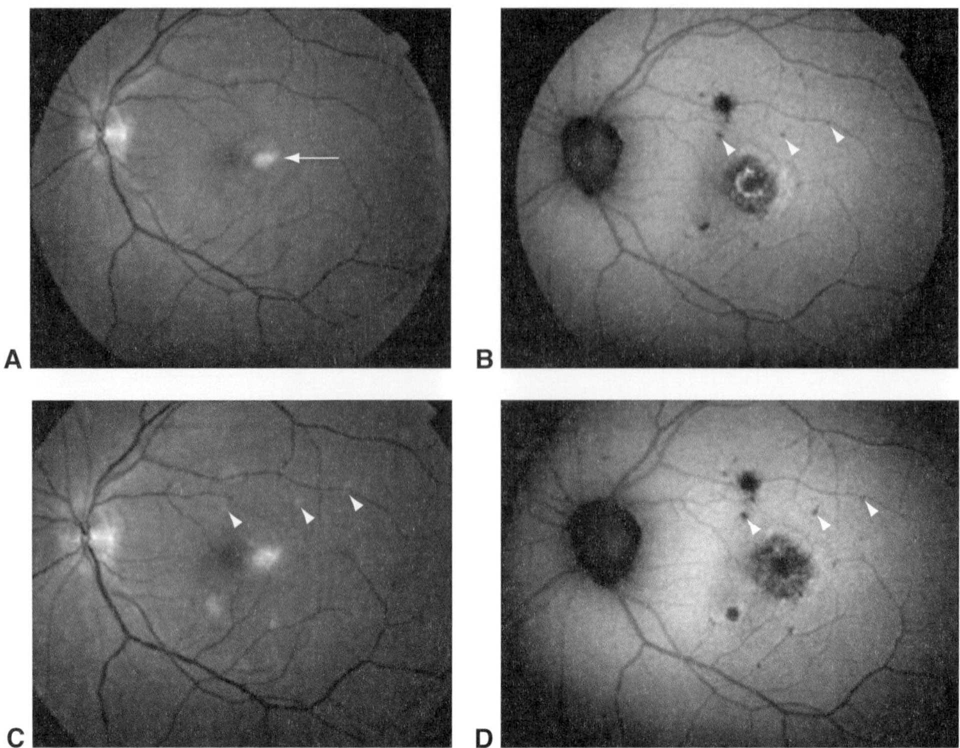

Figure 9-23 Images from a 36-year-old woman with multifocal choroiditis and panuveitis. **A,** Fundus photograph showing an area of choroidal neovascularization *(arrow)* treated with photodynamic therapy 3 years earlier. **B,** Fundus autofluorescence (FAF) image shows multiple hypoautofluorescent spots *(arrowheads)* that did not correspond to ophthalmoscopically visible lesions. **C,** Three years later, fundus photograph shows multiple visible spots *(arrowheads)* corresponding to previously visualized hypoautofluorescent spots. **D,** FAF photograph taken at the same time as **C** shows corresponding hypoautofluorescent spots *(arrowheads)*, which are slightly enlarged from the previous study. *(Reprinted with permission from Haen SP, Spaide RF. Fundus autofluorescence in multifocal choroiditis and panuveitis.* Am J Ophthalmol. *2008;145[5]:850.)*

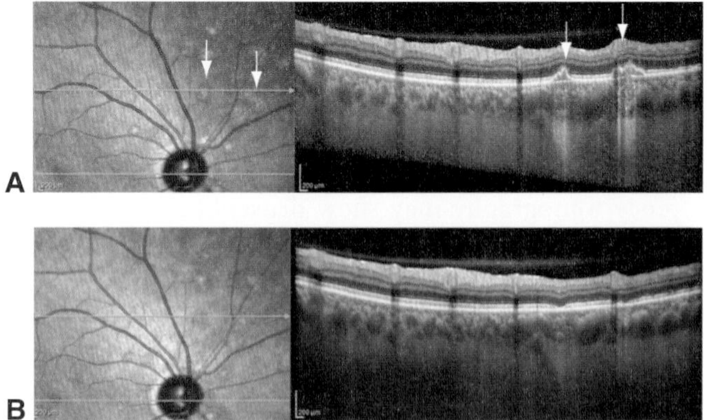

Figure 9-24 Multifocal choroiditis. **A,** Optical coherence tomography (OCT) image through 2 active lesions *(arrows)*. **B,** OCT slice through same area of retina, with resolution of active lesions after treatment. *(Courtesy of Wendy M. Smith, MD.)*

Yeh S, Forooghian F, Wong WT, et al. Fundus autofluorescence imaging of the white dot syndromes. *Arch Ophthalmol.* 2010;128(1):46–56.

Diagnosis The diagnosis is one of exclusion, as many other conditions—such as sarcoidosis, syphilis, and TB—may produce lesions similar in appearance to those of MCP.

Treatment Systemic and periocular corticosteroids may be effective for the treatment of macular edema and have been shown to induce regression of CNV in some patients. Corticosteroid-sparing strategies with IMT are frequently required because of the chronic, recurrent nature of the inflammation; these treatments have been successful in achieving not only inflammatory quiescence but also an 83% reduction in the risk of posterior pole complications (macular edema, ERM, and CNV) and a 92% reduction in the risk of vision loss to 20/200 or worse in affected eyes. The intravitreal fluocinolone acetonide implant is also a potential treatment option for patients who cannot tolerate systemic therapy. Intravitreal anti-VEGF drugs are important adjuncts for the treatment of CNV. However, active inflammation can stimulate neovascularization and blunt the effectiveness of these treatments, so it is important that inflammation also be well controlled. This concept applies to any uveitic entity complicated by CNV.

Haen SP, Spaide RF. Fundus autofluorescence in multifocal choroiditis and panuveitis. *Am J Ophthalmol.* 2008;145(5):847–853.

Michel SS, Ekong A, Baltatzis S, Foster CS. Multifocal choroiditis and panuveitis: immunomodulatory therapy. *Ophthalmology.* 2002;109(2):378–383.

Spaide RF, Goldberg N, Freund KB. Redefining multifocal choroiditis and panuveitis and punctate inner choroidopathy through multimodal imaging. *Retina.* 2013;33(7):1315–1324.

Prognosis The visual prognosis is guarded, with permanent vision loss in at least 1 eye occurring in up to 75% of patients as a result of the complications associated with chronic, recurrent inflammation. In one study, the incidence of vision loss to 20/200 or worse was 12% per eye-year in the affected eye.

Thorne JE, Wittenberg S, Jabs DA, et al. Multifocal choroiditis with panuveitis: incidence of ocular complications and loss of visual acuity. *Ophthalmology.* 2006;113(12):2310–2316.

Punctate inner choroiditis

Punctate inner choroiditis is an idiopathic inflammatory disorder that, like MCP, predominantly occurs in otherwise healthy myopic White women, but it presents at a younger median age (29 vs 45 years, respectively).

Manifestations Patients with PIC can present with metamorphopsia, paracentral scotomata, photopsias, and asymmetric loss of central acuity. In contrast to the lesions of MCP, those of PIC are smaller (100–200 μm), rarely extend to the midperiphery, and are never associated with vitritis (Fig 9-25). They progress to atrophic scars, sometimes leaving a halo of pigmentation, and appear deeper and more punched-out than those of MCP. Macular edema is rarely seen in this condition, although serous retinal detachments may be found over confluent PIC lesions. With the exception of CNV, patients with PIC have

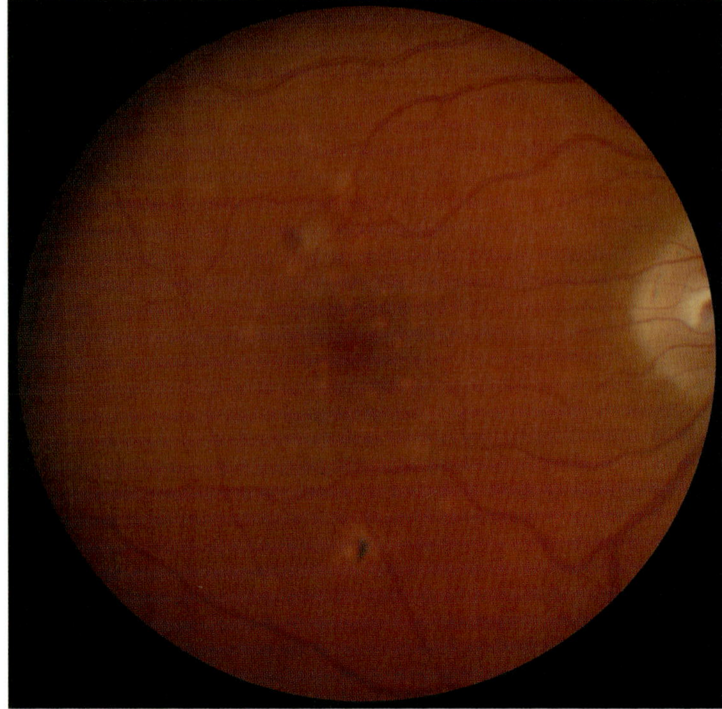

Figure 9-25 Punctate inner choroiditis. Fundus photograph. *(Courtesy of Bryn M. Burkholder, MD.)*

few structural complications (cataract, macular edema, or ERM) at presentation, unlike patients with MCP, a difference undoubtedly related to the presence of chronic intraocular inflammation in MCP. Choroidal neovascularization, a common vision-threatening complication in both entities, may be more frequent at presentation in patients with PIC (79%) than with MCP (28%), but patients with MCP are more likely to have bilateral visual impairment of visual acuity 20/50 or worse.

Fluorescein angiography studies in patients with PIC show early hypofluorescence of the inflammatory lesions with late staining, although early hyperfluorescence can also occur, especially if CNV is present (Figs 9-26, 9-27). Indocyanine green angiography displays midphase hypocyanescence throughout the posterior pole in a peripapillary distribution that may exceed the lesions apparent on FA and clinical examination (Fig 9-28); these imaging studies may be employed to delineate disease extent and monitor its activity. OCT findings are similar to those seen in MCP and may be useful in identifying CNV (Fig 9-29).

Kedhar SR, Thorne JE, Wittenberg S, Dunn JP, Jabs DA. Multifocal choroiditis with panuveitis and punctate inner choroidopathy: comparison of clinical characteristics at presentation. *Retina*. 2007;27(9):1174–1179.

Leung TG, Moradi A, Liu D, et al. Clinical features and incidence rate of ocular complications in punctate inner choroidopathy. *Retina*. 2014;34(8):1666–1674.

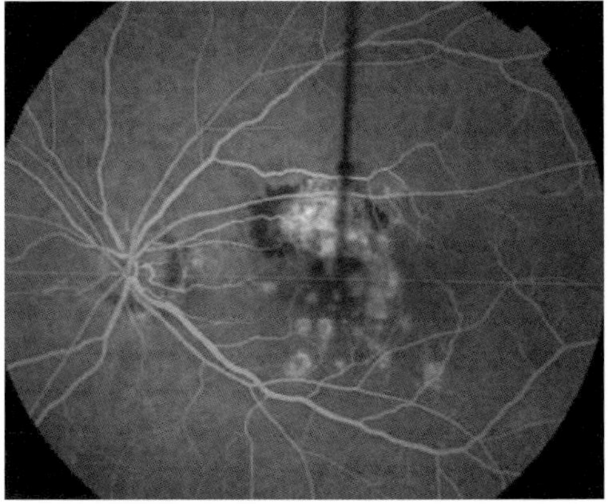

Figure 9-26 Punctate inner choroiditis. Fluorescein angiogram showing early hyperfluorescence of lesions and choroidal neovascularization. *(Courtesy of Albert T. Vitale, MD.)*

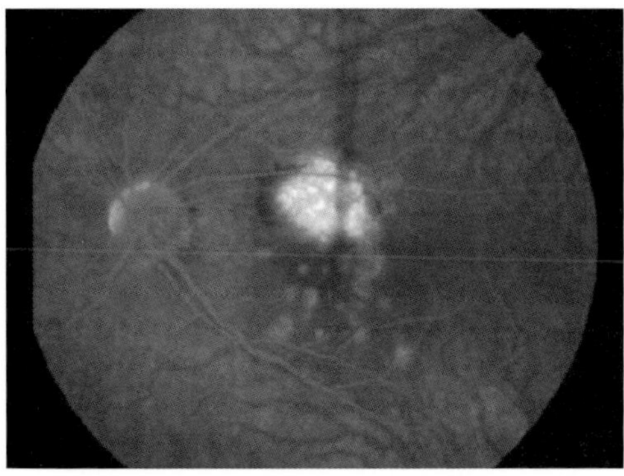

Figure 9-27 Punctate inner choroiditis. Fluorescein angiogram showing late staining of lesions with leakage from choroidal neovascularization. *(Courtesy of Albert T. Vitale, MD.)*

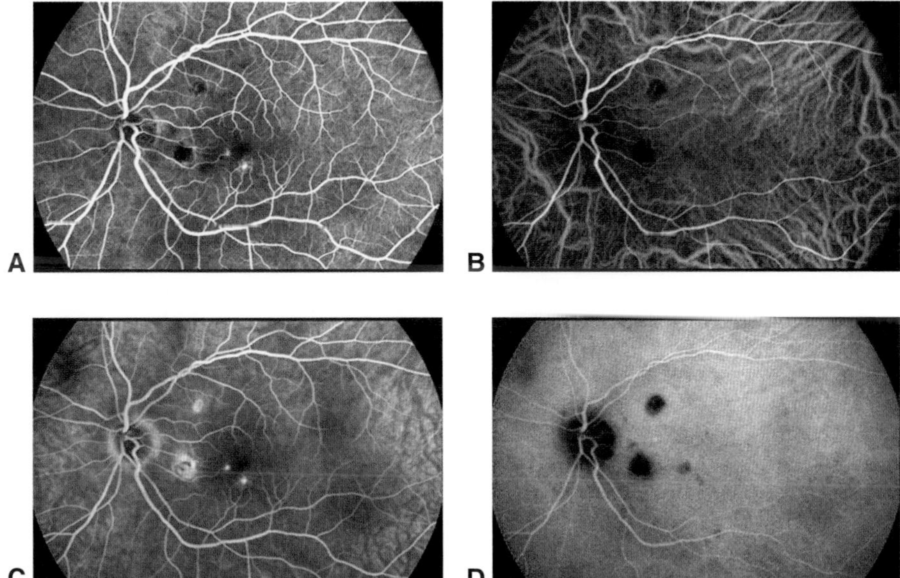

Figure 9-28 Punctate inner choroiditis (PIC). Fluorescein angiograms demonstrating early hyperfluoresence **(A)** and late staining **(C)** of PIC lesions. Corresponding early **(B)** and late **(D)** indocyanine green angiography demonstrating multiple hypocyanescent spots. *(Courtesy of Wendy M. Smith, MD.)*

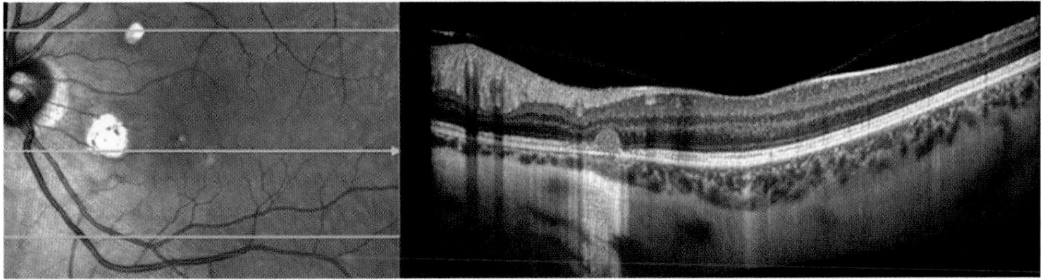

Figure 9-29 Optical coherence tomography scan through an active punctate inner choroiditis lesion. *(Courtesy of Wendy M. Smith, MD.)*

Treatment Treatment should target both inflammation and its complications. Options include local and systemic corticosteroids and IMT. Depending on disease severity, some eyes may be carefully observed without treatment. Intravitreal anti-VEGF drugs may be considered in eyes with CNV. The visual prognosis is favorable in eyes without CNV involving the foveal center.

Subretinal fibrosis and uveitis syndrome

Subretinal fibrosis and uveitis syndrome is an extremely uncommon panuveitis of unknown etiology affecting otherwise healthy myopic females between the ages of 20 and 40 years.

Manifestations and differential diagnosis Significant anterior segment inflammation and mild to moderate vitritis are typically present bilaterally, with white-yellow lesions (50–500 μm) located in the posterior pole to midperiphery at the level of the RPE. These lesions may fade without RPE alterations, become atrophic, or enlarge and coalesce into large, white, stellate zones of subretinal fibrosis (Figs 9-30, 9-31). Serous neurosensory retinal detachment, macular edema, and CNV may also be observed.

Histopathologic studies of eyes with this disease reveal a lymphocytic granulomatous infiltration of the choroid with marked gliosis of the retina and subretinal fibrosis. It has been theorized that this is an immune-driven destruction of RPE, which is replaced by fibrotic tissue.

Fluorescein angiography shows multiple areas of blocked choroidal fluorescence and hyperfluorescence in the early stages of the study; in the late phase, staining of the lesions without leakage is observed. Optical coherence tomography shows variable retinal edema, subretinal fluid, and subretinal fibrosis. The differential diagnosis includes sarcoidosis, OHS, APMPPE, syphilis, TB, birdshot chorioretinopathy, pathologic myopia, sympathetic ophthalmia, and toxoplasmosis.

Kim MK, Chan CC, Belfort R Jr, et al. Histopathologic and immunohistopathologic features of subretinal fibrosis and uveitis syndrome. *Am J Ophthalmol.* 1987;104(1):15–23.

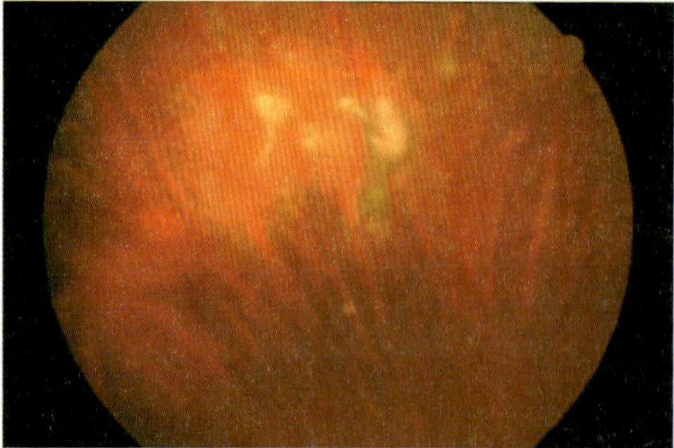

Figure 9-30 Subretinal fibrosis and uveitis syndrome. Fundus photograph showing multifocal white subretinal lesions. *(Courtesy of E. Mitchel Opremcak, MD.)*

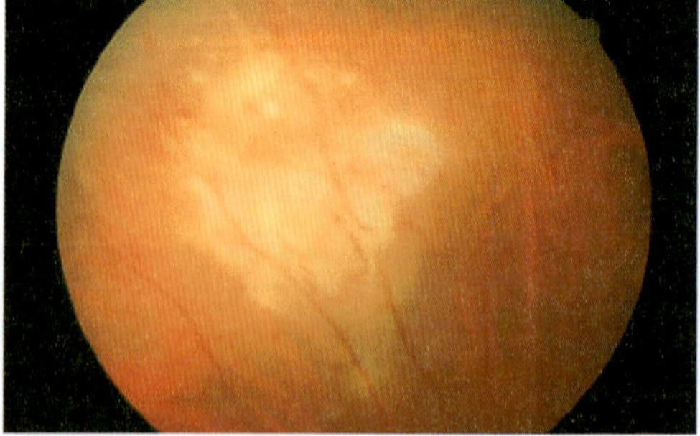

Figure 9-31 Subretinal fibrosis and uveitis syndrome. Fundus photograph from the same patient as in Figure 9-30, showing progressive subretinal fibrosis. *(Courtesy of E. Mitchel Opremcak, MD.)*

Disease course and treatment The course of the disease is marked by chronic recurrent inflammation, and the visual prognosis is guarded. Treatment with systemic corticosteroids and IMT has shown variable success. Recent reports suggest that biologic agents may have some efficacy.

Adán A, Sanmarti R, Burés A, Casaroli-Marano RP. Successful treatment with infliximab in a patient with diffuse subretinal fibrosis syndrome. *Am J Ophthalmol.* 2007;143(3):533–534.

Brown J Jr, Folk JC, Reddy CV, Kimura AE. Visual prognosis of multifocal choroiditis, punctate inner choroidopathy, and the diffuse subretinal fibrosis syndrome. *Ophthalmology.* 1996;103(7):1100–1105.

Cornish KS, Kuffova L, Forrester JV. Treatment of diffuse subretinal fibrosis uveitis with rituximab. *Br J Ophthalmol.* 2015;99(2):153–154.

Multiple evanescent white dot syndrome

Multiple evanescent white dot syndrome (MEWDS) is an uncommon idiopathic inflammatory condition of the retina that typically affects otherwise healthy, young, moderately myopic females in the second to fourth decades of life.

Manifestations In MEWDS, patients present with acute, unilateral decreased vision, photopsias, and central or paracentral scotomata. An antecedent viral prodrome occurs in approximately one-third of cases. Funduscopy during the acute phase of the disease reveals multiple, discrete, white-to-orange spots (100–200 µm) at the level of the RPE or deep retina, typically in a perifoveal location (Fig 9 32), but can be found in the midperiphery and peripheral retina as well. These spots are transitory and frequently missed. A granular macular pigmentary change is usually present—a pathognomonic finding that can be very useful in making the diagnosis when patients present with symptoms after the white dots have faded. Bilateral disease has been reported in rare cases. There may be variable degrees of vitreous inflammation, mild blurring of the optic disc, and, in rare instances, isolated vascular sheathing.

Fluorescein angiography reveals characteristic, late-staining punctate hyperfluorescent lesions in a wreath-like configuration surrounding the fovea (Fig 9-33).

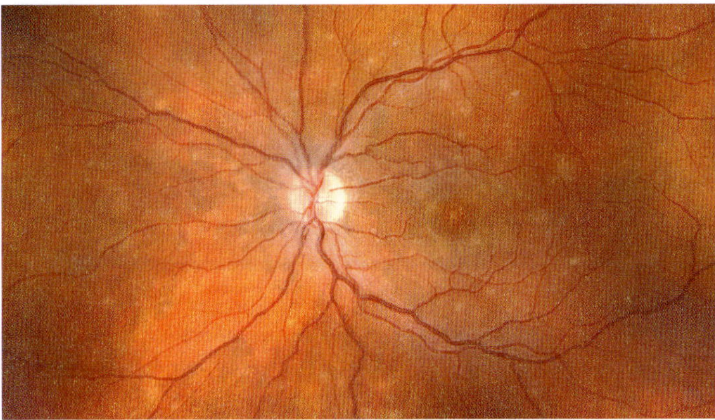

Figure 9-32 Multiple evanescent white dot syndrome. Multiple discrete, punctate, yellowish perifoveal dots. *(Courtesy of Wendy M. Smith, MD.)*

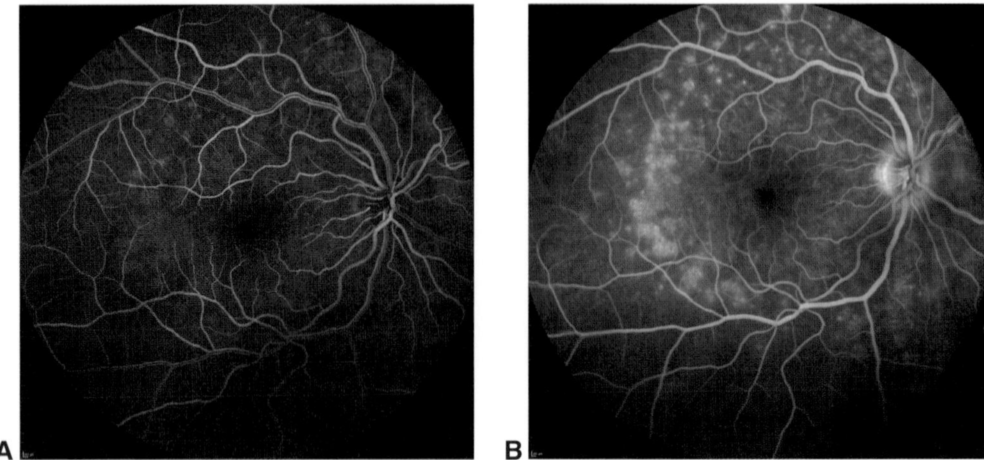

Figure 9-33 Multiple evanescent white dot syndrome. Fluorescein angiogram. **A,** Early phase with multiple punctate hyperfluorescent lesions surrounding the fovea. **B,** The lesions stain late in a wreath-like configuration. *(Courtesy of Bryn M. Burkholder, MD.)*

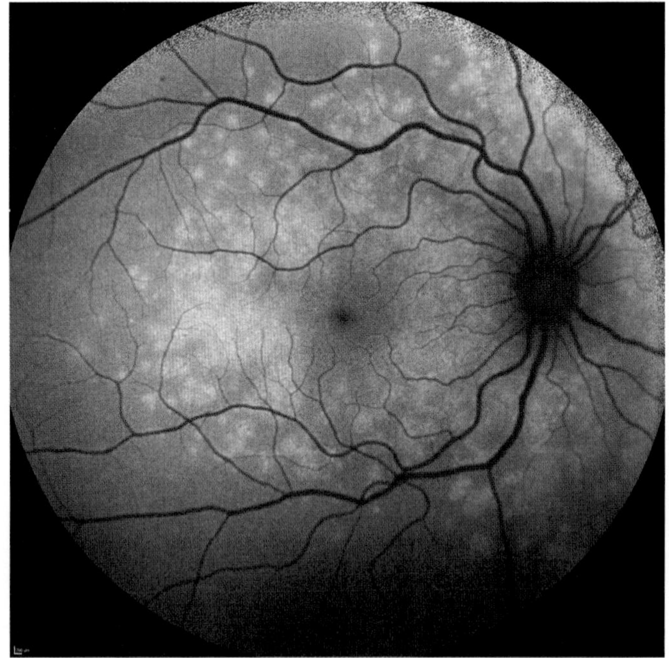

Figure 9-34 Multiple evanescent white dot syndrome. Fundus autofluorescence image of the same patient as in Figure 9-33, showing multiple hypoautofluorescent spots in the same configuration as seen on the angiogram. *(Courtesy of Bryn M. Burkholder, MD.)*

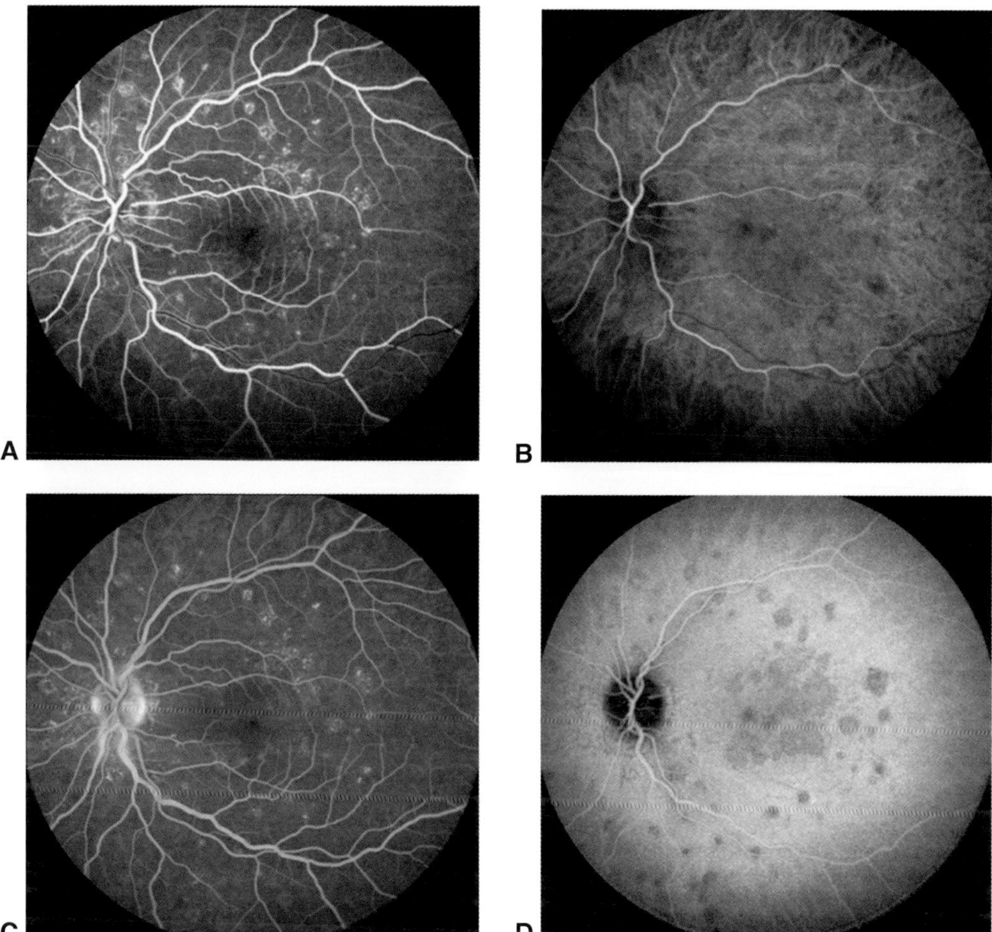

Figure 9-35 Multiple evanescent white dot syndrome (MEWDS). Fluorescein angiogram demonstrating early hyperfluoresence **(A)** and late staining **(C)** of wreath-like configurations of MEWDS lesions. Corresponding early **(B)** and late **(D)** indocyanine green angiograms demonstrating multiple hypocyanescent lesions. *(Courtesy of Wendy M. Smith, MD.)*

Fundus autofluorescence imaging shows hyperfluorescent spots corresponding to and exceeding those found on clinical examination (Fig 9-34) and may also show small, punctate hypoautofluorescent areas localized around the optic disc and posterior pole. The lesions on FAF may show delayed resolution than clinically apparent lesions. Indocyanine green angiography shows multiple hypocyanescent lesions that are more numerous than those apparent on clinical examination or FA and that typically fade with resolution of the disease (Fig 9-35).

Visual field abnormalities are variable and include generalized depression, paracentral or peripheral scotomata, and enlargement of the blind spot. The ERG reveals diminished a-wave and early receptor potential (ERP) amplitudes, both of which are reversible. Results of the multifocal ERG (mfERG) and electro-oculogram (EOG) localize the disease process to the RPE–photoreceptor complex rather than to the choroid.

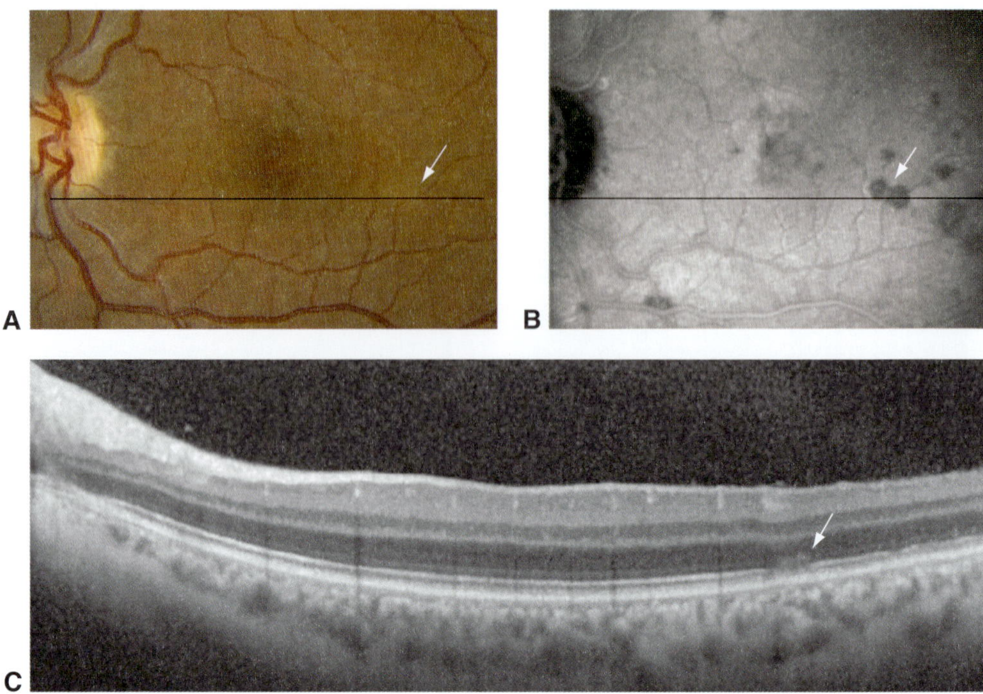

Figure 9-36 Multiple evanescent white dot syndrome. **A,** Color fundus photograph shows subtle spots *(arrow)* and foveal granularity. **B,** Indocyanine green angiogram shows more spots *(arrow)* than are apparent on the color photograph. **C,** Spectral-domain optical coherence tomography image of the spots (positioned at *horizontal lines* in **A** and **B**) shows disruption of the inner/outer segment line (ellipsoid zone) *(arrow)*. *(Courtesy of Janet L. Davis, MD, and Charles Wycoff, MD.)*

Further support for localization of the disease process to the RPE–photoreceptor complex comes from the demonstration of abnormal photoreceptor inner/outer segment line (ellipsoid zone) reflectivity on spectral-domain optical coherence tomography (SD-OCT), the corresponding findings of hypocyanescent spots visualized on ICG angiography, and changes in microperimetry sensitivity (Fig 9-36). These abnormalities completely resolve during the course of the disease.

Hangai M, Fujimoto M, Yoshimura N. Features and function of multiple evanescent white dot syndrome. *Arch Ophthalmol.* 2009;127(10):1307–1313.

Thomas BJ, Albini TA, Flynn HW Jr. Multiple evanescent white dot syndrome: multimodal imaging and correlation with proposed pathophysiology. *Ophthalmic Surg Lasers Imaging Retina.* 2013;44(6):584–587.

Prognosis The prognosis is excellent, with recovery of vision within 2–10 weeks without treatment; however, residual symptoms including photopsias and enlargement of the blind spot may persist for months. Recurrences are uncommon (10%–15% of patients) and have a similarly good prognosis.

Disease associations The syndrome has been reported in association with MCP, acute zonal occult outer retinopathy, and acute macular neuroretinopathy (AMN). The last is a rare condition that affects otherwise healthy young women. It is characterized by the acute onset of visual impairment and multiple scotomata that correspond to reddish-brown, flat, wedge-shaped lesions in the macula that are best appreciated on infrared imaging. Associated risk factors suggest microvascular etiology. AMN has been associated with nonspecific febrile illness, use of oral contraceptives, and epinephrine/ephedrine use.

Acute retinal pigment epitheliitis

Acute retinal pigment epitheliitis, or Krill disease, is a benign, self-limited inflammatory disorder of the RPE of unknown etiology. It typically presents in otherwise healthy young adults between the ages of 16 and 40 years with acute unilateral vision loss, central metamorphopsia, and scotomata. No treatment is required, as the lesions resolve without sequelae over 6–12 weeks.

Manifestations Ophthalmoscopic findings include clusters of small, discrete, hyperpigmented lesions, typically with a yellow halo, in the posterior pole, without associated vitritis (Fig 9-37A). Fluorescein angiography shows early hyperfluorescence of the pinpoint dots with a surrounding halo of hyperfluorescence and late staining (Fig 9-37B). Fundus autofluorescence results have been variable, with some reports of normal autofluorescence and some with hypoautofluorescent spots, corresponding to the fundus lesions. Visual field testing shows central scotomata. Abnormal EOG findings, in the setting of a normal ERG, localize the disease process to the RPE. Optical coherence tomography shows transient disruption of the ellipsoid zone, along with wider disruption of the RPE inner band.

Aydoğan T, Güney E, Akçay Bİ, Bozkurt TK, Ünlü C, Ergin A. Acute retinal pigment epitheliitis: spectral domain optical coherence tomography, fluorescein angiography, and autofluorescence findings. *Case Rep Med.* 2015;2015:149497.

Baillif S, Wolff B, Paoli V, Gastaud P, Mauget-Faÿsse M. Retinal fluorescein and indocyanine green angiography and spectral-domain optical coherence tomography findings in acute retinal pigment epitheliitis. *Retina.* 2011;31(6):1156–1163.

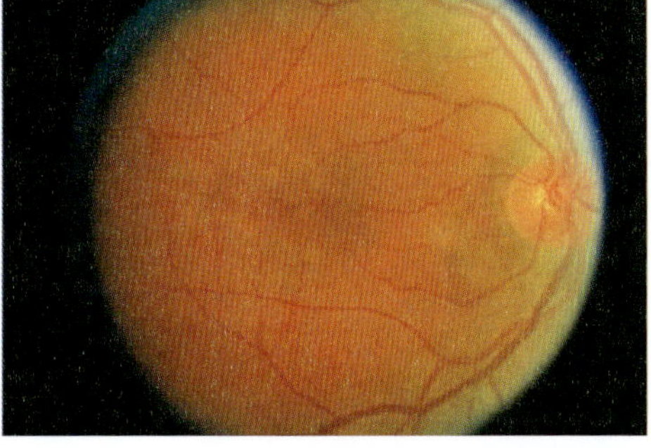

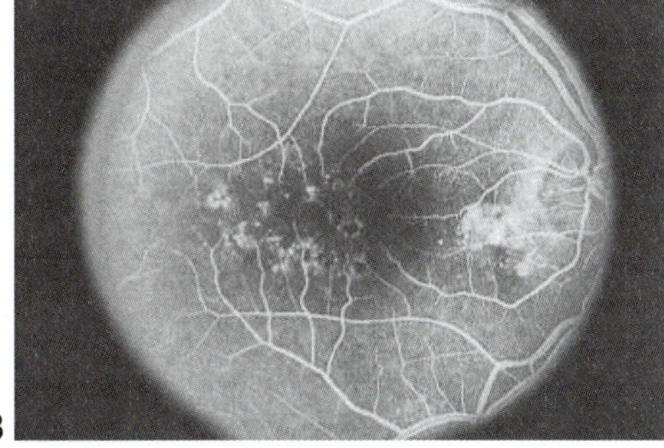

Figure 9-37 Acute retinal pigment epitheliitis. **A,** Fundus photograph. **B,** Fluorescein angiogram showing honeycomb lesions at the level of the retinal pigment epithelium. *(Courtesy of E. Mitchel Opremcak, MD.)*

Cho HJ, Han SY, Cho SW, et al. Acute retinal pigment epitheliitis: spectral-domain optical coherence tomography findings in 18 cases. *Invest Ophthalmol Vis Sci.* 2014;55(5):3314–3319.

Acute zonal occult outer retinopathy

Acute zonal occult outer retinopathy (AZOOR) is typified by acute loss of 1 or more zones of outer retinal function associated with photopsias and visual field loss, often in the setting of a normal-appearing fundus. Patients are typically young, myopic women who present with acute unilateral visual disturbances, sometimes associated with a mild vitritis (50%), and visual acuity in the 20/40 range.

Manifestations Electrophysiological studies demonstrate abnormality not only at the photoreceptor–RPE complex but also at the inner retinal level. Essentially, this dysfunction consists of a delayed 30-Hz flicker ERG and a reduction in the EOG light rise, which, when present with classic symptomatology, may be helpful diagnostically. Visual field changes include paracentral defects and enlargement of the blind spot, even in the absence of any visible fundus changes.

With disease progression, subtle RPE changes may develop, with depigmentation in areas of vision loss (Fig 9-38). Occasionally a demarcation line can be seen at the edge of active disease expansion. In later stages of disease, vessel attenuation, late pigment migration, and focal perivenous sheathing may be seen.

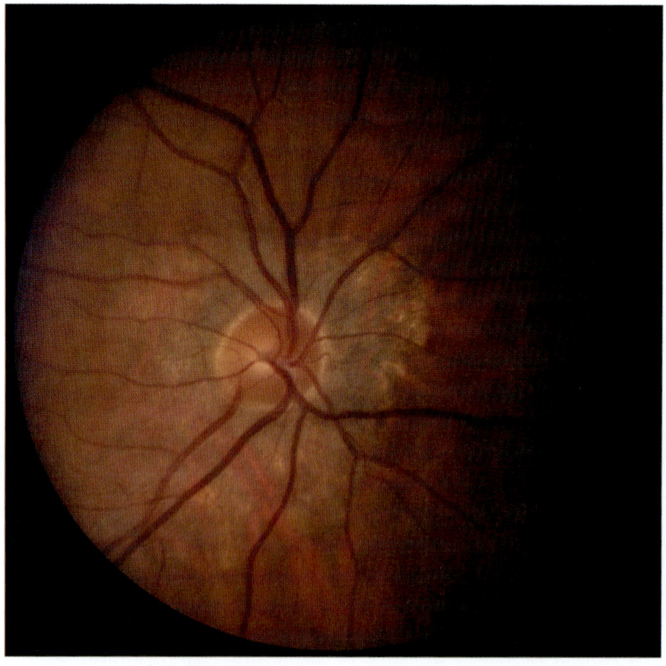

Figure 9-38 Acute zonal occult outer retinopathy. Fundus photograph demonstrates peripapillary changes in the retinal pigment epithelium, which are more apparent in the fundus autofluorescence image (see Figure 9-40). *(Courtesy of Bryn M. Burkholder, MD.)*

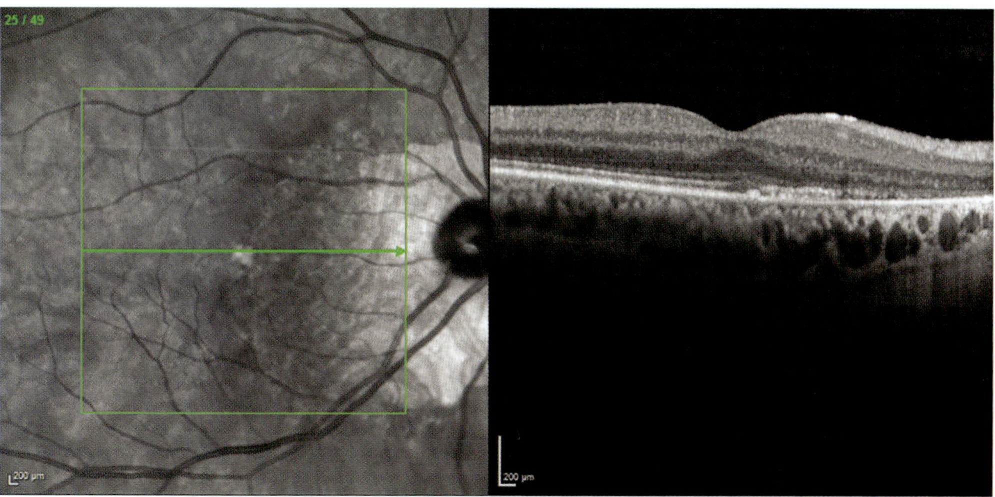

Figure 9-39 Acute zonal occult outer retinopathy. Optical coherence tomography scan from the patient in Figure 9-38 demonstrates loss of the peripapillary ellipsoid zone. *(Courtesy of Bryn M. Burkholder, MD.)*

Optical coherence tomography demonstrates areas of loss or irregularity of the ellipsoid zone, corresponding to the visual field defects, and suggests that photoreceptor outer segment dysfunction and/or degeneration is the primary lesion in AZOOR (Fig 9-39).

During the early disease stages, FA findings may be essentially normal, showing only a prolonged retinal circulation time. With disease progression, however, diffuse areas of hyperfluorescence due to window defects, corresponding to zones of RPE derangement, may develop.

Fundus autofluorescence imaging may be particularly useful in monitoring patients with AZOOR, as it reveals conspicuous areas of central hypoautofluorescence corresponding to RPE and choriocapillary atrophy; peripheral hyperautofluorescence is found at the border of the expanding lesion, due to the presence of lipofuscin-laden cells that presage RPE cell death (Fig 9-40). There may also be diffuse zones of speckled hyperautofluorescence in areas of subacute disease activity. These evolve into areas of speckled hypoautofluorescence as atrophic changes ensue.

Francis PJ, Marinescu A, Fitzke FW, Bird AC, Holder GE. Acute zonal occult outer retinopathy: towards a set of diagnostic criteria. *Br J Ophthalmol.* 2005;89(1):70–73.

Mrejen S, Khan S, Gallego-Pinazo R, Jampol LM, Yannuzzi LA. Acute zonal occult outer retinopathy: a classification based on multimodal imaging. *JAMA Ophthalmol.* 2014;132(9):1089–1098.

Disease course and differential diagnosis With extended follow-up, most patients are found to develop bilateral disease, with recurrences in approximately one-third. Visual field abnormalities typically stabilize in approximately 75% of patients and partially improve in about 25%. Visual acuity remains in the 20/40 range in 68% of patients; however, legal blindness has been reported in as many as 18% with long-term follow-up.

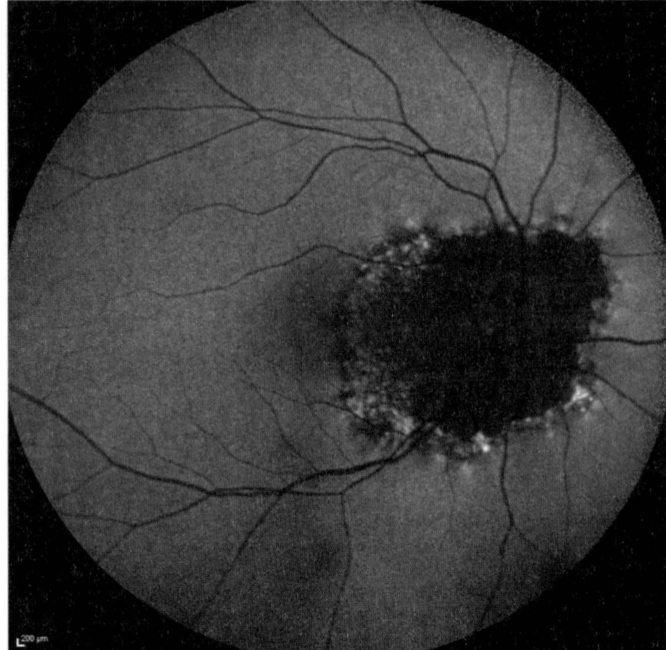

Figure 9-40 Acute zonal occult outer retinopathy. Fundus autofluorescence image of the patient in Figure 9-38, with broad areas of peripapillary hypoautofluorescence, corresponding to atrophy of the retinal pigment epithelium–choriocapillaris. Intense hyperautofluorescence at the outer border of the lesion represents accumulation of large amounts of lipofuscin. *(Courtesy of Bryn M. Burkholder, MD.)*

Cancer-associated retinopathy and retinitis pigmentosa should be considered in the differential diagnosis of AZOOR. It is unclear whether treatment with systemic corticosteroids or IMT alters the disease course or vision outcome.

The considerable similarities between AZOOR and other white dot syndromes—namely, MEWDS, MCP, OHS, PIC, acute macular neuroretinopathy, and acute idiopathic blind spot enlargement syndrome—have led some investigators to group these entities together in the so-called *AZOOR complex* of diseases. Although an infectious etiology has been postulated, systemic autoimmune disease has been observed in 28% of these patients, supporting the notion that these diseases are of an inflammatory etiology and arise in patients with a common non–disease-specific genetic background, possibly triggered by some exogenous agent.

Monson DM, Smith JR. Acute zonal occult outer retinopathy. *Surv Ophthalmol.* 2011;56(1):23–35.

Autoimmune retinopathy

Autoimmune retinopathy (AIR) can be broadly categorized into paraneoplastic retinopathy and nonparaneoplastic retinopathy. Paraneoplastic retinopathy can be further subdivided into cancer-associated retinopathy (CAR) and melanoma-associated retinopathy (MAR).

AIR is a rare and poorly understood immune-mediated disease that is characterized by antiretinal antibodies, photoreceptor dysfunction, and resultant visual field loss.

Manifestations AIR typically presents with progressive, bilateral vision loss, scotomata, photopsias, nyctalopia, and dyschromatopsias. About 50% of patients with nonparaneoplastic AIR will have a systemic autoimmune disease. The fundus may initially appear normal, but arteriolar attenuation, RPE mottling, and diffuse retinal and optic nerve atrophy may develop as the disease progresses. Inflammatory cells are rare or absent. Both visual field testing and ERG are typically abnormal, often markedly so. While the ERG in CAR typically demonstrates depressed cone responses, the ERG in MAR most commonly shows a normal photoreceptor response, followed by an attenuated b-wave. Visual prognosis is variable but generally poor.

Pathophysiology and diagnosis The pathophysiology of AIR is thought to be related to an immune response to retinal proteins, some of which have been identified as potential targets. Recoverin, a photoreceptor-specific calcium-binding protein, is the most commonly associated antibody target in paraneoplastic retinopathy but has also been implicated in nonparaneoplastic retinopathy. The role of testing for antiretinal antibodies is unclear at this point, as these antibodies are nonspecific, and it is not well understood which of them cause disease. Additionally, no standardized laboratory detection techniques for antiretinal antibodies exist at this time, so test results between laboratories may vary widely.

The diagnosis is one of exclusion; importantly, workup should include a thorough search for malignancy. The most common malignancy associated with CAR is small cell lung cancer.

Faez S, Loewenstein J, Sobrin L. Concordance of antiretinal antibody testing results between laboratories in autoimmune retinopathy. *JAMA Ophthalmol.* 2013;131(1):113–115.

Treatment As with many other rare diseases, the treatment for AIR is not well established and based primarily on anecdotal evidence. Corticosteroids and nonbiologic IMT are generally first-line therapy, although randomized, controlled trials are needed to determine whether these treatments are efficacious. Biologic agents and intravenous immunoglobulin have also been used in nonparaneoplastic AIR. Refer also to discussion of paraneoplastic and autoimmune retinopathies in BCSC Section 5, *Neuro-Ophthalmology*, and BCSC Section 12, *Retina and Vitreous.*

Ferreyra HA, Jayasundera T, Khan NW, He S, Lu Y, Heckenlively JR. Management of autoimmune retinopathies with immunosuppression. *Arch Ophthalmol.* 2009;127(4):390–397.

Fox AR, Gordon LK, Heckenlively JR, et al. Consensus on the diagnosis and management of nonparaneoplastic autoimmune retinopathy using a modified Delphi approach. *Am J Ophthalmol.* 2016;168:183–190.

Panuveitis

By definition, *panuveitis* requires involvement of all anatomical compartments of the eye—namely, the anterior chamber, vitreous, and retina or choroid—with no single predominant site of inflammation. As with posterior uveitis, structural complications (eg, macular edema, retinal or choroidal neovascularization, and peripheral vasculitis) are not considered essential features in the anatomical classification of panuveitis. Generally, panuveitis is bilateral, although one eye may be affected first, and disease severity may be asymmetric. The discussion of panuveitis in this chapter is limited to the noninfectious entities.

Sarcoidosis

Sarcoidosis is a multisystem granulomatous disorder of unknown etiology with protean systemic and ocular manifestations. Although pulmonary manifestations are most common (90%), other sites frequently involved include the lymph nodes, skin, eyes, CNS, bones and joints, liver, and heart. Ocular involvement may be present in up to 50% of patients with systemic disease, and uveitis is the most frequent manifestation. In most large series, sarcoidosis accounts for up to 10% of all cases of uveitis. The basic lesion of sarcoidosis is a noncaseating granuloma without histologic evidence of infection or foreign body (Fig 9-41). See BCSC Section 4, *Ophthalmic Pathology and Intraocular Tumors,* for a more detailed description of the pathology of sarcoidosis.

Sarcoidosis has a worldwide distribution and affects all ethnic groups; the highest prevalence is in the northern European countries (40 cases per 100,000 people). In the United States, the disease is up to 20 times more prevalent among African Americans than Whites. Both sexes are affected, albeit with a slight female predominance. Although onset usually occurs between the ages of 20 and 50 years, sarcoidosis is also an important diagnostic consideration in older patients. In a recent review, sarcoidosis was a common cause of newly diagnosed uveitis among patients ages 60 years and older. Patients with late-onset sarcoidosis may be more likely to have uveitis and less likely to have asymptomatic chest radiograph abnormalities than younger patients with the disease.

Pediatric involvement is uncommon, and the clinical course is atypical. Children with early-onset sarcoidosis (younger than 5 years) are less likely than adults to manifest

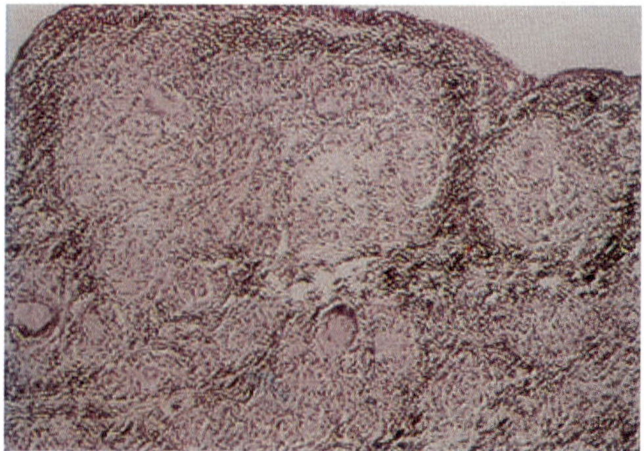

Figure 9-41 Sarcoidosis. Histologic view of conjunctival biopsy. Note the giant cells and granulomatous inflammation.

pulmonary disease and far more likely to have cutaneous and articular involvement; the disease course in older children (8–15 years) approximates that in adults.

Although numerous environmental, infectious, and genetic factors have been implicated in causing the disease, no single etiologic agent or genetic locus has been clearly identified in the pathogenesis of sarcoidosis. For instance, the ACCESS (A Case Control Etiologic Study of Sarcoidosis) project suggested that exposure to microbe-rich environments may modestly increase the risk of developing sarcoidosis; however, no dominant factor could be determined. Molecular studies of tissue specimens provide evidence suggesting that mycobacteria and, less convincingly, propionibacteria may be important etiologic factors. A genetic predisposition for the disease is suggested by familial clustering; siblings of patients have a fivefold-increased risk of developing the disease.

Chen ES, Moller DR. Etiology of sarcoidosis. *Clin Chest Med.* 2008;29(3):365–377.

Manifestations

Systemic sarcoidosis may present acutely, frequently with associated anterior uveitis in young patients, and spontaneously remit within 2 years of onset. One form of acute sarcoidosis, called *Löfgren syndrome,* consists of erythema nodosum, febrile arthropathy, bilateral hilar adenopathy, and acute iritis. This syndrome is quite responsive to systemic corticosteroids and has a good long-term prognosis. Another, termed *Heerfordt syndrome* (uveoparotid fever), is characterized by uveitis, parotitis, fever, and facial nerve palsy. Chronic sarcoidosis presents insidiously and is characterized by persistent disease of more than 2 years' duration, frequently with pulmonary involvement and chronic uveitis. Extended corticosteroid therapy may be required. Pulmonary disease is the major cause of morbidity; overall mortality from sarcoidosis approaches 5% but may be as high as 10% with neurosarcoidosis.

Sarcoidosis can affect any ocular tissue, including the orbit and adnexa. Cutaneous involvement is frequent, and orbital and eyelid granulomas are common (Fig 9-42). Palpebral and bulbar conjunctival nodules may also be observed and provide a readily accessible site for tissue biopsy (Fig 9-43). Lacrimal gland infiltration may cause dacryoadenitis and keratoconjunctivitis sicca.

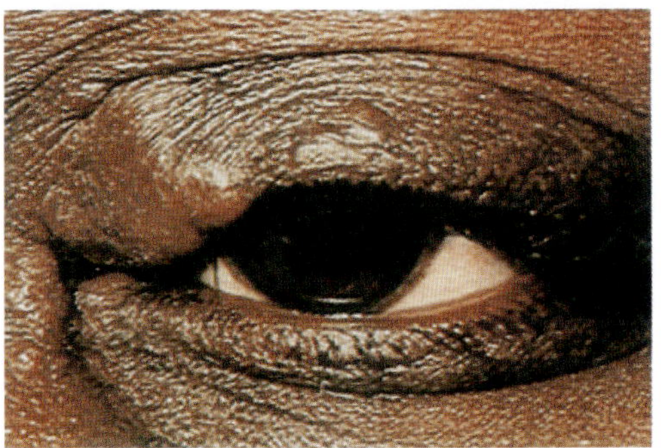

Figure 9-42 Sarcoidosis. Skin lesions.

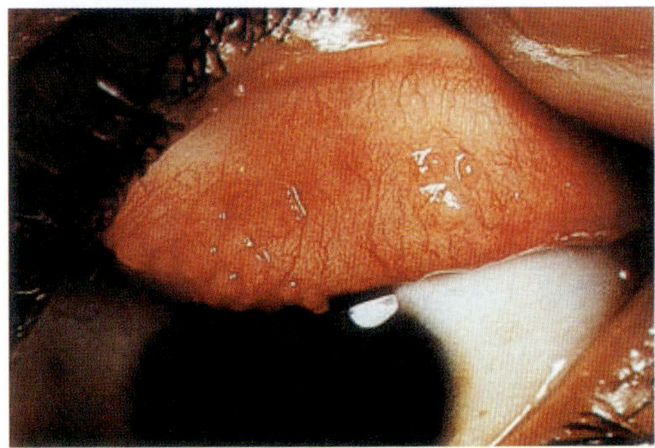

Figure 9-43 Sarcoidosis. Conjunctival nodules.

Anterior uveitis, presenting either acutely or as a chronic granulomatous uveitis, is the most common ocular manifestation, occurring in approximately two-thirds of patients with ocular sarcoidosis. Symptoms of uveal involvement are variable and frequently include mild-to-moderate blurring of vision and aching around the eyes. Typical biomicroscopic findings include

- mutton-fat keratic precipitates (KPs; Fig 9-44), including those involving the anterior chamber angle
- Koeppe and Busacca iris nodules at the pupil margin and in the iris stroma, respectively (Fig 9-45)
- white clumps of cells ("snowballs") in the anterior vitreous, typically settling inferiorly

Although the cornea is infrequently involved, nummular corneal infiltrates and inferior corneal endothelial opacification may be present; band keratopathy may develop as a result of either chronic uveitis or hypercalcemia. Large iris granulomas may also be noted. Extensive posterior synechiae may lead to iris bombé and angle-closure glaucoma. Peripheral anterior synechiae may also be extensive, encompassing the entire angle in advanced cases. Secondary glaucoma, together with sarcoid uveitis, may be severe and portends a poor prognosis with associated severe vision loss.

Posterior segment manifestations occur in up to 20% of patients with ocular sarcoidosis. Vitreous involvement is common and often presents as clumps of snowballs with or without diffuse cellular infiltration. Vitreous cells may also form linear strands known as "strings of pearls." Nodular granulomas measuring from ¼ to 1 disc diameter may be present on the optic nerve, in both the retina and the choroid, either posteriorly or peripherally (Fig 9-46). Perivascular sheathing is also common, appearing most commonly as either a linear or segmental periphlebitis (Fig 9-47). Retinal artery macroaneurysms can occur. Irregular nodular granulomas along venules have been termed *candlewax drippings* or *taches de bougie.* Occlusive retinal vascular disease, especially branch retinal vein occlusion and, less commonly, central retinal vein occlusion, together with peripheral retinal capillary nonperfusion, may lead to retinal neovascularization and vitreous hemorrhage. Macular edema is frequently present, and optic disc edema without granulomatous invasion of the optic nerve may be observed in patients with papilledema and

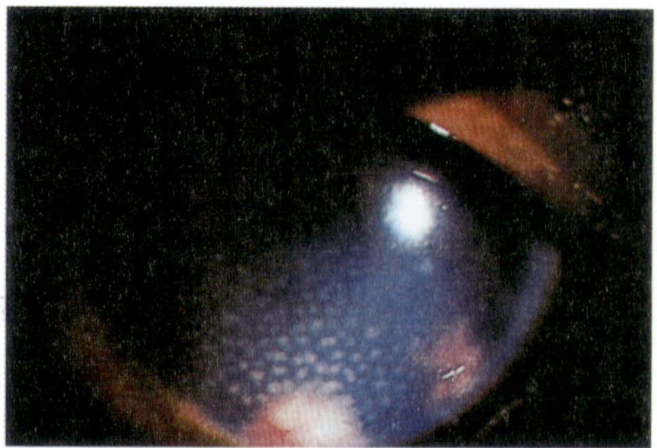

Figure 9-44 Sarcoidosis with keratic precipitates and anterior uveitis.

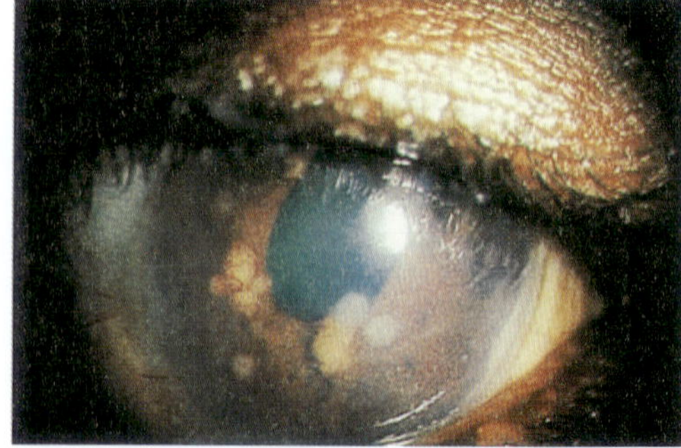

Figure 9-45 Sarcoidosis. Iris nodules (Koeppe and Busacca nodules).

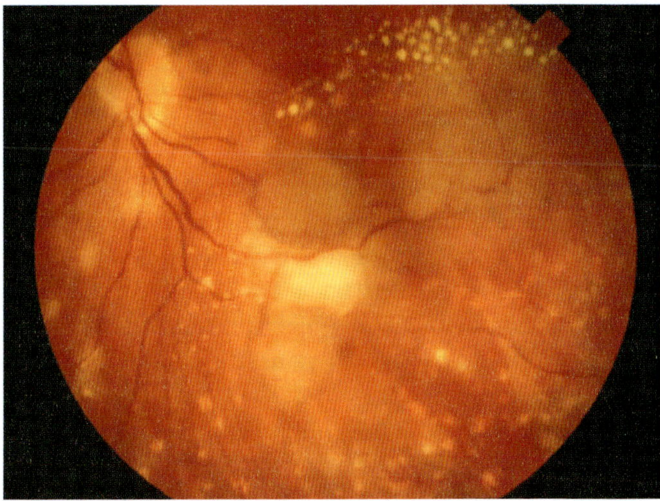

Figure 9-46 Fundus photograph showing numerous retinal and choroidal nodular granulomas, perivasculitis with candlewax drippings, and vitritis in a patient with sarcoidosis-associated posterior segment involvement. *(Courtesy of Albert T. Vitale, MD.)*

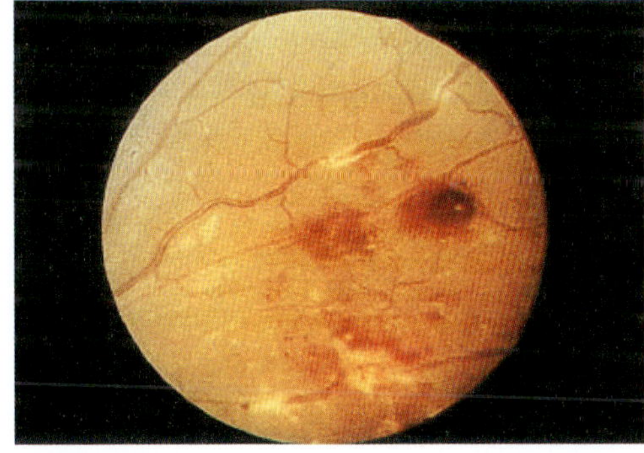

Figure 9-47 Sarcoidosis. Fundus photograph showing retinal vascular sheathing.

neurosarcoidosis. In addition, sarcoidosis may be associated with an inflammatory optic neuropathy, with or without concurrent intraocular inflammation.

Acharya NR, Browne EN, Rao N, Mochizuki M; International Ocular Sarcoidosis Working Group. Distinguishing features of ocular sarcoidosis in an international cohort of uveitis patients. *Ophthalmology*. 2018;125(1):119–126.

Kidd DP, Burton BJ, Graham EM, Plant FT. Optic neuropathy associated with systemic sarcoidosis. *Neurol Neuroimmunol Neuroinflamm*. 2016;3(5):e270.

Diagnosis

Given its heterogeneous presentation, sarcoidosis should be considered in the differential diagnosis of any patient presenting with intraocular inflammation. Early-onset sarcoidosis in children (5 years of age or younger) must be differentiated from JIA-associated anterior uveitis and from familial juvenile systemic granulomatosis (Blau syndrome), given the overlap of ocular and articular involvement. Familial juvenile systemic granulomatosis, an autosomal dominantly inherited syndrome with 100% phenotypic correspondence to mutations in the *NOD2* gene (also known as *CARD15*), may produce ocular disease that is virtually identical to sarcoidosis and should be suspected in patients with a family history of granulomatous disease.

Chest radiograph abnormalities are present at some point in up to 90% of sarcoid patients, but these abnormalities do not persist throughout the disease course and thus may be absent at the time of workup. High-resolution chest computed tomography is a more sensitive imaging modality and may be particularly valuable in patients with a normal appearance on chest radiograph but for whom a high clinical index of suspicion remains; the risk of increased radiation must be weighed against the clinical utility of the information gained in such cases.

Although the serum angiotensin-converting enzyme (ACE) and lysozyme levels may be abnormally elevated, neither result is diagnostic nor specific; rather, they are reflective of total-body granuloma content and, as such, may be useful in tracking active disease. (Note that the ACE levels may be artificially low in patients taking ACE-inhibitor medications.) Other laboratory evaluations that may have utility include serum and urinary calcium levels and liver function tests; they are not specific for sarcoidosis but may suggest more widespread involvement in patients likely to have the disease.

Gallium scanning has been used to check for occult disease activity, but it has limited sensitivity. Fluorine-18-fluorodeoxyglucose positron emission tomography is considered more accurate in pulmonary and extrapulmonary sarcoidosis, but its utility in ophthalmic sarcoidosis is not well defined. The finding of mononuclear alveolitis with increased $CD4^+$ lymphocytes, as revealed by bronchoalveolar lavage, can also help support the diagnosis.

The traditional approach for suspected ophthalmic involvement with sarcoidosis is to obtain a chest radiograph, possibly along with ACE and lysozyme levels. The additional tests mentioned above can then supplement the workup, depending on the degree of suspicion and/or preference of the managing physician.

Ultimately, the diagnosis of sarcoidosis is made histologically from tissue obtained from the lungs, mediastinal lymph nodes, skin, peripheral lymph nodes, liver, conjunctiva, minor salivary glands, or lacrimal glands. Readily accessible and clinically evident lesions (such as those on the skin, palpable lymph nodes, and nodules on the conjunctiva) should be sought for biopsy, because they are associated with a high yield and low morbidity and may obviate the need for more invasive transbronchial biopsy.

Currently, there is no gold standard for diagnosing ocular sarcoidosis. Diagnostic criteria for ocular sarcoidosis were proposed in an international workshop of ophthalmologists in 2009. These criteria consist of diagnostic grades ranging from "definitive" (based on tissue biopsy), to "presumed" (based on typical ocular findings in combination with bilateral hilar adenopathy), to "probable" or "possible" disease (with supporting ancillary evidence). When these criteria were evaluated using a large group of patients with uveitis, there was no clinical sign or test that was highly sensitive in the diagnosis of sarcoidosis, with the exception of bilateral hilar adenopathy; in fact, a large percentage (40%) of clinician-suspected cases did not meet any of the criteria.

Treatment

Topical, periocular, and systemic corticosteroids are the mainstays of therapy for ocular sarcoidosis. Cycloplegia is useful for comfort and prevention of synechiae. Vision-threatening posterior segment disease generally requires, and is responsive to, systemic corticosteroids. Intravitreal corticosteroids, including the fluocinolone acetonide and dexamethasone implants, are potential treatment options for patients intolerant of systemic therapy, but they do not treat systemic disease.

Systemic IMT with methotrexate, azathioprine, mycophenolate mofetil, or cyclosporine can provide good control of the disease while minimizing the risks of long-term corticosteroid therapy. The TNF-α inhibitors infliximab and adalimumab have been shown to be effective in the treatment of sarcoidosis-associated uveitis. Paradoxically, the TNF-α inhibitor etanercept has been reported to cause a sarcoid-like syndrome in some patients. The likelihood of significant visual improvement is substantially increased with systemic therapy; patients with chronic vision-threatening sarcoidosis seem to respond better to IMT than to management with intermittent local or systemic corticosteroids.

Prognostic factors associated with vision loss in patients with ocular sarcoidosis include chronic intermediate or posterior uveitis, glaucoma, and a delay in presentation to a uveitis specialist of more than 1 year.

Baughman RP, Lower EE, Ingledue R, Kaufman AH. Management of ocular sarcoidosis. *Sarcoidosis Vasc Diffuse Lung Dis.* 2012;29(1):26–33.

Dana MR, Merayo-Lloves J, Schaumberg DA, Foster CS. Prognosticators for visual outcome in sarcoid uveitis. *Ophthalmology.* 1996;103(11):1846–1853.

Herbort CP, Rao NA, Mochizuki M; members of Scientific Committee of First International Workshop on Ocular Sarcoidosis. International criteria for the diagnosis of ocular sarcoidosis: results of the first International Workshop on Ocular Sarcoidosis (IWOS). *Ocul Immunol Inflamm.* 2009;17(3):160–169.

Sympathetic Ophthalmia

Sympathetic ophthalmia (SO) is a rare, bilateral, diffuse, granulomatous, nonnecrotizing panuveitis that may develop after either surgical or accidental trauma to 1 eye (called the *exciting eye*), followed by a latent period and the appearance of uveitis in the uninjured fellow eye (the *sympathizing eye*). Although the precise incidence of SO is difficult to ascertain because of its rarity, significant improvements in the management of ocular trauma have led to an overall decrease. Earlier estimates of the incidence of SO ranged from 0.01% after intraocular surgery to 0.5% in eyes with nonsurgical trauma. Although the most recent minimum incidence estimate is low (0.03/100,000), SO remains a disease with a persistent and potentially devastating presence.

Accidental penetrating ocular trauma was once the most common precipitating event for SO. Ocular surgery—particularly vitreoretinal surgery—has emerged as the main risk for the development of SO. In the early 1980s, the prevalence of SO in patients who had undergone pars plana vitrectomy was reported to be 0.01%, increasing to 0.06% when the procedure was performed in the context of other penetrating ocular injuries. More recent studies suggest that the risk of developing SO following pars plana vitrectomy is more than twice this figure and may be significantly higher than the risk of infectious endophthalmitis after vitrectomy. Improved access to emergency surgical care following penetrating ocular trauma and improved microsurgical technique have undoubtedly influenced this etiologic shift from penetrating injury to surgical trauma.

Similarly, the demographic of SO has changed from earlier reports, in which there was higher prevalence among men, children, and older patients (due to their presumed increased risk of accidental trauma), to more recent studies, which show no sex predominance and a lower risk in children (resulting in part from a reduced incidence of pediatric ocular injuries), as well as an increased risk in older patients (likely stemming from an increased frequency of ocular surgery and retinal detachment in this population).

In addition, although SO has traditionally been reported to develop in 80% of patients within 3 months of injury and in 90% within 1 year, these time intervals may actually be longer than previously thought. In a recent series, only one-third of patients developed SO within 3 months, and less than one-half did so within 1 year of injury.

Chu XK, Chan CC. Sympathetic ophthalmia: to the twenty-first century and beyond. *J Ophthalmic Inflamm Infect*. 2013;3(1):49.

Galor A, Davis JL, Flynn HW Jr, et al. Sympathetic ophthalmia: incidence of ocular complications and vision loss in the sympathizing eye. *Am J Ophthalmol.* 2009;148(5):704–710.

Manifestations

Patients with SO typically present with asymmetric bilateral panuveitis, in which the exciting eye exhibits more severe inflammation than the sympathizing eye, at least initially. Signs and symptoms vary in their severity and onset. Anterior segment findings include mutton-fat KPs, thickening of the iris from lymphocytic infiltration, and posterior synechiae formation. Intraocular pressure (IOP) may be elevated, due to trabeculitis, or low as a result of ciliary body shutdown.

Posterior segment findings include moderate to severe vitritis with characteristic yellowish white, midperipheral choroidal lesions (*Dalen-Fuchs nodules*) that may become confluent. Peripapillary choroidal lesions and exudative retinal detachment may also develop (Fig 9-48). Structural complications of SO include cataract, chronic macular edema, peripapillary and macular CNV, and optic atrophy. In a recent study, complications in the sympathizing eye at presentation were frequent (up to 47%); cataract and optic nerve abnormalities were most often associated with decreased vision and the further development of new complications, which occurred at a rate of 40% per person-year. Furthermore, a history of traumatic injury, the presence of active intraocular inflammation, and exudative retinal detachment correlated with poorer vision in the sympathizing eye. Extraocular findings similar to those observed with VKH syndrome, including cerebral spinal fluid pleocytosis, sensory neural hearing disturbance, alopecia, poliosis, and vitiligo, may be noted, although they are uncommon.

During the acute stage of the disease, FA reveals multiple hyperfluorescent sites of leakage during the early phase, which persists into the late phase of the study (Fig 9-49). Pooling of dye is observed in areas of exudative neurosensory retinal detachment. Multiple

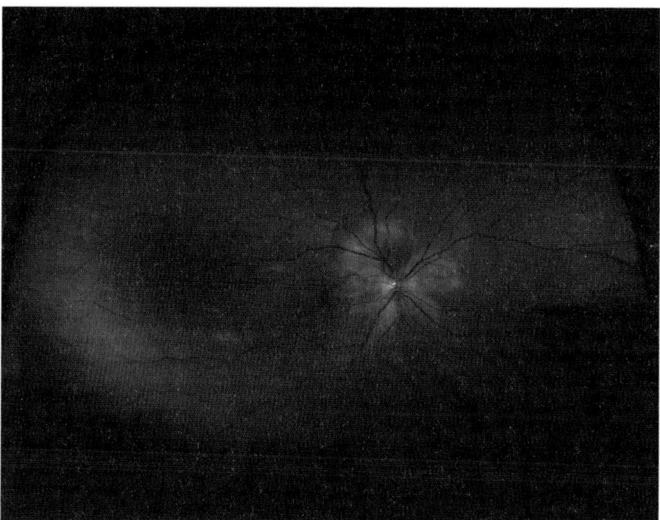

Figure 9-48 Sympathetic ophthalmia. Fundus photograph showing peripapillary and multifocal choroiditis (yellowish subretinal inflammatory infiltrates) with associated exudative retinal detachments. *(Courtesy of Bryn M. Burkholder, MD.)*

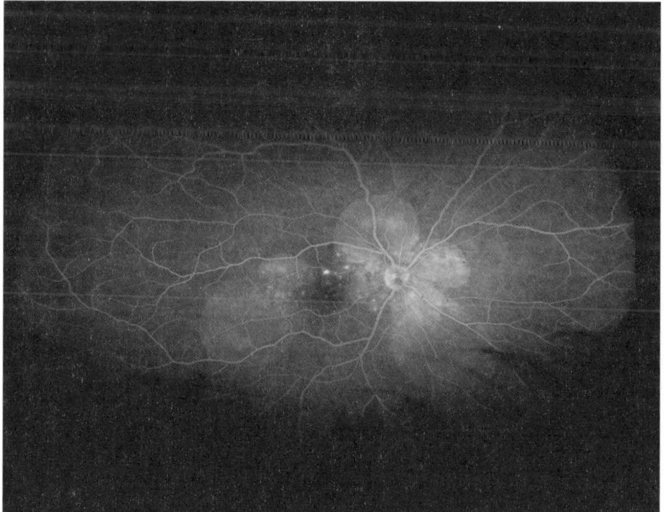

Figure 9-49 Sympathetic ophthalmia. Wide-field angiogram of the patient in Figure 9-48 demonstrates multiple hyperfluorescent points of leakage with late pooling of dye in areas of serous detachment. *(Reprinted with permission from Burkholder BM, Dunn JP. Multiple serous retinal detachments seen on wide-field imaging in a patient with sympathetic ophthalmia.* JAMA Ophthalmol. *2014;132[10]:1220.)*

chorioretinal lesions may be present and appear hypofluorescent in early phases, simulating the pattern seen in APMPPE, or hyperfluorescent with late staining. Indocyanine green angiography reveals numerous hypocyanescent foci, which are best visualized during the intermediate phase of the angiogram; some of these foci may become less visible in the late stage of the study (Fig 9-50). Optical coherence tomography may demonstrate a shallow,

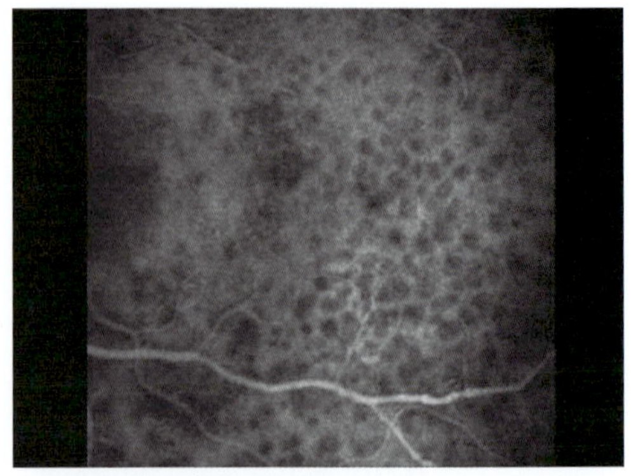

Figure 9-50 Sympathetic ophthalmia. Indocyanine green angiogram demonstrating multiple midphase hypocyanescent foci corresponding to, and more numerous than, the choroidal lesions found on clinical exam or fluorescein angiography.

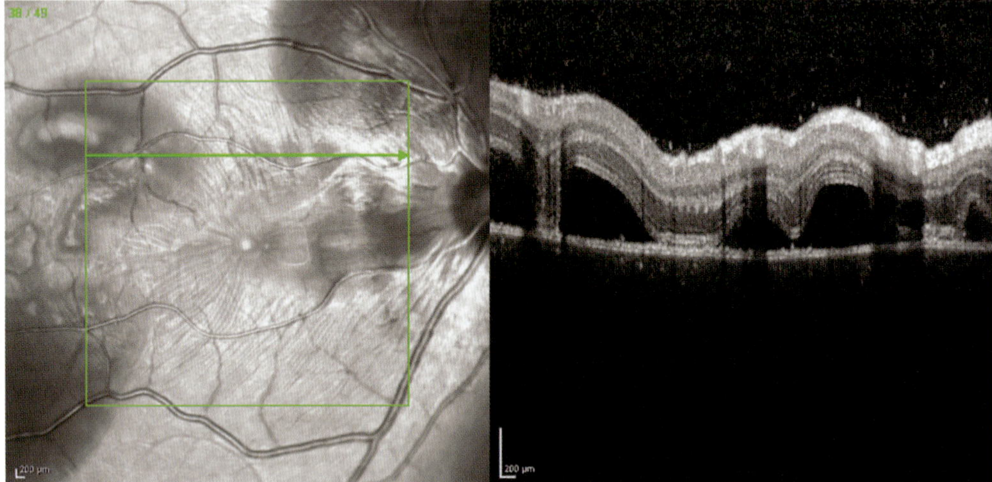

Figure 9-51 Sympathetic ophthalmia. Optical coherence tomography scan of patient in Figure 9-48 demonstrates multiple serous retinal detachments throughout the macula. *(Reprinted with permission from Burkholder BM, Dunn JP. Multiple serous retinal detachments seen on wide-field imaging in a patient with sympathetic ophthalmia.* JAMA Ophthalmol. *2014;132[10]:1220.)*

serous retinal detachment and/or intraretinal edema, and monitoring these findings can help determine the efficacy of treatment (Fig 9-51). B-scan ultrasonography frequently reveals choroidal thickening.

The histologic features of SO are similar for both the exciting and sympathizing eyes. Findings include diffuse, granulomatous, nonnecrotizing infiltration of the choroid that classically spares the choriocapillaris in the early stage. Dalen-Fuchs nodules, which are clusters of epithelioid cells located between the RPE and Bruch membrane, are present in about one-third of patients. The nodules are not specific to SO and can also be found in VKH syndrome and sarcoidosis (see BCSC Section 4, *Ophthalmic Pathology and Intraocular Tumors*).

Castiblanco C, Adelman RA. Imaging for sympathetic ophthalmia: impact on the diagnosis and management. *Int Ophthalmol Clin*. 2012;52(4):173–181.

Diagnosis

The precise etiology of SO is unknown; however, in the overwhelming majority of patients, there is a history of surgery or penetrating ocular injury complicated by incarceration of uveal tissue. The disorder may result from altered T-lymphocyte responses to previously sequestered ocular antigens derived from the RPE or choroid. The penetrating wound itself may facilitate exposure of uveoretinal antigens to conjunctival lymphatic channels and thereby initiate this immunopathologic response. Furthermore, there may be a genetic predisposition to the development of the disease, as patients with SO are more likely to express HLA-DR4, -DRw53, and -DQw3 haplotypes. It should be noted that the immunogenetics of SO and VKH syndrome are virtually identical, as the same associations have been found in both diseases.

The diagnosis of SO is clinical, and the disorder should be suspected in the presence of bilateral uveitis following any ocular trauma or surgery. Differential diagnosis includes other causes of panuveitis, including TB, sarcoidosis, syphilis, and fungal infections, as well as traumatic or postoperative endophthalmitis. Lens-associated uveitis has been reported with SO in up to 25% of cases and may present with a similar clinical picture. The clinical presentations of SO and VKH syndrome may be strikingly similar; however, a history of prior ocular injury is by definition absent in patients with VKH syndrome.

Treatment

The course of SO is chronic, with frequent exacerbations; however, it is a treatable condition, and in cases with penetrating trauma, every attempt should be made to salvage eyes with a reasonable prognosis for useful vision. Enucleation within 2 weeks of injury to prevent the development of SO should be considered in patients with grossly disorganized globes and no discernible visual potential. Although controversial, enucleation may still be preferred to evisceration as the operation of choice for the removal of ocular contents in severely injured eyes, because it eliminates the possibility of residual uveal tissue, which may predispose to the development of sympathetic disease. BCSC Section 7, *Oculofacial Plastic and Orbital Surgery,* discusses the advantages and disadvantages of enucleation and evisceration in greater detail. Regardless of visual potential, once SO has developed, enucleation of the exciting eye has not been shown to be beneficial in altering the disease course of the sympathizing eye. In fact, the exciting eye may eventually become the better-seeing eye.

The initial treatment of SO involves systemic corticosteroids, with the frequent addition of corticosteroid-sparing drugs such as azathioprine, methotrexate, mycophenolate mofetil, cyclosporine, chlorambucil, and cyclophosphamide, as chronic therapy is anticipated in most patients. Topical corticosteroids are essential in the treatment of the acute anterior uveitis associated with SO. Periocular and intravitreal corticosteroids, including the intravitreal fluocinolone acetonide implant, are options for patients intolerant of systemic corticosteroid therapy. With prompt and aggressive systemic therapy, the visual prognosis of SO is good; 60% of patients achieve a final visual acuity of 20/40, although up to 25% may decline to 20/200 or worse in the sympathizing eye.

Lubin JR, Albert DM, Weinstein M. Sixty-five years of sympathetic ophthalmia. A clinicopathologic review of 105 cases (1913–1978). *Ophthalmology.* 1980;87(2):109–121.

Vogt-Koyanagi-Harada Syndrome

Vogt-Koyanagi-Harada syndrome is a multisystem disease of presumed autoimmune etiology that is characterized by chronic, bilateral, diffuse, granulomatous panuveitis with accompanying integumentary, neurologic, and auditory involvement. Although the disease more commonly affects some of the more darkly pigmented ethnic groups—including people of Asian, Hispanic, Native American, and Middle Eastern ancestry—and is uncommon among Whites, VKH syndrome is also rare among sub-Saharan Africans, suggesting that additional factors, other than skin pigmentation, are important in its pathogenesis. The incidence of VKH syndrome varies geographically, accounting for up to 4% of all uveitis referrals in the United States and 8% in Japan. In Brazil and Saudi Arabia, it is the most commonly encountered cause of noninfectious uveitis.

The precise etiology and pathogenesis of VKH syndrome are unknown, but current clinical and experimental evidence suggests a cell-mediated autoimmune process driven by T lymphocytes directed against self-antigens associated with melanocytes of all organ systems in genetically susceptible individuals. A genetic predisposition for the development of the disease is further supported by the strong association with HLA-DR4 among Japanese patients and with HLA-DR1 or HLA-DR4 among Hispanic patients from southern California.

Fang W, Yang P. Vogt-Koyanagi-Harada syndrome. *Curr Eye Res.* 2008;33(7):517–523.
Rao NA. Pathology of Vogt-Koyanagi-Harada disease. *Int Ophthalmol.* 2007;27(2–3):81–85.

Histologic findings

There are 4 clinically distinct stages of VKH syndrome: (1) prodromal, (2) acute uveitic, (3) convalescent, and (4) chronic recurrent. Histologic findings vary depending on the stage.

During the acute uveitic stage, there is a diffuse, nonnecrotizing, granulomatous inflammation virtually identical to that seen in SO, consisting of lymphocytes and macrophages admixed with epithelioid and multinucleate giant cells, with preservation of the choriocapillaris. Proteinaceous fluid exudates are observed in the subretinal space between the detached neurosensory retina and the RPE. Although the peripapillary choroid is the predominant site of granulomatous inflammatory infiltration, the ciliary body and iris may also be affected.

The convalescent stage is characterized by nongranulomatous inflammation, with uveal infiltration of lymphocytes, few plasma cells, and the absence of epithelioid histiocytes. The number of choroidal melanocytes decreases with loss of melanin pigment, which corresponds with the characteristic clinical feature known as *sunset-glow fundus.* In addition, the appearance of numerous nummular chorioretinal scars in the peripheral retina histologically corresponds to the focal loss of RPE cells with chorioretinal adhesions.

The chronic recurrent stage is characterized by granulomatous choroiditis with damage to the choriocapillaris. The numerous clinical, pathologic, and genetic similarities between SO and VKH syndrome suggest that they share a similar immunopathogenesis, albeit with different triggering events and modes of sensitization.

Manifestations

The clinical features of VKH syndrome also vary depending on the stage of the disease. The prodromal stage is marked by flulike symptoms. Several days preceding the onset of ocular symptoms, patients may present with headache, nausea, meningismus, dysacusia, tinnitus, fever, orbital pain, photophobia, and hypersensitivity of the skin to touch. Focal neurologic signs, although rare, may include cranial neuropathies, hemiparesis, aphasia, transverse myelitis, and ganglionitis. Cerebrospinal fluid analysis reveals lymphocytic pleocytosis with normal levels of glucose in more than 80% of patients; this finding may persist for up to 8 weeks. Central dysacusia, usually involving higher frequencies, occurs in approximately 30% of patients early in the disease course, typically improving within 2–3 months; however, persistent deficits may remain.

The acute uveitic stage is heralded by the onset of sequential blurring of vision in both eyes, 1–2 days after the onset of CNS signs, and is marked by bilateral granulomatous anterior uveitis, a variable degree of vitritis, thickening of the posterior choroid, edema of the optic nerve, and multiple serous retinal detachments (Fig 9-52). The focal serous retinal detachments are often shallow, exhibiting a cloverleaf pattern around the posterior pole, but they may coalesce and evolve into large, bullous, exudative detachments. Profound vision loss may occur during this phase. Less commonly, mutton-fat KPs and iris nodules at the pupillary margin may be observed. IOP may be elevated, and the anterior chamber may be shallow because of forward displacement of the lens–iris diaphragm as the result of ciliary body edema or annular choroidal detachment. Alternatively, IOP may be low, secondary to ciliary body shutdown.

The convalescent stage occurs several weeks later and is marked by resolution of the exudative retinal detachments and gradual depigmentation of the choroid, resulting in

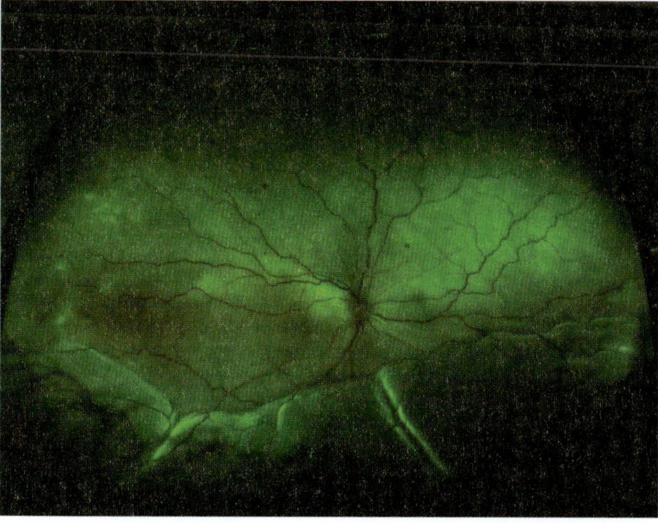

Figure 9-52 Vogt-Koyanagi-Harada syndrome. Wide-field photograph shows disc hyperemia and diffuse choroiditis with large exudative detachments in the acute uveitic stage. *(Reprinted with permission from Burkholder BM. Vogt-Koyanagi-Harada disease.* Curr Opin Ophthalmol. *2015;26[6]:506–511.)*

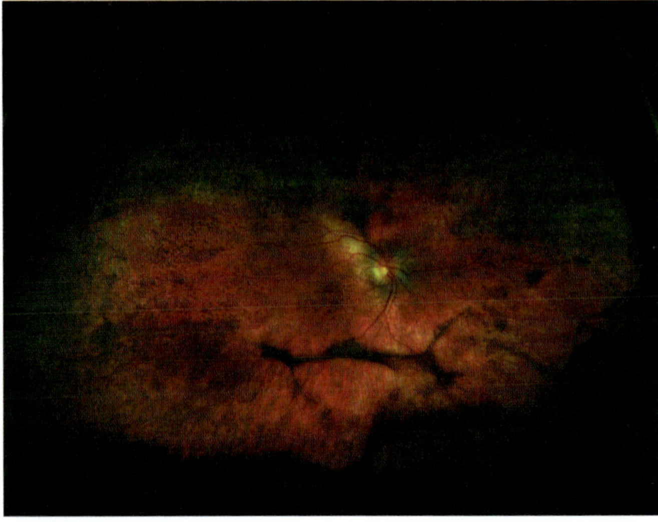

Figure 9-53 Vogt-Koyanagi-Harada syndrome. Fundus photograph of the patient in Figure 9-52 showing sunset-glow fundus appearance with pigment migration in the convalescent stage. *(Reprinted with permission from Burkholder BM. Vogt-Koyanagi-Harada disease.* Curr Opin Ophthalmol. *2015;26[6]:506–511.)*

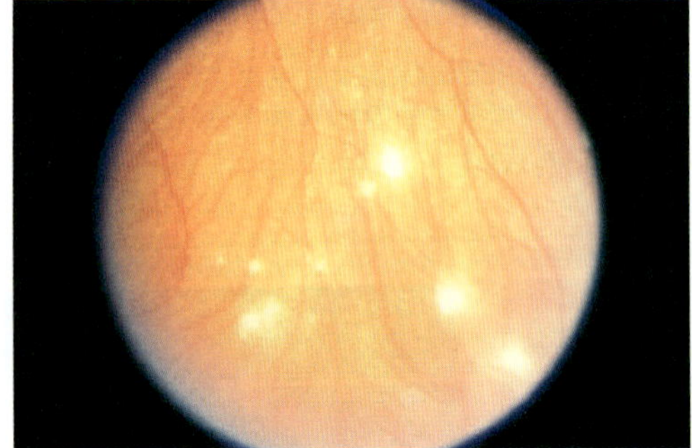

Figure 9-54 Vogt-Koyanagi-Harada syndrome. Fundus photograph showing multiple inferior, peripheral, punched-out chorioretinal lesions in a patient in the convalescent stage. *(Courtesy of Ramana S. Moorthy, MD.)*

the classic orange-red discoloration, or sunset-glow fundus (Fig 9-53). In addition, small, round, discrete depigmented lesions develop in the inferior peripheral fundus (Fig 9-54). Juxtapapillary depigmentation may also be seen (Fig 9-55). The sunset-glow fundus may show focal areas of retinal hyper- or hypopigmentation. Perilimbal vitiligo (Sugiura sign) may be present in up to 85% of Japanese patients but is rarely observed among White patients (Fig 9-56). Integumentary changes, including vitiligo, alopecia, and poliosis, typically appear during the convalescent stage in about 30% of patients and correspond with the development of fundus depigmentation (Fig 9-57). In general, skin and hair changes occur weeks to months after the onset of ocular inflammation, but in some cases, they may appear simultaneously. Between 10% and 63% of patients develop vitiligo, depending on ethnic background; among Hispanic patients, the incidence of cutaneous and other extraocular manifestations is relatively low.

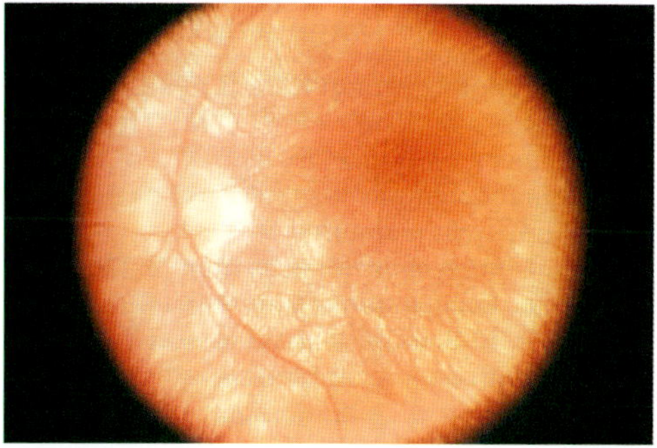

Figure 9-55 Vogt-Koyanagi-Harada syndrome. Fundus photograph showing sunset-glow fundus appearance with juxtapapillary detachment in a Hispanic patient in the convalescent stage. *(Reprinted with permission from Moorthy RS, Inomata H, Rao NA. Vogt-Koyanagi-Harada syndrome.* Surv Ophthalmol. *1995;39[4]:272.)*

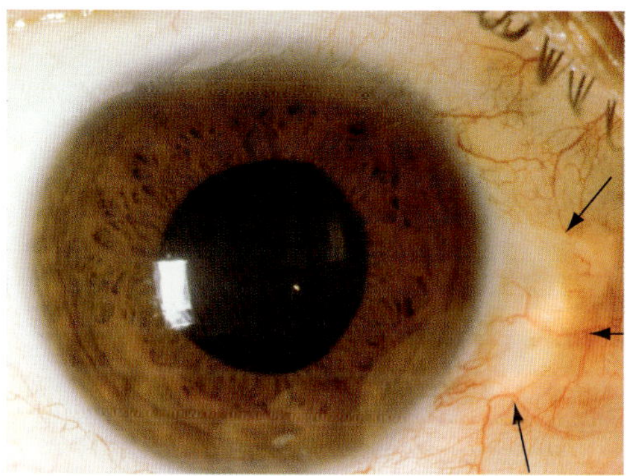

Figure 9-56 Perilimbal vitiligo (Sugiura sign) (arrows). *(Courtesy of Albert T. Vitale, MD.)*

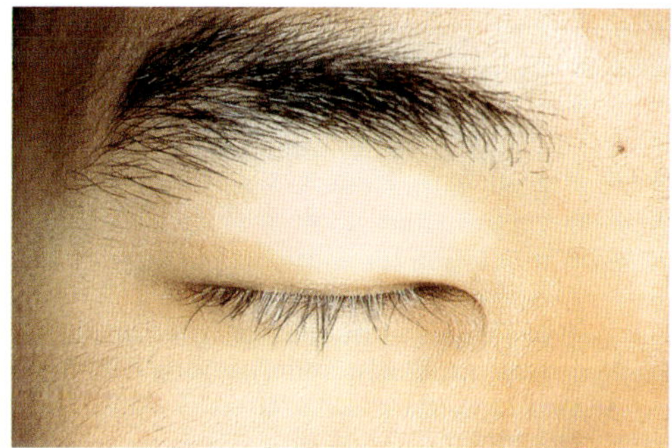

Figure 9-57 Vogt-Koyanagi-Harada syndrome. Vitiligo of the upper eyelid and marked poliosis in the convalescent stage. *(Courtesy of Ramana S. Moorthy, MD.)*

The chronic recurrent stage is marked by repeated bouts of granulomatous anterior uveitis, with the development of KPs, posterior synechiae, iris nodules, iris depigmentation, and stromal atrophy. Recurrent posterior segment inflammation can occur but is uncommon during this stage. Visually debilitating sequelae of chronic inflammation develop during this stage and include posterior subcapsular cataract, glaucoma, CNV, and subretinal fibrosis.

Rao NA, Gupta A, Dustin L, et al. Frequency of distinguishing clinical features in Vogt-Koyanagi-Harada disease. *Ophthalmology.* 2010;117(3):591–599.

Read RW, Holland GN, Rao NA, et al. Revised diagnostic criteria for Vogt-Koyanagi-Harada disease: report of an international committee on nomenclature. *Am J Ophthalmol.* 2001;131(5):647–652.

Diagnosis

Based on the clinical features and their distinctive appearance within the overall disease course, comprehensive diagnostic criteria for the complete, incomplete, and probable forms of VKH syndrome were revised in 2001 (Table 9-2). Regardless of the form of the disease, essential features for the diagnosis of VKH syndrome include bilateral

Table 9-2 Revised Diagnostic Criteria for Vogt-Koyanagi-Harada Syndrome

Complete Vogt-Koyanagi-Harada syndrome

I. No history of penetrating ocular trauma or surgery
II. No clinical or laboratory evidence of other ocular or systemic disease
III. Bilateral ocular disease (either A or B below must be met):
  A. Early manifestations
    1. Diffuse choroiditis as manifested by either:
      a. Focal areas of subretinal fluid, or
      b. Bullous serous subretinal detachments
    2. With equivocal fundus findings, then both:
      a. Fluorescein angiography showing focal delayed choroidal perfusion, pinpoint leakage, large placoid areas of hyperfluorescence, pooling of dye within subretinal fluid, and optic nerve staining
      b. Ultrasonography showing diffuse choroidal thickening without evidence of posterior scleritis
  B. Late manifestations
    1. History suggestive of findings from IIIA, and either both 2 and 3 below, or multiple signs from 3
    2. Ocular depigmentation
      a. Sunset-glow fundus, or
      b. Sugiura sign
    3. Other ocular signs
      a. Nummular chorioretinal depigmentation scars, or
      b. Retinal pigment epithelium clumping and/or migration, or
      c. Recurrent or chronic anterior uveitis
IV. Neurologic/auditory findings (may have resolved by time of examination):
  A. Meningismus
  B. Tinnitus
  C. Cerebrospinal fluid pleocytosis
V. Integumentary findings (not preceding central nervous system or ocular disease)
  A. Alopecia
  B. Poliosis
  C. Vitiligo

Incomplete Vogt-Koyanagi-Harada syndrome
Criteria I to III and either IV or V from above

Probable Vogt-Koyanagi-Harada syndrome
Criteria I to III from above must be present
Isolated ocular disease

Adapted from Read RW, Holland GN, Rao NA, et al. Revised diagnostic criteria for Vogt-Koyanagi-Harada disease: report of an international committee on nomenclature. *Am J Ophthalmol.* 2001;131(5):647–652.

involvement, no history of penetrating ocular trauma, and no evidence of other ocular or systemic disease.

The diagnosis of VKH syndrome is essentially clinical; exudative retinal detachment during the acute disease and sunset-glow fundus during the chronic phase are highly specific to this entity. In patients presenting without extraocular manifestations, FA, ICG angiography, OCT, FAF imaging, lumbar puncture, and ultrasonography may be useful confirmatory tests. During the acute uveitic stage, FA typically reveals numerous punctate hyperfluorescent foci in the early stage of the study, followed by pooling of dye in the

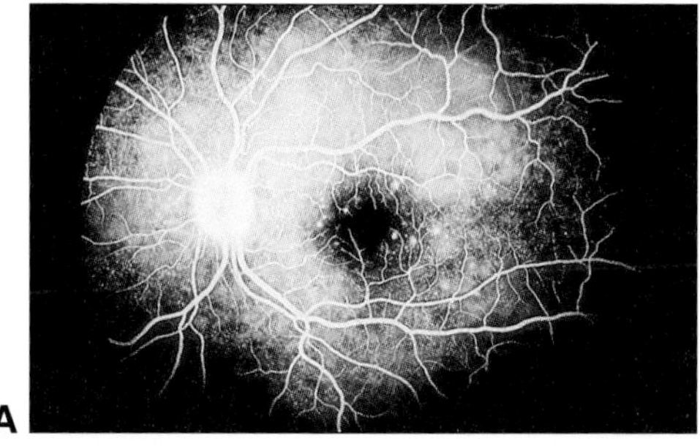
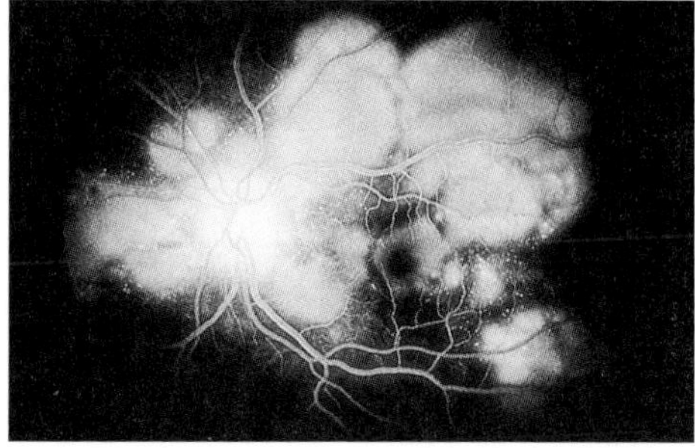

Figure 9-58 Vogt-Koyanagi-Harada syndrome. **A,** Early arteriovenous phase fluorescein angiogram showing multiple pinpoint foci of hyperfluorescence in the posterior pole of the left eye of a patient in the acute uveitic stage. **B,** Late arteriovenous phase fluorescein angiogram showing fluorescein pooling in multiple serous retinal detachments in the posterior pole in the same eye. *(Courtesy of Ramana S. Moorthy, MD.)*

subretinal space in areas of neurosensory detachment (Fig 9-58). The vast majority of patients show disc leakage, but macular edema and retinal vascular leakage are uncommon. In the convalescent and chronic recurrent stages, focal RPE loss and atrophy produce multiple hyperfluorescent window defects without progressive staining.

Indocyanine green angiography highlights the choroidal pathology, demonstrating a delay in choroidal perfusion, early choroidal hypercyanescence and leakage, multiple hypocyanescent spots throughout the fundus (thought to correspond to foci of lymphocytic infiltration), and hypercyanescent pinpoint changes within areas of exudative retinal detachment. The hypocyanescent spots may be present even when the funduscopic and FA findings are unremarkable; thus, they serve as sensitive markers for the detection and monitoring of subclinical choroidal inflammation.

Ultrasonography may be helpful in establishing the diagnosis, especially in the presence of media opacity. Findings include diffuse, low to medium reflective thickening of the posterior choroid that is most prominent in the peripapillary area, with extension to the equatorial region, exudative retinal detachment, vitreous opacification, and posterior thickening of the sclera.

Optical coherence tomography may be useful in the diagnosis and monitoring of serous macular detachments, macular edema, and choroidal neovascular membranes. Patients may have characteristic fibrin bands extending from the retina to the RPE in the acute phase (Fig 9-59). Enhanced-depth OCT imaging demonstrates choroidal thickening in the acute phase that decreases with treatment. The combined use of OCT and FAF imaging, which shows granular hyperautofluorescence in areas of inflammation, offers a noninvasive assessment of RPE and outer retinal inflammation that may not be apparent on clinical examination in patients with chronic VKH syndrome.

In highly atypical cases—particularly patients presenting early in the course of the disease with prominent neurologic signs and a paucity of ocular findings—a lumbar puncture, revealing lymphocytic pleocytosis, may be useful diagnostically. However, in

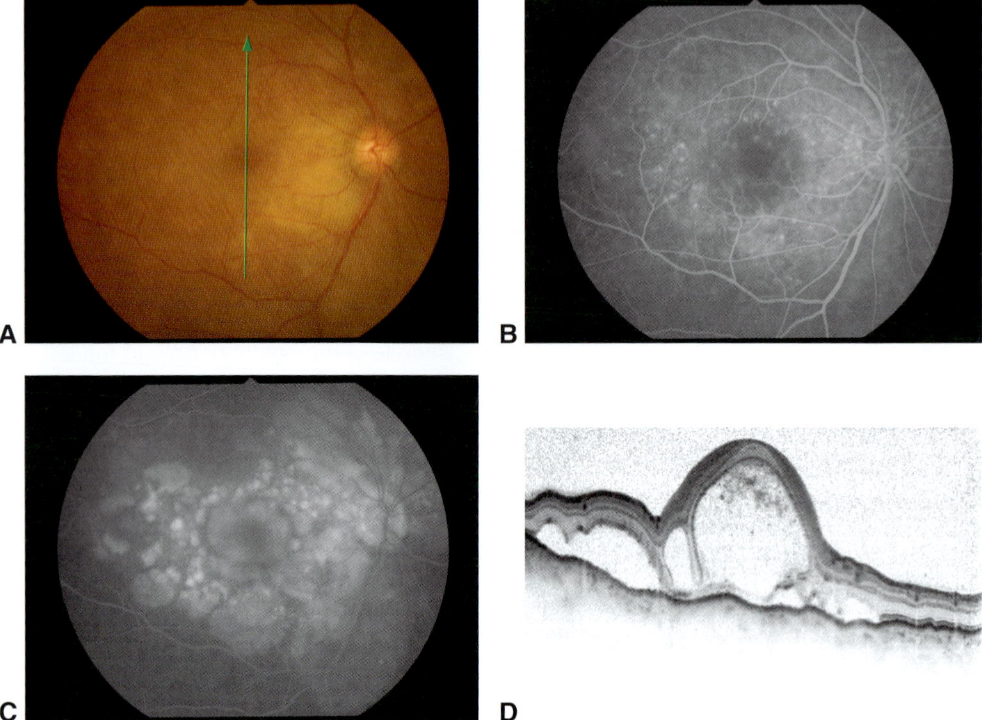

Figure 9-59 Vogt-Koyanagi-Harada syndrome. **A,** Color photograph showing multiple serous retinal detachments. **B, C,** Fluorescein angiograms showing early punctate hyperfluorescence **(B)** followed by late filling of the subretinal spaces with dye **(C)**. **D,** Optical coherence tomography scan showing characteristic loculated spaces of subretinal fluid, with bands extending from the retina to the retinal pigment epithelium. The location of the optical coherence tomography scan is indicated by the *green arrow* in **A**. *(Courtesy of Annabelle Okada, MD.)*

the vast majority of cases, the history and clinical examination, together with results of FA and/or ultrasonography, are sufficient to establish the diagnosis.

The differential diagnosis of VKH syndrome includes SO, uveal effusion syndrome, posterior scleritis, primary intraocular lymphoma, uveal lymphoid infiltration, APMPPE, bilateral diffuse uveal melanocytic proliferation, TB-associated uveitis, and sarcoidosis. These entities may be differentiated from VKH syndrome by a thorough history, review of systems, and examination, together with a directed laboratory evaluation.

Jap A, Chee SP. Imaging in the diagnosis and management of Vogt-Koyanagi-Harada disease. *Int Ophthalmol Clin.* 2012;52(4):163–172.

Jap A, Chee SP. The role of enhanced depth imaging optical coherence tomography in chronic Vogt-Koyanagi-Harada disease. *Br J Ophthalmol.* 2017;101(2):186–189.

Vasconcelos-Santos DV, Sohn EH, Sadda S, Rao NA. Retinal pigment epithelial changes in chronic Vogt-Koyanagi-Harada disease: fundus autofluorescence and spectral domain-optical coherence tomography findings. *Retina.* 2010;30(1):33–41.

Treatment and prognosis

The acute stage of VKH syndrome is responsive to early and aggressive treatment with corticosteroids. Initial dosages typically are 1–1.5 mg/kg/day of oral prednisone or up to 1 g of intravenous methylprednisolone daily for 3 days, followed by high-dose oral corticosteroids. Oral versus intravenous routes of administration show no demonstrable differences in visual acuity outcomes or the development of visually significant complications. For patients intolerant of systemic therapy, use of intravitreal corticosteroids, including the intravitreal fluocinolone acetonide and dexamethasone implants, is an option. Systemic corticosteroids are tapered slowly according to the clinical response, on average over a 6–12-month period, in an effort to prevent progression of the disease to the chronic recurrent stage and to minimize the incidence and severity of extraocular manifestations. Tapering corticosteroids too soon can result in early recurrence.

Despite adequate initial treatment with systemic corticosteroids, many patients experience recurrent episodes of inflammation. This risk has led many experts to initiate IMT earlier to achieve more prompt inflammatory control and to facilitate more rapid tapering of corticosteroids. The overall visual prognosis for patients treated in this fashion is fair, with up to 70% of patients retaining visual acuity of 20/40 or better.

Structural complications associated with ocular morbidity include cataract formation (50%), glaucoma (33%), CNV (up to 15%), and subretinal fibrosis, the development of which is associated with increased disease duration, more frequent recurrences, and an older age at disease onset.

The use of either oral corticosteroids or IMT with extended follow-up has been shown to reduce the risk of vision loss and the development of some structural complications. Specifically, oral corticosteroids reduced the risk of CNV and subretinal fibrosis by 82% and the risk of visual acuity decline to 20/200 or worse (in better-seeing eyes) by 67%. IMT was associated with risk reductions of 67% for vision loss to 20/50 or worse and 92% for vision loss to 20/200 or worse in better-seeing eyes.

Bykhovskaya I, Thorne JE, Kempen JH, Dunn JP, Jabs DA. Vogt-Koyanagi-Harada disease: clinical outcomes. *Am J Ophthalmol.* 2005;140(4):674–678.

Greco A, Fusconi M, Gallo A, et al. Vogt-Koyanagi-Harada syndrome. *Autoimmun Rev.* 2013;12(11):1033–1038.

Read RW, Rechodouni A, Butani N, et al. Complications and prognostic factors in Vogt-Koyanagi-Harada disease. *Am J Ophthalmol.* 2001;131(5):599–606.

Behçet Disease

Behçet disease (BD) is a chronic, relapsing, multisystem inflammatory disorder of unknown etiology. It can affect both the anterior and the posterior segments of the eye, often simultaneously. The disease symptoms have been described for more than 2500 years. They were formally characterized in the early 20th century by Adamantiades and Behçet as a triad of aphthous ulceration, genital lesions, and recurrent uveitis. It is now known to affect almost any organ system and occurs in a variety of ethnic populations all over the world. It is most common in the Northern Hemisphere in the countries of the eastern Mediterranean and on the eastern rim of Asia, particularly along the ancient Silk Road.

Table 9-3 Diagnostic System for Behçet Disease (Japan)

Major criteria
- Recurrent oral aphthous ulcers
- Skin lesions (erythema nodosum, acneiform pustules, folliculitis)
- Recurrent genital ulcers
- Ocular inflammatory disease

Minor criteria
- Arthritis
- Gastrointestinal ulceration
- Epididymitis
- Systemic vasculitis or associated complications
- Neuropsychiatric symptoms

Types of Behçet disease
- Complete (4 major criteria)
- Incomplete (3 major criteria or ocular involvement with 1 other major criterion)
- Suspect (2 major criteria with no ocular involvement)
- Possible (1 major criterion)

Information from Behçet's Disease Research Committee of Japan. Behçet's disease: guide to diagnosis of Behçet's disease. *Jpn J Ophthalmol.* 1974;18:291–294.

Table 9-4 Diagnostic System for Behçet Disease (International Study Group for Behçet's Disease)

Recurrent oral aphthous ulcers (at least 3 or more times per year) plus 2 of the following criteria:
1. Recurrent genital ulcers
2. Ocular inflammation
3. Skin lesions
4. Positive cutaneous pathergy test

Adapted from International Study Group for Behçet's Disease. Criteria for diagnosis of Behçet's disease. *Lancet.* 1990;335(8697):1078–1080.

The prevalence of BD varies from as high as 20–421 cases per 100,000 inhabitants in Turkey to 8–13.5 per 100,000 in Japan and 5.2 per 100,000 in the United States. The age of onset is typically in the third and fourth decades but can also occur after age 50 or in childhood. Both genders are affected equally, but BD may have a more severe course in males. Although there have been some familial cases of BD, most are sporadic.

The diagnosis of BD is clinical and is based on the presence of multiple systemic findings. The diagnostic system for BD in Table 9-3 was suggested by researchers in Japan, and another diagnostic system was suggested by the International Study Group for Behçet's Disease (Table 9-4). Although BD is a multisystem disease, it can have its predominant effect on a single system; thus, special clinical types of BD occur—namely, neuro-BD, ocular BD, intestinal BD, and vascular BD. However, importantly, being free from major organ involvement early in the disease does not protect against its development later on. Epidemiologic studies also report significant regional variability in organ-specific disease expression.

Kitaichi N, Miyazaki A, Iwata D, Ohno S, Stanford MR, Chams H. Ocular features of Behçet's disease: an international collaborative study. *Br J Ophthalmol.* 2007;91(12):1579–1582.

Tugal-Tutkun I, Onal S, Altan-Yaycioglu R, Huseyin Altunbas H, Urgancioglu M. Uveitis in Behçet disease: an analysis of 880 patients. *Am J Ophthalmol.* 2004;138(3):373–380.
Yazici H, Seyahi E, Hatemi G, Yazici Y. Behçet syndrome: a contemporary view. *Nat Rev Rheumatol.* 2018;14(2):107–119.

Nonocular systemic manifestations

Recurrent, painful oral aphthae are the most frequent finding and often the presenting sign in BD (Fig 9-60). They can occur on the lips, gums, palate, tongue, uvula, and posterior pharynx. They are discrete, rounded, white ulcerations with red rims varying in size from 2 to 15 mm. They typically last 7–10 days and heal with little scarring unless large.

Genital ulcers appear grossly similar to oral aphthous ulcers, but tend to be deeper and larger and heal with more scarring. In male patients, they can occur on the scrotum or penis. In female patients, they can appear on the vulva and vaginal mucosa. Genital scarring may be apparent on examination even if patients have no acute symptoms.

Skin lesions can include painful or recurrent erythema nodosum, often over extensor surfaces such as the tibia, but also on the face, neck, and buttocks. Acne vulgaris or folliculitis-like skin lesions may frequently appear on the upper thorax and face. Skin lesions may disappear spontaneously with minimal or no scarring. Nearly 40% of patients with BD exhibit cutaneous pathergy, which is characterized by the development of a sterile pustule at the site of a venipuncture or an injection but is not pathognomonic of BD.

Systemic vasculitis affecting any size artery or vein in the body may occur in up to 25% of patients with BD. Common manifestations are arterial occlusions and aneurysms, and superficial or deep venous occlusions and varices. Cardiac involvement can include granulomatous endocarditis, myocarditis, endomyocardial fibrosis, coronary arteritis, and pericarditis. Gastrointestinal lesions, such as ulcers involving the esophagus, stomach, and intestines, may be seen in over 50% of BD patients in Japan, where it is a significant cause of morbidity. Pulmonary involvement is mainly pulmonary arteritis with aneurysmal dilatation of the pulmonary artery. Fifty percent of patients with BD develop arthritis, commonly of the knee, elbow, hand, or ankle.

Neurologic involvement is among the most serious of all manifestations of BD. Lesions of the white matter of the brain and brainstem may lead to motor dysfunction, stroke, and cognitive/behavioral changes. Headaches and aseptic meningitis have been

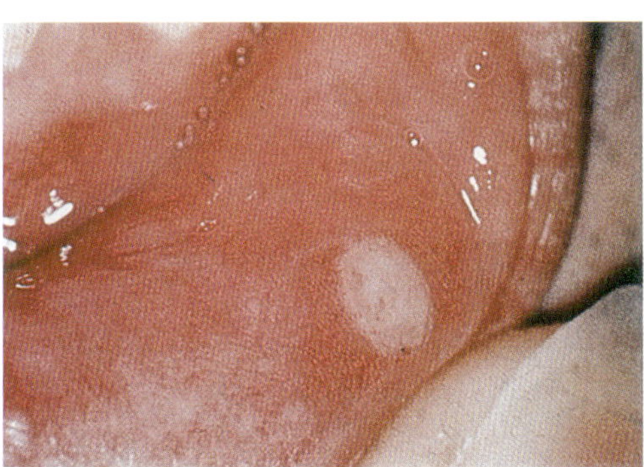

Figure 9-60 Behçet disease. Mucous membrane ulcers (oral aphthae).

associated with CNS vasculitis and meningeal involvement, respectively. Ten percent of patients with neuro-BD can have ocular disease, and 30% of patients with ocular BD may have neurologic involvement. Mortality has previously been reported to be as high as 10% in patients with neuro-BD, but it may be lower currently, especially with the use of IMT. Neuro-ophthalmic involvement can include cranial nerve palsies, papillitis, and papilledema resulting from thrombosis of the superior sagittal sinus or other venous sinuses.

Ocular manifestations

Ocular manifestations affect up to 70% of patients with BD. They carry serious implications because they are often recurrent and relapsing, resulting in permanent ocular damage. Severe vision loss can occur in up to 25% of patients with BD. Ocular disease most often presents as panuveitis that appears to be more severe and more common in men; over 80% of cases are bilateral. Ocular involvement as an initial presenting problem is relatively uncommon, and there may be a delay of years between presenting signs in other organs and the first occurrence of uveitis. The intraocular inflammation is characterized by a nongranulomatous, necrotizing, obliterative vasculitis that can affect any or all portions of the uveal tract.

In a minority of cases, anterior uveitis may be the only ocular manifestation of BD, classically described as the sudden onset of a hypopyon that disappears over weeks with or without treatment (Fig 9-61). The anterior uveitis may be accompanied by redness, pain, photophobia, and blurred vision, though occasionally there is a striking lack of inflammatory signs and symptoms, manifesting as a relatively quiet eye, despite the presence of hypopyon. On clinical examination, the hypopyon can shift with the patient's head position or disperse with head shaking, and it may not be visible unless viewed by gonioscopy. With relapses, posterior synechiae, iris bombé, and angle-closure glaucoma may all develop. Other less-common anterior segment findings of BD include cataract, episcleritis, scleritis, conjunctival ulcers, and corneal immune ring opacities.

Posterior segment manifestations of ocular BD are often profoundly sight threatening. The essential finding is an occlusive retinal vasculitis affecting both arteries and veins, which may be associated with multifocal areas of chalky white retinitis (Fig 9-62). Posterior and panuveitis are the most common types of BD ocular inflammation, seen in

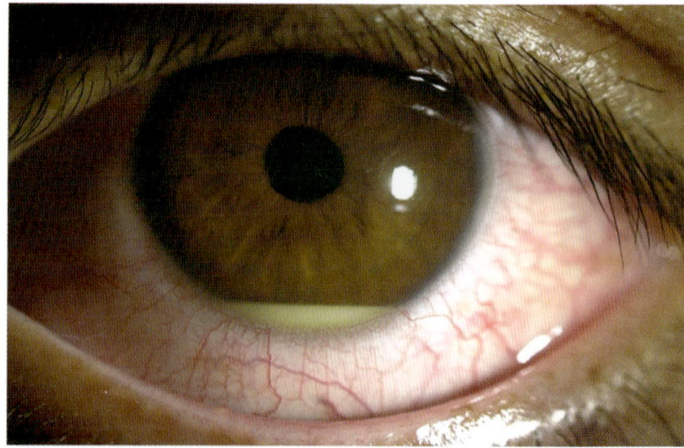

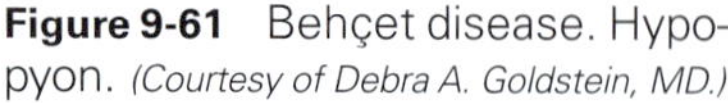

Figure 9-61 Behçet disease. Hypopyon. *(Courtesy of Debra A. Goldstein, MD.)*

50%–80% of cases of BD patients with uveitis. Other posterior manifestations can include retinal artery and vein occlusions, vascular sheathing with variable amounts of vitritis, and associated uveitic macular edema. Retinal ischemia can lead to the development of retinal and iris neovascularization with neovascular glaucoma. After repeated episodes of retinal vasculitis and vascular occlusions, retinal vessels may become white and sclerotic. The ischemic nature of the vasculitis and accompanying retinitis may produce a funduscopic appearance that may be confused with acute retinal necrosis syndrome or other necrotizing herpetic entities (Fig 9-63 and Chapter 11). The optic nerve is affected in 25% of patients with BD. Optic papillitis can occur, but progressive optic atrophy may occur as a result of the vasculitis affecting the arterioles that supply blood to the optic nerve.

Pathogenesis

Many environmental factors have been suggested as potential causes of BD, but none has been proven. No infectious agent or microorganism has been reproducibly isolated from the lesions of patients with BD. The disorder is clinically and experimentally unlike other autoimmune diseases.

HLA associations have been found in 2 systemic forms of BD: HLA-B12 with mucocutaneous lesions and HLA-B51 with ocular lesions. These associations are not reproducible in all populations, and testing lacks the sensitivity and specificity to support its use for diagnosis. Histologically, BD lesions resemble those of delayed-type hypersensitivity reactions early on; late lesions resemble those of immune-complex–type reactions. Histopathology may show an inflammatory occlusive vasculitis (Fig 9-64).

Diagnosis

Laboratory tests—for example, HLA typing, cutaneous pathergy testing, and blood tests for ESR and CRP—are of little value in confirming the diagnosis.

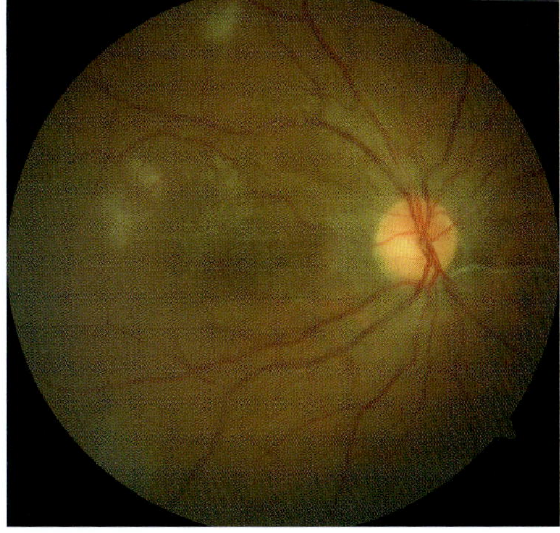

Figure 9-62 Behçet disease. Fundus photograph of retinitis and vasculitis. *(Courtesy of Didar Ucar, MD.)*

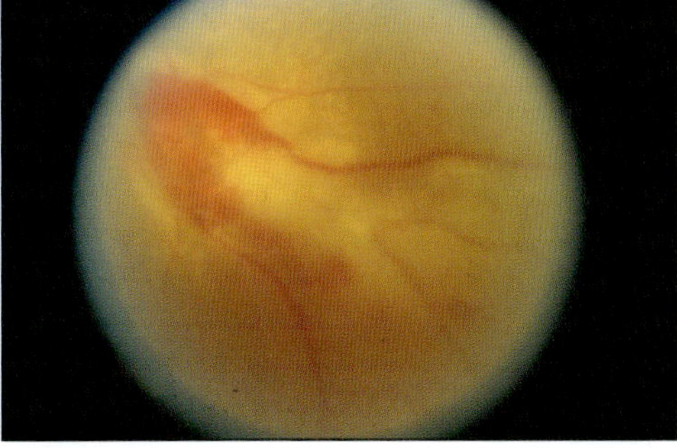

Figure 9-63 Behçet disease. Fundus photograph of retinitis and vasculitis with retinal hemorrhage. The retinitis shown here appears similar to necrotizing herpetic retinitis with retinal whitening and occlusive retinal vasculitis. *(Courtesy of Ramana S. Moorthy, MD.)*

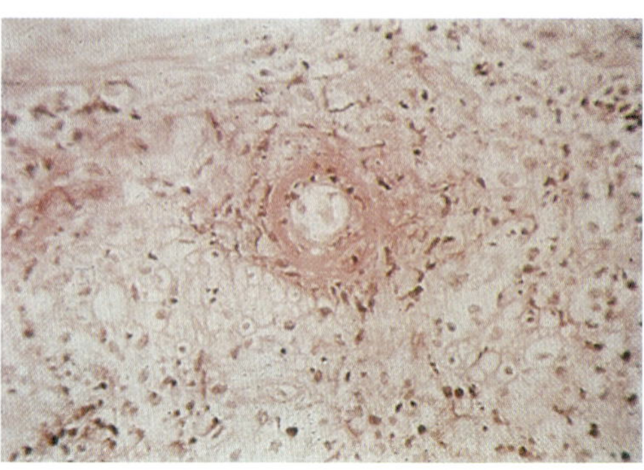

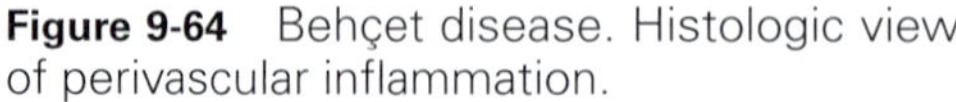
Figure 9-64 Behçet disease. Histologic view of perivascular inflammation.

Fluorescein angiography demonstrates marked dilatation and occlusion of retinal capillaries with perivascular staining, evidence of retinal ischemia, leakage of fluorescein into the macula with the development of macular edema, and retinal neovascularization that may leak (Fig 9-65). Subtle vascular leakage may be present on FA even during periods of clinical quiescence. Adjusting therapy in response to this leakage may prevent the development of inflammatory damage.

Because of the transient nature of posterior segment inflammatory episodes in BD, serial color photography may be of benefit in diagnosis.

OCT imaging can show structural alterations caused by the vasculitis in the form of macular edema and disruption of the retinal architecture (see Fig 9-65). Systemic investigations may be helpful, as indicated by clinical presentation.

Kaçmaz RO, Kempen JH, Newcomb C, et al; Systemic Immunosuppressive Therapy for Eye Diseases Cohort Study Group. Ocular inflammation in Behçet disease: incidence of ocular complications and of loss of visual acuity. *Am J Ophthalmol.* 2008;146(6):828–836.

Tugal-Tutkun I, Ozdal P, Oray M, Onal S. Review for diagnostics of the year: multimodal imaging in Behçet uveitis. *Ocul Immunol Inflamm.* 2017;25(1):7–19.

Differential diagnosis

The differential diagnosis for BD includes HLA-B27–associated anterior uveitis, reactive arthritis syndrome, sarcoidosis, Susac syndrome, and systemic vasculitides including systemic lupus erythematosus, PAN, and GPA. Necrotizing herpetic retinitis can also mimic occlusive BD retinal vasculitis.

Tugal-Tutkun I, Gupta V, Cunningham ET. Differential diagnosis of Behçet uveitis. *Ocul Immunol Inflamm.* 2013;21(5):337–350.

Treatment of ocular Behçet disease

The goal of treatment is not only to treat the explosive onset of acute disease with systemic corticosteroids but also to control chronic inflammation and prevent or decrease the number of relapses of ocular inflammation with IMT. Posterior segment ocular BD is an absolute indication for prompt initiation of IMT.

An American expert panel has recommended TNF inhibitor therapy with infliximab (good-quality evidence) or adalimumab (moderate-quality evidence) as first- or second-line corticosteroid-sparing therapy. A European League Against Rheumatism panel has

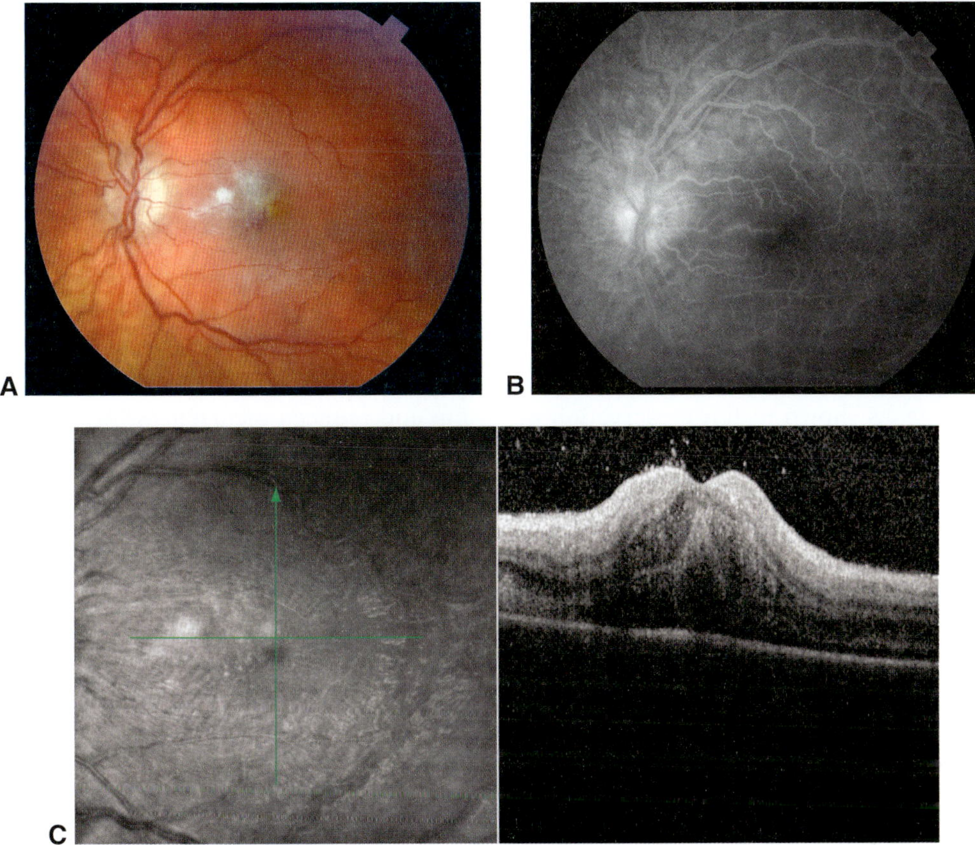

Figure 9-65 Behçet disease. **A,** Color fundus photograph indicating vasculitis and localized retinitis. **B,** Fluorescein angiogram showing disc staining and perivascular leakage. **C,** Optical coherence tomography scan revealing macular edema and inflammatory disruption of the retinal microarchitecture. *(Courtesy of David J. Browning, MD, PhD.)*

recommended using azathioprine (with corticosteroids) as first-line IMT for ocular BD and cyclosporine or infliximab as second-line treatment. When other major organs are involved, close collaboration with specialists in other fields is necessary, as treatment modifications based on severity and type of BD may be required.

Corticosteroids Systemic corticosteroids (eg, 1.0–1.5 mg/kg/day of prednisone with a gradual taper) are extremely useful in controlling acute inflammation. Periocular and intravitreal steroids may also be a useful adjunct in selected patients. Corticosteroid monotherapy should be avoided in sight-threatening BD uveitis, as severe rebound attacks may occur during tapering.

Nonbiologic IMT Only azathioprine and cyclosporine have undergone randomized clinical trials indicating effectiveness in reducing uveitis recurrence and preserving vision. Uncontrolled trials have shown benefit with mycophenolate mofetil and tacrolimus as steroid-sparing agents; alkylating agents, while effective, are used less frequently due to serious side effects. Chlorambucil administration can help achieve a durable remission in ocular BD. Cyclophosphamide is an alternative to chlorambucil and can be used orally or as pulsed intravenous therapy. Both of these alkylating agents have been shown to be more effective than cyclosporine in the management of posterior segment ocular BD but carry a greater risk of systemic complications and require complex hematologic monitoring. The availability of biologic drugs has led most experts to reserve the use of alkylating agents for patients with severe refractory disease.

Biologic agents The use of systemic TNF inhibitors has heralded a new era in the treatment of ocular BD. A substantial body of literature has emerged demonstrating the long-term efficacy and relative safety of systemic infliximab use in severe refractory ocular BD, often achieving rapid and complete control of disease, with reduction in retinal vascular leakage, as shown in FA; preservation of vision; and reduced recurrences. Additional data suggest greater benefit of infliximab therapy when initiated early on in the disease course. Adalimumab has been studied to a lesser extent, although preliminary data are promising, including a cohort studied prospectively as a part of the phase 3 clinical trials of adalimumab for noninfectious posterior uveitis. Interferon alfa is a naturally occurring cytokine involved in immune regulation, which, when administered in ocular BD as interferon alfa-2a, has been shown in a number of observational studies to be a safe and effective therapy. Combined with its lower cost and compatibility with concomitant latent tuberculosis infection, some experts prefer it as first-line therapy specific to ocular BD.

Hatemi G, Silman A, Bang D, et al; EULAR Expert Committee. EULAR recommendations for the management of Behçet disease. *Ann Rheum Dis.* 2008;67(12):1656–1662.

Keino H, Okada AA, Watanabe T, Nakayama M, Nakamura T. Efficacy of infliximab for early remission induction in refractory uveoretinitis associated with Behçet disease: a 2-year follow-up study. *Ocul Immunol Inflamm.* 2017;25(1):46–51.

Levy-Clarke G, Jabs DA, Read RW, Rosenbaum JT, Vitale A, Van Gelder RN. Expert panel recommendations for the use of anti–tumor necrosis factor biologic agents in patients with ocular inflammatory disorders. *Ophthalmology.* 2014;121(3):785–796.

Zierhut M, Abu El-Asrar AM, Bodaghi B, Tugal-Tutkun I. Therapy of ocular Behçet disease. *Ocul Immunol Inflamm.* 2014;22(1):64–76.

Prognosis

The prognosis for vision is guarded in patients with BD. Nearly 25% of patients worldwide with chronic ocular BD have visual acuity less than 20/200, most commonly caused by macular edema, occlusive retinal vasculitis, optic atrophy, and glaucoma. Adult men tend to have poorer vision outcomes. Patients appear to have a better visual prognosis because of earlier and more aggressive use of IMT. The presence of posterior synechiae, persistent inflammation, elevated IOP, and hypotony are all statistically significant predictive factors for vision loss. The chronic relapsing nature of this disease, with frequent exacerbations after long periods of remission, makes it difficult to predict visual outcomes.

CHAPTER 10

Infectious Uveitis: Bacterial Causes

This chapter includes a related video, which can be accessed by scanning the QR code provided in the text or going to www.aao.org/bcscvideo_section09.

Highlights

- Bacterial uveitis most commonly presents as posterior uveitis. Causative organisms include *Treponema pallidum, Mycobacterium tuberculosis*, and less frequently, *Borrelia burgdorferi* and *Bartonella* species, among others.
- Syphilis is reemerging globally and should be considered in the differential diagnosis of every individual with uveitis.
- Tuberculous uveitis can arise in the absence of detectable active systemic disease, with the diagnosis being presumptive in most cases.
- Ocular involvement occurs in 5%–10% of individuals with cat-scratch disease, and may manifest as neuroretinitis, focal/multifocal retinitis, and, less frequently, Parinaud oculoglandular syndrome.

Syphilis

Syphilis is a reemerging multisystem, chronic bacterial infection caused by the spirochete *Treponema pallidum*. It is associated with numerous ocular manifestations in both the acquired and congenital forms of the disease. Transmission occurs most often through sexual contact; however, transplacental infection of the fetus is also possible, mainly after the tenth week of pregnancy. Having reached an all-time low in the year 2000 in the United States, the incidence rate of syphilis at any disease stage has been rising in the last 2 decades, not only in men, particularly those having sex with men, but also among women. This rise is associated with an almost twofold increase in the incidence of congenital syphilis in the United States (from 9.4 to 15.7 per 100,000 live births).

Although syphilis is thought to be responsible for less than 2% of all uveitis cases, it is one of the great masqueraders in medicine and should always be considered in the differential diagnosis of any intraocular inflammatory disease. It is one of the few entities that can be cured with appropriate antimicrobial therapy, even in patients with human immunodeficiency virus (HIV) coinfection. Delay in the diagnosis of syphilitic uveitis may lead not only to permanent vision loss but also to significant neurologic and cardiac morbidity, which may have been averted with early treatment.

Centers for Disease Control and Prevention. *Sexually Transmitted Disease Surveillance 2016.* Atlanta: US Department of Health and Human Services; 2017. Available at www.cdc.gov/std/stats16/CDC_2016_STDS_Report-for508WebSep21_2017_1644.pdf. Accessed November 16, 2020.

Congenital Syphilis

The prevalence of congenital syphilis is increasing in the United States in parallel to higher rates of infection in young women, associated with limited to late or even absent prenatal care, without proper serologic screening. Primary or secondary syphilis in the mother is more likely to be transmitted to the baby than is latent syphilis; the longer the mother had syphilis, the less likely is the transmission. Systemic findings in patients with early congenital syphilis (age 2 years or younger) include hepatosplenomegaly, characteristic changes of the long bones on radiographic examination, abdominal distention, desquamative skin rash, low birth weight, pneumonia, and severe anemia. Late manifestations (age 3 years or older) result from scarring during early systemic disease. These include Hutchinson teeth, mulberry molars, abnormal facies, cranial nerve VIII deafness, bony changes such as saber shins and perforations of the hard palate, cutaneous lesions such as rhagades, and neurosyphilis. Cardiovascular complications are unusual in late congenital syphilis. For further discussion of ocular manifestations of congenital syphilis, see BCSC Section 6, *Pediatric Ophthalmology and Strabismus.*

Ocular inflammatory signs of congenital syphilis may present at birth or decades later and include uveitis, interstitial keratitis, optic neuritis, glaucoma, and congenital cataract. Multifocal chorioretinitis and, less commonly, retinal vasculitis are the most frequent uveitic manifestations of early congenital infection. They may result in a bilateral salt-and-pepper fundus, which affects the peripheral retina, posterior pole, or even a single quadrant. These changes are not progressive, and the patient may have normal vision. A less commonly described fundus finding is that of a bilateral secondary degeneration of the retinal pigment epithelium (RPE), which may mimic retinitis pigmentosa, with narrowing of the retinal and choroidal vessels, optic disc pallor with sharp margins, and morphologically variable deposits of pigment.

Nonulcerative stromal interstitial keratitis, often accompanied by anterior uveitis, is the most common inflammatory sign of untreated late congenital syphilis, occurring in up to 50% of cases, most commonly in girls (Fig 10-1). Intraocular inflammation in this setting is thought to be reactive to *T pallidum* in the cornea (keratouveitis). Symptoms include intense pain and photophobia. Blood vessels invade the cornea, and late stages show deep “ghost” (nonperfused) stromal vessels and corneal opacities. Left untreated, corneal inflammation may regress but leave the cornea focally or diffusely opaque, with reduced vision, even to the level of light perception only. Anterior uveitis accompanying interstitial keratitis may be difficult to observe because of corneal haze. Glaucoma may also occur. The constellation of interstitial keratitis, cranial nerve VIII deafness, and Hutchinson teeth is called the *Hutchinson triad.*

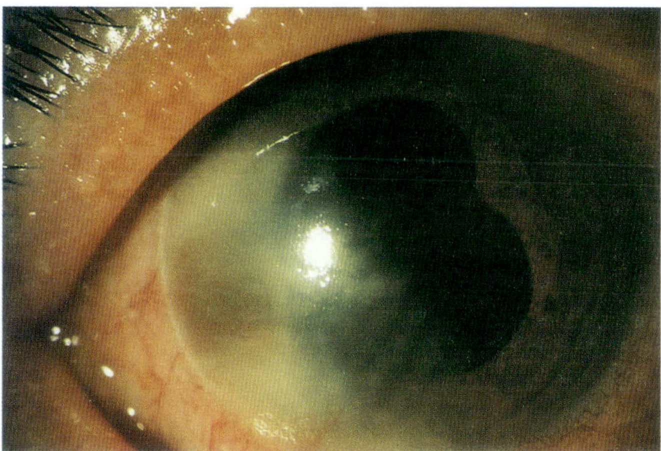

Figure 10-1 Active syphilitic interstitial keratitis.

Acquired Syphilis

Primary syphilis

Primary syphilis follows an incubation period of approximately 3 weeks and is characterized by a chancre, a painless, solitary lesion that originates at the site of inoculation, resolving spontaneously within 12 weeks regardless of treatment. The central nervous system (CNS) may be seeded with treponemes during this period, often in the absence of neurologic findings.

Secondary syphilis

Secondary syphilis occurs 6–8 weeks later and is heralded by the appearance of lymphadenopathy and a generalized maculopapular rash that may be prominent on the palms and soles. Uveitis occurs in approximately 10% of cases. This phase is followed by a latent period ranging from 1 year (early latency) to decades (late latency).

Tertiary syphilis

Approximately one-third of untreated patients incur *tertiary syphilis,* which may be further subcategorized as benign tertiary syphilis (the characteristic lesion being gumma, most frequently found on the skin and mucous membranes but also in the choroid and iris), cardiovascular syphilis, and neurosyphilis. Although uveitis may occur in up to 5% of patients whose disease has progressed to tertiary syphilis, it can occur at any stage of infection, including primary disease. Because the eye is an extension of the CNS, ocular syphilis is best regarded as a variant of neurosyphilis, a notion that has important diagnostic and therapeutic implications.

Ocular Involvement

Ocular manifestations of syphilis are protean and may affect all structures, including conjunctiva, sclera, cornea, lens, uveal tract, retina, optic nerve, cranial nerves, and pupillomotor pathways. Patients present with pain, redness, photophobia, blurred vision, and floaters. Intraocular inflammation may be granulomatous or nongranulomatous, unilateral or bilateral, and it may affect the anterior or posterior segment. Anterior segment findings can include iris roseola, vascularized papules (iris papulosa), larger red nodules (iris nodosa), and gummata. Interstitial keratitis, posterior synechiae, lens dislocation, and iris atrophy can also occur.

Posterior segment findings of acquired syphilis include vitritis, chorioretinitis, focal/multifocal retinitis, necrotizing retinochoroiditis, retinal vasculitis, exudative retinal detachment, isolated papillitis, and neuroretinitis. A focal or multifocal chorioretinitis, usually associated with a variable degree of vitritis, is the most common manifestation (Fig 10-2). These lesions are typically small, grayish yellow, and located in the postequatorial fundus, but they may become confluent. Retinal vasculitis and disc edema, with exudates appearing around the disc and the retinal arterioles, together with serous retinal detachment, may accompany the chorioretinitis. A syphilitic posterior placoid chorioretinitis has been described, the clinical appearance and angiographic characteristics of which are thought to be pathognomonic of secondary syphilis (Fig 10-3 and Video 10-1). Solitary or multifocal, macular or papillary, placoid, yellowish gray lesions at the level of the RPE, often with accompanying vitritis, display corresponding early hypofluorescence and late staining, along with retinal perivenous staining on fluorescein angiography (FA). Indocyanine green (ICG) angiography shows hypofluorescent spots corresponding to the lesions. Optical coherence tomography (OCT) displays irregularities at the level of the RPE, with corresponding disorganization of outer retinal layers.

Less common posterior segment involvement includes focal retinitis, periphlebitis, and, infrequently, exudative retinal detachment. Syphilis may present as a focal retinitis (Fig 10-4) or as a peripheral necrotizing retinochoroiditis that may resemble acute retinal necrosis or progressive outer retinal necrosis. Punctate inner retinal infiltrates have also

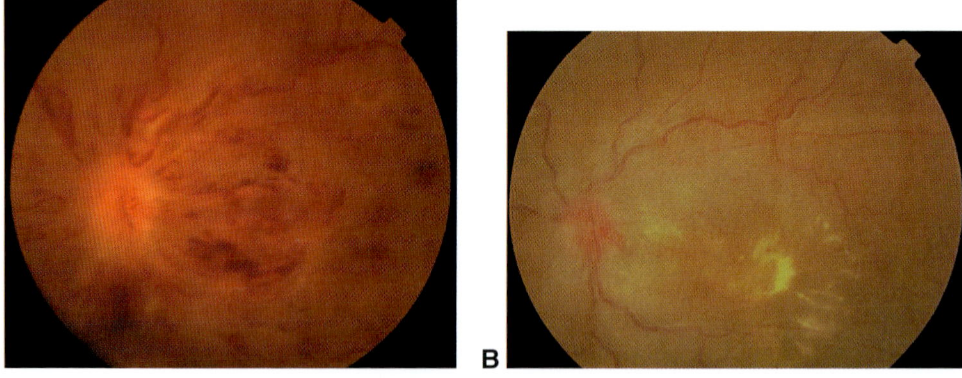

Figure 10-2 Syphilitic chorioretinitis. **A,** Fundus photograph of acute syphilitic chorioretinitis. Note diffuse edema of the disc, retina, and choroid in the posterior pole. **B,** Fundus photograph showing healing chorioretinitis after 2 weeks of intravenous penicillin therapy. Note the subretinal hard exudate that is organizing, as well as the reduction in disc edema and choroidal inflammation. *(Courtesy of Ramana S. Moorthy, MD.)*

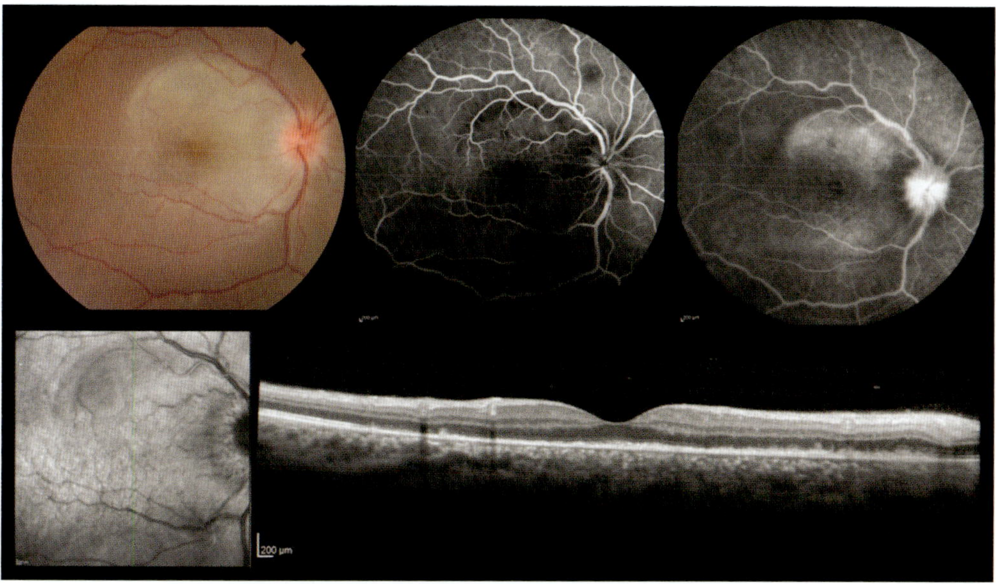

Figure 10-3 Fundus *(top left)*, angiographic *(top middle and top right)*, and optical coherence tomography *(bottom)* features of syphilitic posterior placoid chorioretinitis. Progressive placoid hyperfluorescence is seen on angiography *(top right)*, in correspondence to the yellowish geographic infiltrate in the posterior pole *(top left)*. Spectral-domain optical coherence tomography reveals deep granular changes, with disruption of outer retinal layers and underlying homogeneous hyper-reflectivity of the inner choroid. *(Courtesy of Daniel V. Vasconcelos-Santos, MD, PhD.)*

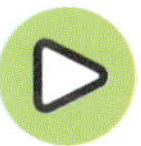

VIDEO 10-1 SD-OCT of syphilitic posterior placoid chorioretinitis.
Courtesy of Daniel V. Vasconcelos-Santos, MD, PhD.
Access the video at www.aao.org/bcscvideo_section09.

been described (Fig 10-5). Although the foci of retinitis may become confluent and are frequently associated with retinal vasculitis, syphilitic retinitis is more slowly progressive and responds dramatically to therapy with intravenous penicillin, often with a good visual outcome. Isolated retinal vasculitis that affects the retinal arterioles, capillaries, and larger arteries or veins (or both) is another feature of syphilitic intraocular inflammation that may best be appreciated on FA. Focal retinal vasculitis may masquerade as a branch retinal vein and/or arterial occlusion.

Syphilis is an important entity to consider in the differential diagnosis of patients with neuroretinitis and papillitis who present with macular star formation. Patients with syphilis who are immunocompromised or who have an HIV infection or AIDS may have atypical or more fulminant ocular disease patterns. Optic neuritis and neuroretinitis are more common in the initial presentation of these patients, and disease recurrences may be noted even after appropriate antibacterial therapy.

Neuro-ophthalmic manifestations of syphilis include the Argyll Robertson pupil, ocular motor nerve palsies, optic neuropathy, and retrobulbar optic neuritis, all of which

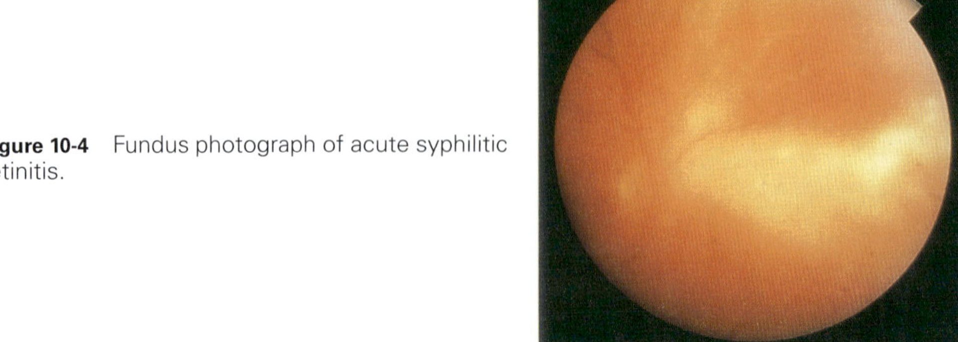

Figure 10-4 Fundus photograph of acute syphilitic retinitis.

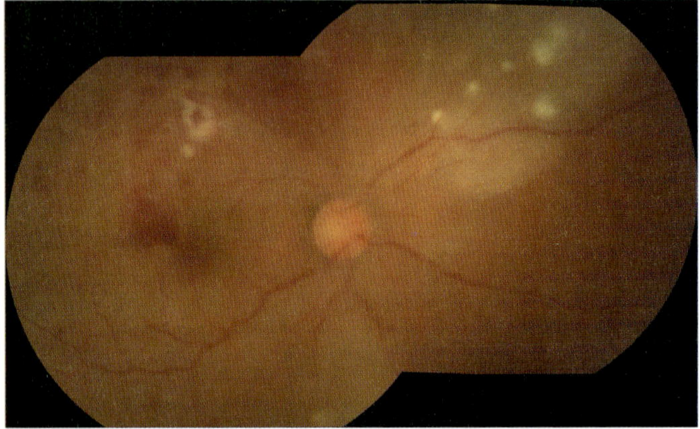

Figure 10-5 Fundus photograph of the right eye of a patient with syphilitic posterior uveitis, disclosing punctate inner retinal infiltrates overlying an area of retinal edema superonasally. *(Courtesy of Daniel V. Vasconcelos-Santos, MD, PhD.)*

appear most often in patients with tertiary syphilis or in neurosyphilis (see BCSC Section 5, *Neuro-Ophthalmology,* for further discussion).

Diagnosis

The diagnosis of syphilitic uveitis is supported by history and clinical presentation. It is confirmed by serologic testing. Primary syphilis may occasionally be diagnosed by direct visualization of spirochetes with dark-field microscopy and by direct fluorescent antibody tests of lesion exudates or tissue. Serodiagnosis is based on the results of both nontreponemal and treponemal antigen tests. Nontreponemal tests include the Venereal Disease Research Laboratory (VDRL) and rapid plasma reagin (RPR) evaluations. Treponemal tests include *T pallidum* antibodies via enzyme immunoassays (EIAs) or chemiluminescence immunoassays (CIAs), the microhemagglutination assay for *T pallidum* antibodies (MHA-TP), and the older fluorescent treponemal antibody absorption (FTA-ABS) assay. The EIA test has become the preferred test for many laboratories.

Van Gelder RN. Diagnostic testing in uveitis. *Focal Points: Clinical Modules for Ophthalmologists.* San Francisco: American Academy of Ophthalmology; 2013, module 4.

Nontreponemal and treponemal antigen tests

Nontreponemal antibody titers correlate with disease activity, generally increasing during primary or secondary syphilis and decreasing when the spirochetes are not active, such as during latent syphilis or after adequate antibiotic treatment. They are useful barometers for monitoring therapy for both systemic and ocular disease. Results of treponemal tests become positive during the secondary stage of syphilis and remain positive throughout the patient's life; as such, they are not useful in assessing therapeutic response.

Testing for HIV infection should be performed in all patients with syphilis, given the high frequency of coinfection. As a result of passive transfer of immunoglobulin G (IgG) across the placenta, VDRL and FTA-ABS IgG test results are positive among infants born to mothers with syphilis. For this reason, serodiagnosis of congenital syphilis is made using the immunoglobulin M (IgM) FTA-ABS test, which indicates infection in the infant.

False-positive nontreponemal test results occur in various medical conditions, including systemic lupus erythematosus (SLE), leprosy, advanced age, intravenous drug abuse, bacterial endocarditis, tuberculosis, vaccinations, infectious mononucleosis, HIV infection, atypical pneumonia, malaria, pregnancy, rickettsial infections, and other spirochetal infections (eg, Lyme disease). False-positive treponemal test results are rare (1%–2%) and may occur with other spirochetal infections (Lyme disease, leptospirosis), autoimmune disease (SLE, primary biliary cirrhosis, and rheumatoid arthritis), leprosy, malaria, and advanced age. Although nontreponemal tests are appropriate for screening large populations with a relatively lower risk for syphilis, specific treponemal tests, such as *T pallidum* antibody via EIA, CIA, MHA-TP, or FTA-ABS, have a higher predictive value in patients with uveitis and should be used in conjunction with nontreponemal tests in diagnosing and treating ocular syphilis. Both the false-positive and false-negative rates of serologic testing may be greater in HIV-infected patients. A lumbar puncture with examination of cerebrospinal fluid (CSF) is warranted in every case of syphilitic uveitis. A positive CSF VDRL result and/or pleocytosis is diagnostic for neurosyphilis, as CSF VDRL may be nonreactive in some cases of active CNS involvement. Although less specific, the CSF FTA-ABS test is highly sensitive and may be useful in excluding neurosyphilis. Follow-up for patients with chorioretinitis and abnormal CSF findings requires spinal fluid examination every 6 months until the cell count, protein, and VDRL results return to normal.

Other techniques

Polymerase chain reaction (PCR)-based DNA amplification techniques may be used on intraocular fluids, cerebrospinal fluids, or fluid taken from swabs of mucosal sites or ulcerative lesions.

Treatment

Parenteral penicillin G is the preferred treatment for all stages of syphilis (Table 10-1). Although the formulation, dose, route of administration, and duration of therapy vary with

Table 10-1 Treatment of Syphilis in Adults

Stage of Disease	Primary Treatment Regimen	Alternative Treatment Regimen
Primary, secondary, or early latent disease	Benzathine penicillin G 2.4 million U intramuscularly as a single dose	Doxycycline 100 mg orally 2 times per day for 2 weeks or tetracycline 500 mg orally 4 times per day for 2 weeks
Late latent or latent syphilis of uncertain duration, tertiary disease in the absence of neurosyphilis	Benzathine penicillin G 2.4 million U inramuscularly, weekly for 3 doses	Doxycycline 100 mg orally 2 times per day for 4 weeks or tetracycline 500 mg orally 4 times per day for 4 weeks
Neurosyphilis	Aqueous penicillin G 18–24 million U/day given intravenously as 3–4 million U every 4 hours or continuous infusion, for 10–14 days	Procaine penicillin 2.4 million U/day intramuscularly *plus* probenecid 500 mg orally 4 times per day, both for 10–14 days

U = units.

Adapted from Centers for Disease Control and Prevention. *Sexually Transmitted Disease Surveillance 2010.* Atlanta: US Department of Health and Human Services; 2011. Available at https://www.cdc.gov/std/stats/archive/surv2010.pdf. Accessed November 16, 2020.

the stage of the disease, patients with syphilitic uveitis should be managed as though they have neurosyphilis, regardless of immune status. The current Centers for Disease Control and Prevention (CDC) recommendation for the treatment of neurosyphilis is 18–24 million units (MU) of aqueous crystalline penicillin G per day, administered as 3–4 MU intravenously every 4 hours or as a continuous infusion for 10–14 days. This may be supplemented with intramuscular benzathine penicillin G, 2.4 MU weekly for 3 weeks. Alternatively, neurosyphilis may be treated with 2.4 MU/day of intramuscular procaine penicillin plus probenecid 500 mg 4 times a day, both for 10–14 days or with either intramuscular or intravenous ceftriaxone 2 g daily for 10–14 days.

The recommended treatment regimen for congenital syphilis in infants during the first months of life is intravenous aqueous crystalline penicillin G, 100,000–150,000 units/kg/day, administered intravenously as 50,000 units/kg/dose every 12 hours during the first 7 days of life and every 8 hours thereafter, for a total of 10 days. Alternatively, procaine penicillin G, 50,000 units/kg/dose, may be administered intramuscularly in a single daily dose for 10 days.

Penicillin remains the first choice for the treatment of neurosyphilis, congenital infection, or disease in pregnant women or patients coinfected with HIV. Patients with penicillin allergy may occasionally require desensitization and then treatment with penicillin. Alternative treatments in penicillin-allergic patients who show no signs of neurosyphilis and who are HIV-seronegative include doxycycline or tetracycline. Ceftriaxone and chloramphenicol have been reported to be effective alternatives in patients with ocular syphilis who are allergic to penicillin.

Patients should be monitored for the development of the Jarisch-Herxheimer reaction, a hypersensitivity response of the host to treponemal antigens that are released in large numbers as spirochetes are killed during the first 24 hours of treatment. Patients present with constitutional symptoms, such as fever, chills, hypotension, tachycardia, and malaise, but they may also experience concomitant worsening of intraocular inflammation that may require local and/or systemic corticosteroids. In most cases, however, supportive care and observation are sufficient.

Topical, periocular, and/or systemic corticosteroids, under appropriate antibiotic cover, may be useful adjuncts for treating the anterior and posterior segment inflammation associated with syphilitic uveitis. According to the CDC, syphilis is designated a nationally "notifiable" disease; thus, appropriate health authorities should be notified according to local regulations. Finally, the sexual contacts of the patient must be identified and treated, as a high percentage of these individuals are at risk for acquiring and transmitting this disease.

Amaratunge BC, Camuglia JE, Hall AJ. Syphilitic uveitis: a review of clinical manifestations and treatment outcomes of syphilitic uveitis in human immunodeficiency virus–positive and negative patients. *Clin Exp Ophthalmol.* 2010;38(1):68–74.

Centers for Disease Control and Prevention. *2015 Sexually Transmitted Diseases Treatment Guidelines.* Atlanta: US Department of Health and Human Services; 2016. Available at https://www.cdc.gov/std/tg2015/toc.htm. Accessed November 16, 2020.

Eandi CM, Neri P, Adelman RA, Yannuzzi LA, Cunningham ET Jr; International Syphilis Study Group. Acute syphilitic posterior placoid chorioretinitis: report of a case series and comprehensive review of the literature. *Retina.* 2012;32(9):1915–1941.

Jumper JM, Randhawa S. Imaging syphilis uveitis. *Int Ophthalmol Clin.* 2012;52(4):121–129.

Lyme Disease

Lyme disease (LD) is the most common tick-borne illness in the United States. It has protean systemic manifestations and is caused by the spirochete *Borrelia burgdorferi*, but intraocular inflammation is rare. Animal reservoirs include deer, horses, cows, rodents, birds, cats, and dogs. The spirochete is transmitted to humans through the bite of infected ticks, *Ixodes scapularis* in the northeast, mid-Atlantic, and midwestern United States and *Ixodes pacificus* in the western United States. Numbers of reported cases of LD have been increasing steadily in the United States, recently peaking at almost 40,000 in 2015. The disease affects men (53%) slightly more often than women and has a bimodal distribution, with peaks in children aged 5–14 years and in adults aged 50–59 years. Whites are affected more commonly than are other races. There is a seasonal variation, with most cases occurring between May and August. Lyme disease may be found worldwide, but outside the United States it is caused by different species of *Borrelia,* such as *B afzelii* and *B garinii.*

Clinical Features

The clinical manifestations of LD are divided into 3 stages; ocular findings vary within each stage.

Stage 1

The most characteristic feature of stage 1, or local disease, is a macular rash known as *erythema chronicum migrans* at the site of the tick bite; it appears within 2–28 days in ~70%

of patients, forming a "bull's-eye" lesion (Fig 10-6). Constitutional symptoms appear at this stage and include fever, malaise, fatigue, myalgias, and arthralgias.

Stage 2

Stage 2, or disseminated disease, occurs several weeks to 4 months after exposure. Spirochetes spread hematogenously to the skin, CNS, joints, heart, and eyes. A secondary erythema chronicum migrans rash may appear at sites remote from the tick bite. Left untreated, up to 80% of patients with erythema chronicum migrans develop joint manifestations, most commonly monoarthritis or oligoarthritis involving the large joints, typically the knee (Fig 10-7). Joint involvement may be the only clinical manifestation of LD in children, and juvenile idiopathic arthritis must be considered in the differential diagnosis.

Neurologic involvement, which occurs in up to 40% of patients, may include meningitis, encephalitis, painful radiculitis, or unilateral or bilateral Bell palsy. In endemic areas, as many as 25% of new-onset cranial nerve VII palsies may be attributed to *B burgdorferi* infection.

Stage 3

The most frequent systemic manifestation of stage 3, or persistent disease, which occurs more than 5 months after the initial infection, is episodic arthritis that may become chronic. Chronic arthritis has been associated with HLA-DR4 and -DR2 haplotypes in North America; individuals expressing HLA-DR4 have a poorer response to antibiotics. Acrodermatitis chronica atrophicans, a bluish red lesion on the extremities that may

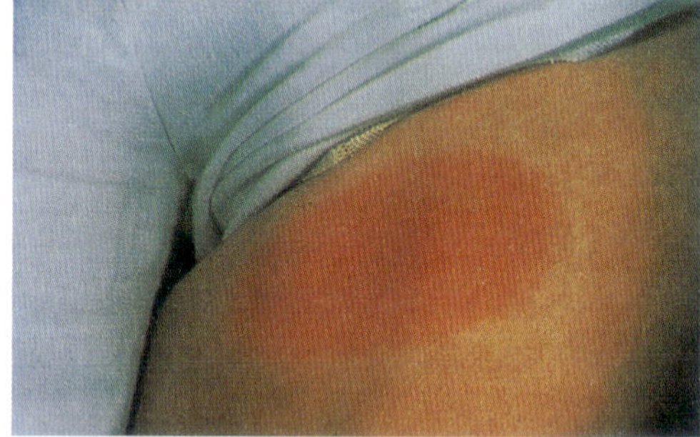

Figure 10-6 Erythema chronicum migrans in a patient with Lyme disease, demonstrating a single dense erythematous lesion. *(Courtesy of Alan B. MacDonald, MD.)*

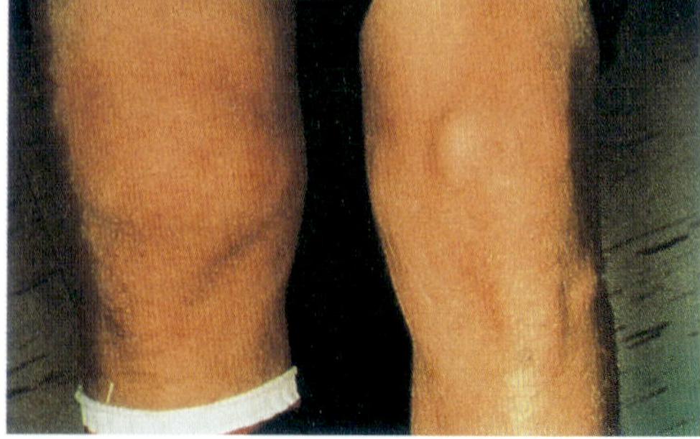

Figure 10-7 Lyme disease arthritis. *(Courtesy of Alan B. MacDonald, MD.)*

progress to fibrous bands and nodules, can occur in some patients, as may chronic neurologic syndromes such as neuropsychiatric disease, radiculopathy, chronic fatigue, peripheral neuropathy, and memory loss.

Ocular Involvement

The spectrum of ocular findings in patients with LD varies with disease stage. The most common ocular manifestation of early stage 1 disease is a follicular conjunctivitis, which occurs in approximately 11% of patients; less commonly present is episcleritis (see BCSC Section 1, *Update on General Medicine,* and Section 8, *External Disease and Cornea,* for further discussion and the differential diagnosis).

Intraocular inflammatory disease is reported most often in stage 2 and, less frequently, in stage 3 disease; it may manifest as anterior uveitis, intermediate uveitis, posterior uveitis, or panuveitis. Intermediate uveitis is one of the most common intraocular presentations. Vitritis may be severe and accompanied by a granulomatous anterior chamber reaction, papillitis, neuroretinitis, choroiditis, retinal vasculitis, and exudative retinal detachment (Fig 10-8).

A distinct clinical entity of peripheral multifocal choroiditis has been described in patients with LD; it is characterized by multiple, small, round, punched-out lesions associated with vitritis, similar to those present in sarcoidosis. Choroidal involvement may lead to pigment epithelial clumping resembling the inflammatory changes that occur with syphilis or rubella. Retinal vasculitis, found in association with peripheral multifocal choroiditis or vasculitic branch retinal vein occlusion, may be more common than previously known.

Neuro-ophthalmic manifestations include involvement of multiple cranial nerves (II, III, IV, V, VI, and, most commonly, VII) unilaterally or bilaterally, either sequentially or simultaneously. Optic nerve findings include optic neuritis, papilledema associated with meningitis, and most commonly papillitis. Horner syndrome has also been reported.

Keratitis is the most common ocular manifestation of stage 3 disease; much less common is episcleritis. Both may present months to years after the onset of infection. Typically, infiltrates are bilateral, patchy, focal, and stromal; subepithelial infiltrates with indistinct borders, peripheral keratitis with stromal edema, and corneal neovascularization can also occur. The keratitis is thought to represent an immune phenomenon rather than an infectious process because it responds to topical corticosteroids alone.

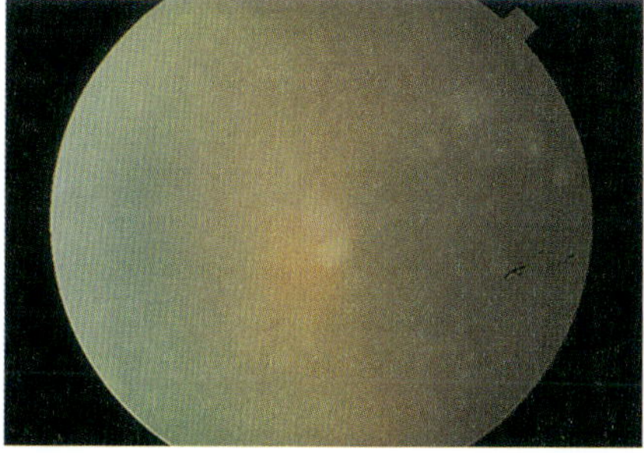

Figure 10-8 Fundus photograph revealing dense vitreous cells and haze in Lyme disease vitritis. *(Courtesy of John D. Sheppard Jr, MD.)*

Diagnosis

The diagnosis of LD is made on the basis of history, clinical presentation, and supportive serology. In the appropriate clinical context, erythema chronicum migrans is diagnostic. However, interpreting serologic data is problematic because of the lack of standardization of the values by which a positive test result is defined—the degree of cross-reactivity with other spirochetes—thus leading to frequent false-positive and false-negative test results. For the diagnosis of active disease or previous infection, the CDC recommends ELISA testing for IgM and IgG, followed by Western immunoblot testing. Assays based on PCR have been used successfully to amplify both genomic and plasmid *B burgdorferi* DNA from a variety of tissues, including ocular fluids, with the highest yields obtained from the skin.

Schwartz AM, Hinckley AF, Mead PS, Hook SA, Kugeler KJ. Surveillance for Lyme disease—United States, 2008–2015. *MMWR Surveill Summ.* 2017;66(22):1–12.

Treatment

Table 10-2 lists treatment recommendations for the various clinical manifestations of LD. For patients with ocular involvement, the route and duration of antibiotic treatment have not been established; however, as with syphilitic uveitis, intraocular inflammation associated with LD is best regarded as a manifestation of CNS involvement and warrants careful neurologic evaluation, including a lumbar puncture. Patients with severe posterior segment manifestations—and certainly those with confirmed CNS involvement—require intravenous antibiotic therapy with neurologic dosing regimens. Likewise, patients with less-severe disease that responds incompletely or relapses when oral antibiotics are discontinued should probably be treated with intravenous drugs as outlined in Table 10-2. Patients with Lyme carditis or who have atrioventricular block should be admitted to the hospital, monitored, and administered treatment with intravenous antibiotics.

After the initiation of appropriate antibiotic therapy, anterior segment inflammation may be treated with topical corticosteroids and mydriatics. The use of systemic corticosteroids has been described as part of the management of LD; however, the routine use of corticosteroids is controversial, as it has been associated with an increase in antibiotic treatment failures. As with syphilis, the Jarisch-Herxheimer reaction may complicate antibiotic therapy. Patients may become reinfected with *B burgdorferi* after successful antibiotic therapy, especially in endemic areas, or they may experience a more severe or chronic course due to concomitant babesiosis (an intraerythrocytic parasitic infection caused by protozoa of the genus *Babesia,* which is also transmitted by *Ixodes* species ticks) or human granulocytic anaplasmosis (previously known as *human granulocytic ehrlichiosis)* and require retreatment with antibiotics. Prevention strategies include avoiding tick-infested habitats, using tick repellents, wearing protective outer garments, removing ticks promptly, and reducing tick populations.

Mikkila E, Smith C, Sood S. The expanding clinical spectrum of ocular Lyme borreliosis. *Ophthalmology.* 2000;107(3):581–587.

Sathiamoorthi S, Smith WM. The eye and tick-borne disease in the United States. *Curr Opin Ophthalmol.* 2016;27(6):530–537.

Table 10-2 Recommended Antimicrobial Regimens for Treatment of Lyme Disease

Drug	Adult Dosage	Pediatric Dosage
Preferred oral regimens		
Amoxicillin	500 mg 3 times per day[a]	50 mg/kg per day in 3 divided doses (maximum, 500 mg per dose)[a]
Doxycycline	100 mg twice per day[b]	Not recommended for children aged <8 years For children aged ≥8 years, 4 mg/kg per day in 2 divided doses (maximum, 100 mg per dose)
Cefuroxime axetil	500 mg twice per day	30 mg/kg per day in 2 divided doses (maximum, 500 mg per dose)
Alternative oral regimen		
Selected macrolides[c]	For recommended dosing regimens, see footnote[d]	For recommended dosing regimens, see footnote[d]
Preferred parenteral regimen		
Ceftriaxone	2 g intravenously once per day	50–75 mg/kg per day intravenously in a single dose (maximum, 2 g)
Alternative parenteral regimens		
Cefotaxime	2 g intravenously every 8 hours[e]	150–200 mg/kg per day intravenously in 3–4 divided doses (maximum, 6 g per day)[e]
Penicillin G	18–24 million U per day intravenously, divided every 4 h[e]	200,000–400,000 U/kg per day divided every 4 hours[e] (not to exceed 18–24 million U per day)

[a] Although a higher dosage given twice per day might be equally as effective, in view of the absence of data on efficacy, twice-daily administration is not recommended.

[b] Tetracyclines are relatively contraindicated in pregnant or lactating women and in children aged <8 years.

[c] Because of their lower efficacy, macrolides are reserved for patients who are unable to take or who are intolerant of tetracyclines, penicillins, and cephalosporins.

[d] For adult patients intolerant of amoxicillin, doxycycline, and cefuroxime axetil, azithromycin (500 mg orally per day for 7–10 days), clarithromycin (500 mg orally twice per day for 14–21 days, if the patient is not pregnant), or erythromycin (500 mg orally 4 times per day for 14–21 days) may be given. Recommended dosages for children: azithromycin 10 mg/kg per day (maximum of 500 mg per day); clarithromycin, 7.5 mg/kg twice per day (maximum of 500 mg per dose); and erythromycin, 12.5 mg/kg 4 times per day (maximum of 500 mg per dose). Patients treated with macrolides should be closely observed to ensure resolution of the clinical manifestations.

[e] Dosage should be reduced for patients with impaired renal function.

Reprinted with permission from Wormser GP, Dattwyler RJ, Shapiro ED, et al. The clinical assessment, treatment, and prevention of Lyme disease, human granulocytic anaplasmosis, and babesiosis: clinical practice guidelines by the Infectious Diseases Society of America. *Clin Infect Dis.* 2006;43(9):1089–1134.

Leptospirosis

Leptospirosis is a zoonotic infection with a worldwide distribution. It occurs most frequently in tropical and subtropical regions and is caused by the gram-negative spirochete *Leptospira interrogans.* The natural reservoirs for *Leptospira* organisms include livestock, horses, dogs, and rodents, which excrete the organism in their urine. Humans contract the disease upon exposure to contaminated soil or water; thus, groups at risk include agricultural workers, sewer workers, veterinarians, fishery and slaughterhouse workers, and military personnel, as well as swimmers, triathletes, and whitewater rafters. The disease is not known to spread from person to person, but maternal–fetal transmission might occur infrequently. It is very rare in the United States, with 100–150 cases being identified annually, half of them in Puerto Rico. Globally, 1 million people are estimated to be infected each year, with almost 60,000 deaths. Since 2013, leptospirosis has been reinstated as a nationally notifiable disease in the United States.

Leptospirosis is frequently a biphasic disease, with the initial, or leptospiremic, phase following an incubation period of 2–4 weeks heralded by the abrupt onset of fever, chills, headache, myalgias, vomiting, and diarrhea. Severe septicemic leptospirosis, also known as *Weil disease,* is characterized by renal and hepatocellular dysfunction; it is rare (occurs in 10%) but can be fatal in 30%. Leptospires may be isolated from the blood and CSF but are cleared rapidly as the disease progresses to the second, or immune, phase of the illness, which is characterized by meningitis, leptospiruria, cranial nerve palsies, myelitis, and uveitis. The organism may persist for longer periods of time in immunologically privileged sites such as the brain and the eye.

Centers for Disease Control and Prevention. Leptospirosis. Atlanta: US Department of Health and Human Services; 2018. Available at www.cdc.gov/leptospirosis/health_care_workers/index.html. Accessed November 16, 2020.

Rathinam SR. Ocular manifestations of leptospirosis. *J Postgrad Med.* 2005;51(3):189–194.

Ocular Involvement

Ocular involvement can occur in both the leptospiremic and immune phases, but there is frequently a prolonged interval between systemic and ocular disease. Circumcorneal conjunctival hyperemia is the earliest and most common sign of ocular leptospirosis. The development of intraocular inflammation, which can range from mild anterior uveitis to panuveitis with retinal vasculitis (in 10%–44% of patients), is the more serious, potentially vision-threatening complication.

Diagnosis

The differential diagnosis includes HLA-B27–associated uveitis, idiopathic pars planitis, Behçet disease, Eales disease, sarcoidosis, tuberculosis, and syphilis. Appropriate history and laboratory evaluation help distinguish these entities from leptospiral uveitis. A definitive diagnosis requires isolation of the organism from bodily fluids. A presumptive diagnosis is made on the basis of serologic assays. Rapid serologic assays such as ELISA and complement-fixation tests for the detection of IgM antibodies against leptospiral antigens are highly sensitive and specific, and PCR-based assays are under evaluation. Leptospirosis may cause a false-positive result on RPR or FTA-ABS tests.

Treatment

Intravenous antibiotic therapy with 1.5 MU of penicillin G every 6 hours or oral doxycycline, 100 mg twice daily for 1 week, may be used for mild or moderate cases. It is not known whether systemic antibiotic treatment is protective with respect to long-term complications such as uveitis. However, systemic antibiotic treatment should be considered for ocular disease that occurs even months after onset of the acute systemic disease. In addition, topical, periocular, or systemic corticosteroids, together with mydriatic and cycloplegic drugs, are routinely used to suppress intraocular inflammation. The visual prognosis of leptospiral uveitis is quite favorable despite severe panuveal inflammation.

Ocular Nocardiosis

Nocardia asteroides is a gram-positive rod with partially acid-fast beaded branching filaments—a bacterium that acts like a fungus. Although ocular involvement in patients with *N asteroides* infection is rare, ocular disease may be the presenting problem in this potentially lethal but treatable systemic disease characterized by pneumonia and disseminated abscesses. The responsible organism is commonly found in soil, and initial infection occurs by ingestion or inhalation, causing an insidious inflammation. Immunocompromised individuals are more likely to be affected.

Garg P. Fungal, mycobacterial, and Nocardia infections and the eye: an update. *Eye (Lond)*. 2012; 26(2):245–251.

Ocular Involvement

Ocular involvement occurs by hematogenous spread of the bacteria, and symptoms may vary from the mild pain and redness of anterior uveitis to the severe pain and decreased vision of panophthalmitis. Nocardia infection can affect essentially any ocular structure, including periorbital tissue and the adnexae. Findings range from keratitis, necrotizing scleritis, or an isolated, unilateral choroidal or subretinal mass (abscess) with minimal vitritis to panuveitis with anterior chamber cell and flare, vitritis, and multiple choroidal abscesses with overlying retinal detachment mimicking fungal endophthalmitis.

Diagnosis

Diagnosis can be established with a culture of the organism taken from tissue or fluid, by vitreous aspiration for Gram stain and culture, or, occasionally, by enucleation and microscopic identification of organisms.

Treatment

Treatment of systemic *N asteroides* infection with systemic sulfonamide (trimethoprim-sulfamethoxazole) may be required for protracted periods of time. Combination therapy with additional antibiotics may be required.

Tuberculosis

Ocular involvement caused by tuberculosis (TB) is uncommon in the United States. In the last 6 decades, the TB incidence rate in the United States has decreased from 52.6 cases per 100,000 persons in 1953 to 2.9 cases per 100,000 in 2016. Worldwide, however, TB remains an important systemic infectious disease, with more than 10.4 million new cases and 1.7 million deaths reported annually. Nearly one-third of the world's population is infected, and 95% of cases occur in resource-limited countries.

In the United States, important risk factors include ethnicity and country of birth, with increased prevalence among Asians, African Americans, and Hispanics, when compared to non-Hispanic Whites. Diabetes mellitus and coninfection with HIV have also emerged as risk factors, in addition to substance abuse or residence in congregate settings, including correctional facilities, military barracks, homeless shelters, refugee camps, dormitories, and nursing homes, among others. Although the frequency of ocular disease parallels the prevalence of TB in general, it remains relatively uncommon both in endemic areas and among institutionalized populations with unequivocal systemic disease. In the United States, the incidence of uveitis attributable to TB at a large tertiary care facility was 0.6%, whereas at major referral centers in India, it ranged from 0.6% to 10%. In similar institutions in Japan and Saudi Arabia, the incidence was 7.9% and 10.5%, respectively.

Mycobacterium tuberculosis is an acid-fast–staining, obligate aerobe most commonly transmitted by aerosolized droplets. The organism has an affinity for highly oxygenated tissues. Tuberculous lesions are commonly found in the apices of the lungs as well as in the choroid, which has the highest blood flow rate in the body. Systemic infection may occur primarily, due to recent exposure; in 90% of patients, however, it occurs secondarily from reactivation of the disease with immune compromise. Widespread hematogenous dissemination of TB, known as *miliary disease,* likewise occurs most often in immunocompromised persons.

Pulmonary TB develops in approximately 80% of patients, whereas extrapulmonary disease occurs in about 20%, with one-half of these patients having a normal-appearing chest radiograph and up to 20% having a negative result on the purified protein derivative (PPD) skin test. Patients coinfected with HIV present more often with extrapulmonary disease, the frequency of which increases with deteriorating immune function. Only 10% of infected individuals develop symptomatic disease; one-half of these manifest illness within the first 1–2 years. Most, however, remain infected but asymptomatic. The classic presentation of symptomatic disease—fever, night sweats, and weight loss—occurs in both pulmonary and extrapulmonary infection. This fact is important to keep in mind when conducting a review of systems in patients suspected of tuberculous uveitis because histologically proven intraocular TB has been found in asymptomatic patients as well as in patients with extrapulmonary disease.

Centers for Disease Control and Prevention. *Reported Tuberculosis in the United States 2016.* Atlanta: US Department of Health and Human Services; 2017. Available at www.cdc.gov/tb/statistics/reports/2016/pdfs/2016_Surveillance_FullReport.pdf. Accessed November 16, 2020.

Yeh S, Sen HN, Colyer M, Zapor M, Wroblewski K. Update on ocular tuberculosis. *Curr Opin Ophthalmol.* 2012;23(6):551–556.

Ocular Involvement

The ocular manifestations of TB may result from either active infection or an immunologic reaction to the organism. External ocular and anterior segment findings include scleritis, phlyctenulosis, interstitial keratitis, corneal infiltrates, anterior chamber and iris nodules, and isolated granulomatous anterior uveitis (Fig 10-9); the last is exceedingly uncommon in the absence of posterior segment disease.

Tuberculous uveitis is classically a chronic granulomatous disease that may affect the anterior and/or posterior segments. It may be replete with mutton-fat keratic precipitates, iris nodules, posterior synechiae, and secondary glaucoma, although nongranulomatous uveitis may also occur. Patients typically experience a waxing and waning course, with accumulation of vitreous opacities and macular edema (Fig 10-10).

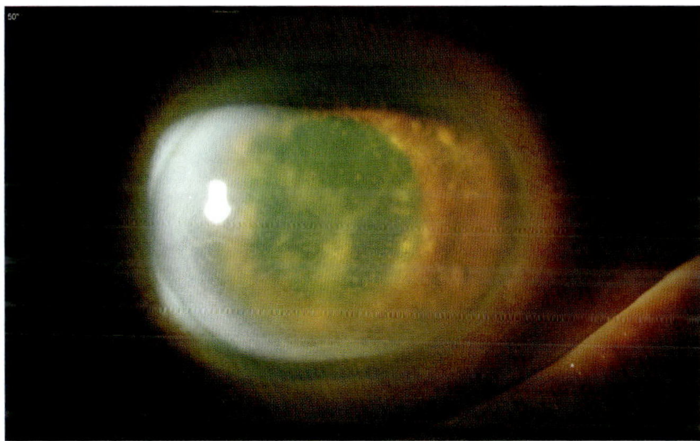

Figure 10-9 Severe fibrinous inflammation and large iris nodules in a patient with ocular tuberculosis. Polymerase chain reaction testing was positive from aqueous. *(Courtesy of H. Nida Sen, MD, National Eye Institute.)*

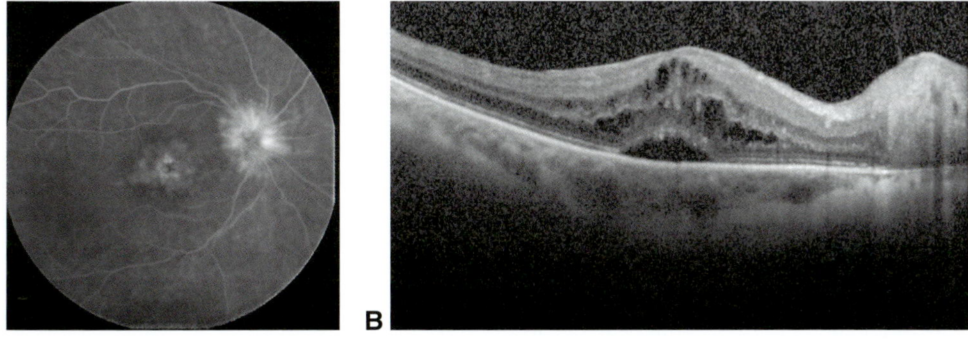

Figure 10-10 Chronic tuberculous uveitis. **A,** Fluorescein angiogram of chronic tuberculous uveitis with disc edema, periphlebitis, and macular edema. **B,** Spectral-domain optical coherence tomography confirms macular edema. *(Courtesy of Daniel V. Vasconcelos-Santos, MD, PhD.)*

Choroidal involvement

Disseminated choroiditis is the most common presentation and is characterized by multiple deep, discrete, yellowish lesions between 0.5 mm and 3.0 mm in diameter and numbering from 5 to several hundred (Fig 10-11). These lesions, or tubercles, are located predominantly in the posterior pole and may be accompanied by disc edema, nerve fiber layer hemorrhages, and varying degrees of vitritis and granulomatous anterior uveitis. Alternatively, they may present as a single, focal, large, elevated choroidal mass (tuberculoma) that varies in size from 4 mm to 14 mm and may be accompanied by neurosensory retinal detachment and macular star formation (Fig 10-12). Choroidal tubercles may be one of the earliest signs of disseminated disease and are more commonly observed among immunocompromised hosts. On FA, active choroidal lesions display early hypo-hyperfluorescence with late leakage, and cicatricial lesions show early blocked fluorescence with late staining. ICG angiography reveals early- and late-stage hypofluorescence corresponding to the choroidal lesions, which are frequently more numerous than those seen on FA or clinical examination (see Fig 10-12). Other manifestations include multifocal choroiditis, frequently with a serpiginoid patter (multifocal serpiginoid choroiditis, also called *serpiginous-like choroiditis;* Fig 10-13). In patients with HIV/AIDS, tuberculous choroiditis may progress despite effective antituberculous therapy.

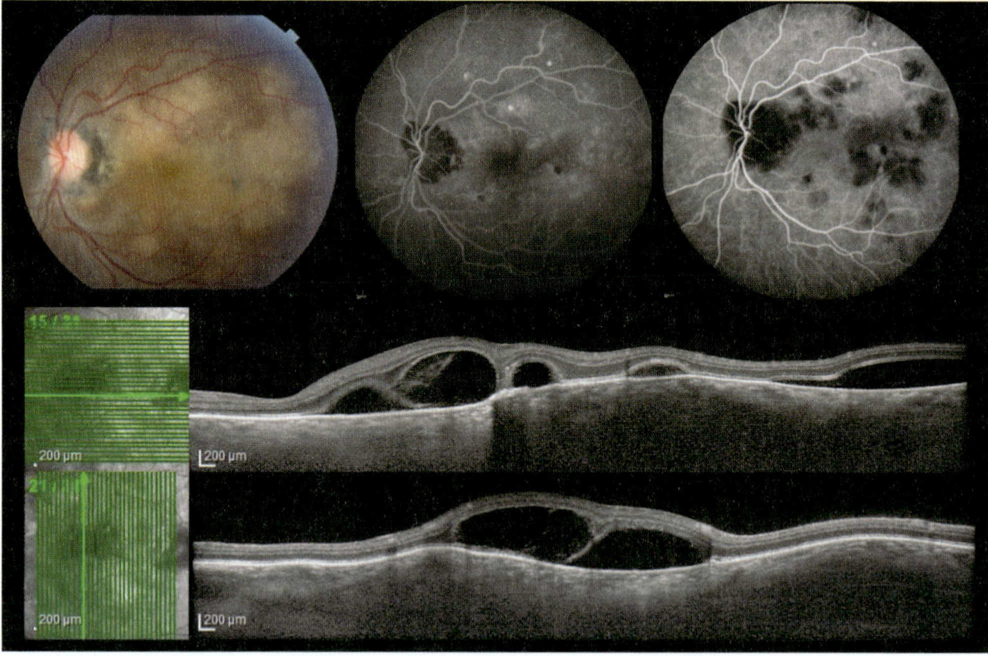

Figure 10-11 Tubercular multifocal choroiditis with serous retinal detachment. Fundus photography shows multiple pockets of subretinal fluid overlying choroidal tubercles *(top left).* Fluorescein angiography reveals multifocal leakage *(top middle),* and indocyanine green angiography delineates hypocyanescence *(top right),* presumably corresponding to areas of choroidal inflammatory infiltration. Choroidal nodules (tubercles) are revealed by spectral-domain optical coherence tomography *(bottom). (Courtesy of Daniel V. Vasconcelos-Santos, MD, PhD.)*

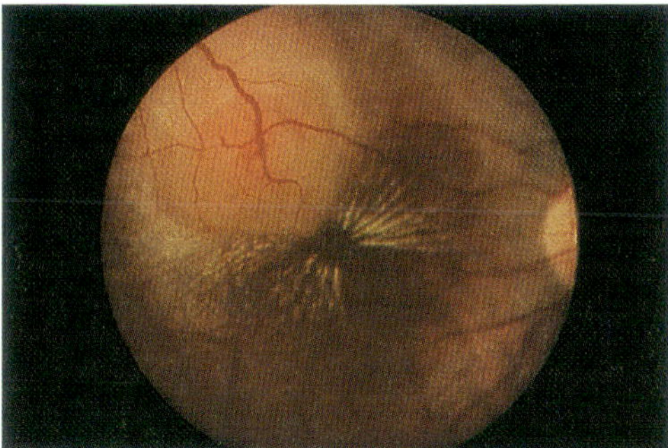

Figure 10-12 Fundus photograph of a choroidal tubercle with a macular star formation (tuberculoma).

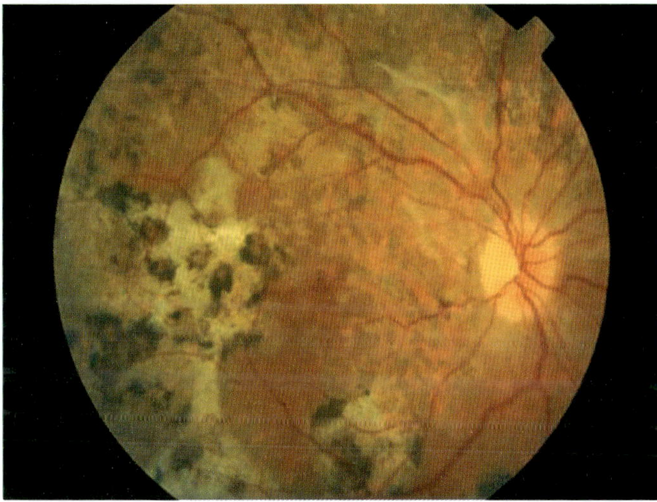

Figure 10-13 Fundus photograph showing tuberculous choroiditis masquerading as atypical serpiginous-like choroiditis. The patient showed progression and recurrence while receiving immunomodulatory drugs; however, after antituberculous treatment was begun, the patient showed improvement in vision and resolution of the vitritis without recurrences. *(Courtesy of Narsing A. Rao, MD.)*

Retinal involvement

Retinal involvement in TB is usually secondary to extension of the choroidal disease or an immunologic response to mycobacteria and should be differentiated from Eales disease, a peripheral retinal perivasculitis that presents in otherwise healthy young men aged 20–40 years with recurrent, unilateral retinal and vitreous hemorrhage and subsequent involvement of the fellow eye. The disease may be associated, at least in part, to some degree of tuberculin hypersensitivity. Interestingly a few studies employing PCR-based assays have detected *M tuberculosis* DNA from aqueous, vitreous, and epiretinal membranes of some patients with Eales disease. Periphlebitis is commonly observed in this setting, and may be accompanied by venous occlusion, peripheral nonperfusion, neovascularization (Fig 10-14), and eventual development of tractional retinal detachment in some cases (see also BCSC Section 12, *Retina and Vitreous,* for additional discussion of Eales disease).

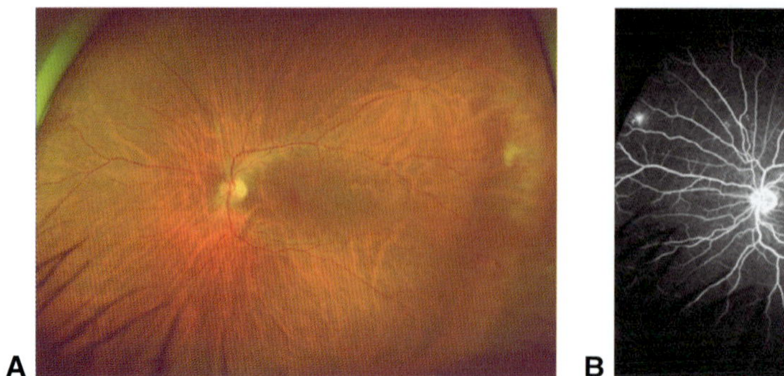

Figure 10-14 Eales disease. **A,** Wide-angle fundus photograph of Eales disease. **B,** Angiographic image shows peripheral retinal nonperfusion and neovascularization (temporally), in addition to perivenular hyperfluorescence (periphlebitis). *(Courtesy of Emilio M. Dodds, MD.)*

Other posterior segment findings of TB include subretinal abscess, CNV, optic neuritis, and panophthalmitis.

Diagnosis

Definitive diagnosis of TB requires direct evidence of mycobacteria in bodily fluids or tissues. In many cases of ocular TB, this confirmation is not possible, and the diagnosis is instead presumptive, based on indirect evidence. A positive result on a tuberculin skin test using PPD (purified protein derivative of *Mycobacterium bovis)* test or an interferon-gamma release assay is indicative of prior exposure to TB but not necessarily of active systemic or ocular infection.

In the United States, an induration of 5 mm or more, read 48–72 hours after intradermal injection of the standard 5-tuberculin-unit (5-TU), or intermediate-strength, test dose is considered a positive result in individuals with HIV infection, those exposed to active TB, or those whose radiographs are consistent with healed tuberculous lesions. An induration of 10 mm or more is considered indicative of a positive result for other high-risk individuals, including patients with diabetes mellitus or renal failure, those on immunomodulatory therapy (IMT), health care workers, and recent immigrants from high-prevalence countries. Patients with no known risks for tuberculosis are considered to have a positive test result if induration is 15 mm or more.

False-negative skin testing results may occur at a rate of up to 25% because of patients with profound acute illness or immune compromise, which can stem from corticosteroid use, advanced age, poor nutrition, and sarcoidosis. False-positive results may arise from patients infected with atypical mycobacteria, immunized with BCG vaccine, and treated with intraluminal BCG injections for bladder carcinoma. Individuals recently immunized with BCG vaccine may have an induration measuring around 10 mm at presentation, but the reaction is usually not sustained and tends to decrease with time compared with the reaction following the skin test after more recent systemic TB exposure. A Bayesian analysis predicts that routine screening of uveitis patients for TB has a low probability of detecting disease in settings where the prevalence of TB is low. It is recommended, therefore, that testing be selectively used for patients in whom the index of suspicion has been heightened by a careful history, review of systems, and clinical examination. Testing for TB is required in patients being considered for treatment with tumor necrosis factor inhibitors or other biologic agents.

A history of recent exposure to TB or a positive TB test result warrants a concerted search for systemic infection, using chest imaging (radiography, computer-assisted tomography and positron emission tomography scanning), and/or microbiologic analysis of sputum, urine, or gastric aspirates, or a cervical lymph node biopsy for acid-fast bacilli. Failure to demonstrate systemic disease does not, however, exclude the possibility of intraocular infection.

For cases of suspected ocular TB in which the results of the above-mentioned testing for systemic infection are negative, the patient is asymptomatic, or the infection is thought to be extrapulmonary, definitive diagnosis may require intraocular fluid analysis or tissue biopsy. Nucleic acid amplification techniques, with either transcription-mediated amplification of 16S ribosomal RNA or PCR amplification of unique DNA sequences of *M tuberculosis,* have been successfully used in some cases to diagnose intraocular TB, though the yield may be low because of a thick cell wall and possibly low bacterial load in the vitreous. Chorioretinal biopsy used in conjunction with PCR testing and routine histologic examination may be necessary in atypical cases where the differential diagnosis and therapeutic options are widely divergent. Recently, antibodies against purified cord factor, the most antigenic and abundant cell wall component of tubercle bacilli, have been detected by ELISA and may be useful for rapid serodiagnosis of pulmonary TB, in addition to providing supportive data for the diagnosis of ocular infection.

Ang M, Vasconcelos-Santos DV, Sharma K, et al. Diagnosis of ocular tuberculosis. *Ocul Immunol Inflamm.* 2018;26(2):208–216.
Gupta A, Gupta V. Tubercular posterior uveitis. *Int Ophthalmol Clin.* 2005;45(2):71–88.
Lewinsohn DM, Leonard MK, LoBue PA, et al. Official American Thoracic Society/Infectious Diseases Society of America/Centers for Disease Control and Prevention Clinical Practice Guidelines: diagnosis of tuberculosis in adults and children. *Clin Infect Dis.* 2017; 64(2):111–115.

Treatment

Systemic antitubercular therapy is clearly indicated for patients with uveitis whose TB test results have recently converted to positive, patients with an abnormal-appearing chest radiograph suggestive of tuberculosis, or persons with positive mycobacterial culture or PCR results to *M tuberculosis.* Multidrug therapy is recommended because of the increasing incidence of resistance to isoniazid as well as adherence problems associated with long-term therapy. These problems, together with the extremely slow growth rate of TB, contribute to the acquisition of multidrug-resistant tuberculosis (MDRTB). Patients at risk for MDRTB include nonadherent patients receiving single-drug therapy; migrant or indigent populations; immunocompromised patients, including those with HIV infection; and recent immigrants from countries where isoniazid and rifampin are available over the counter.

In brief, treatment entails an initial 2-month induction course of isoniazid, rifampin, pyrazinamide, and ethambutol administered daily, followed by a continuation phase of 4–7 months with 2 drugs. More than 95% of immunocompetent patients may be successfully treated with a full course of therapy, provided they adhere to this regimen. Directly observed therapy plays a crucial role in ensuring this success and is now the standard of care in the treatment of tuberculosis. Treatment protocols have been standardized and are available from the CDC.

More difficult is the treatment approach to patients with uveitis consistent with TB, normal chest radiograph appearance, and positive TB test result. In this situation, a diagnosis of extrapulmonary TB may be entertained and treatment initiated, particularly in cases with medically unresponsive uveitis or other findings supportive of the diagnosis, such as recent exposure to or inadequate treatment of the disease, a large area of induration, or skin test result recently converted to positive. Topical and even systemic corticosteroids may be used in conjunction with antimicrobial therapy to treat the inflammatory component of the disease. Because intensive corticosteroid treatment administered without appropriate coverage with antituberculosis treatment may lead to progressive worsening of ocular disease, any patient suspected of harboring TB should undergo appropriate testing before beginning such therapy.

Patients with a positive TB test result or abnormal chest film appearance for whom systemic corticosteroid treatment is being considered, or patients who have received corticosteroids for longer than 2 weeks at doses greater than 15 mg/day, may benefit from prophylactic treatment with isoniazid for 6 months to 1 year based on infectious disease specialist evaluation. Likewise, patients with latent TB in whom IMT (particularly with tumor necrosis factor inhibitors) is being considered should be treated with isoniazid prophylaxis beginning at least 3 weeks before the first administration.

Agrawal R, Gunasekeran DV, Grant R, et al; Collaborative Ocular Tuberculosis Study (COTS)–1 Study Group. Clinical features and outcomes of patients with tubercular uveitis treated with antitubercular therapy in the Collaborative Ocular Tuberculosis Study (COTS)-1. *JAMA Ophthalmol.* 2017;135(12):1318–1327.

Nazari Khanamiri H, Rao NA. Serpiginous choroiditis and infectious multifocal serpiginoid choroiditis. *Surv Ophthalmol.* 2013;58(3):203–232.

Ocular Bartonellosis

Bartonella henselae (formerly *Rochalimaea henselae),* a small, fastidious, gram-negative rod, initially isolated from the tissue of patients with bacillary angiomatosis of AIDS, is now known to be the principal etiologic agent of cat-scratch disease (CSD) and is associated with an expanding spectrum of ocular manifestations. Cat-scratch disease is a feline-associated zoonotic disease found worldwide, with an estimated annual incidence rate in the United States of 9.3 cases per 100,000 persons. The highest age-specific incidence is among children younger than 10 years of age. Cats are the primary mammalian reservoir of *B henselae* and *B quintana,* and the cat flea is an important vector for the transmission of the organism among cats. The disease follows a seasonal pattern, occurring predominantly in the fall and winter, and is most prevalent in the southern states, California, and Hawaii. The disease is transmitted to humans by the scratches, licks, and bites of domestic cats, particularly kittens.

Systemic manifestations of CSD include a mild to moderate flulike illness associated with regional adenopathy that usually precedes the ocular manifestations of the disease. An erythematous papule, vesicle, or pustule usually forms at the primary site of cutaneous injury 3–10 days after primary inoculation and 1–2 weeks before the onset of lymphadenopathy and constitutional symptoms. Less commonly, more severe and disseminated disease may develop that is associated with encephalopathy, aseptic meningitis, osteomyelitis, hepatosplenic disease, pneumonia, and pleural and pericardial effusions.

Biancardi AL, Curi AL. Cat-scratch disease. *Ocul Immunol Inflamm.* 2014;22(2):148–154.
Roe RH, Jumper JM, Fu AD, Johnson RN, McDonald HR, Cunningham ET. Ocular bartonella infections. *Int Ophthalmol Clin.* 2008;48(3):93–105.

Ocular Involvement

Ocular involvement, which occurs in 5%–10% of patients with CSD, includes Parinaud oculoglandular syndrome (unilateral granulomatous conjunctivitis and regional lymphadenopathy) in approximately 5% of patients and a wide array of posterior segment and neuro-ophthalmic findings. Entities to be considered in the differential diagnosis of Parinaud oculoglandular syndrome include tularemia, tuberculosis, syphilis, sporotrichosis, and acute *Chlamydia trachomatis* infection (see also BCSC Section 8, *External Disease and Cornea,* for discussion on Parinaud oculoglandular syndrome).

The best-known posterior segment manifestation of *B henselae* infection is neuroretinitis, a constellation of findings that includes abrupt vision loss, unilateral optic disc swelling, and macular star formation. This syndrome, formerly known as *idiopathic stellate maculopathy* and later renamed *Leber idiopathic stellate neuroretinitis,* is now known to be caused by *B henselae* infection in approximately two-thirds of cases. It occurs in 1%–2% of patients with CSD. Focal or multifocal retinitis may also be identified. Table 10-3 lists other entities that may cause neuroretinitis. Visual acuity loss varies between 20/25 and 20/200 or worse and follows the onset of constitutional symptoms by approximately 2–3 weeks. Although the presentation is most often unilateral, bilateral cases of neuroretinitis have been reported and are frequently asymmetric. Optic disc edema, associated with peripapillary serous retinal detachment, has been observed 2–4 weeks before the appearance of the macular star and may be a sign of systemic *B henselae* infection. The development of the macular star is variable (Fig 10-15) and may be partial or incomplete, usually resolving in approximately 8–12 weeks.

Patients with *Bartonella*-associated neuroretinitis may exhibit some degree of anterior chamber inflammation and vitritis. Discrete, focal, or multifocal retinal and/or choroidal lesions measuring 50–300 μm are common posterior segment findings. Both arterial and venous occlusive disease, as well as localized neurosensory macular detachments, have been described in association with focal retinitis. Other posterior segment ocular complications include epiretinal membranes, inflammatory mass of the optic nerve head, peripapillary angiomatosis, intermediate uveitis, retinal white dot syndromes, orbital abscess, isolated optic

Table 10-3 Differential Diagnosis of Neuroretinitis

Infectious
Bartonellosis *(Bartonella henselae)*
Syphilis
Lyme disease
Tuberculosis
Diffuse unilateral subacute neuroretinitis (DUSN) *(Ancylostoma caninum, Baylisascaris procyonis)*
Toxoplasmosis
Toxocariasis
Leptospirosis
Salmonella
Chickenpox (varicella)
Mumps
Herpes simplex
Ehrlichiosis
Rocky Mountain spotted fever
Noninfectious
Sarcoidosis
Acute systemic hypertension
Diabetes mellitus
Idiopathic intracranial hypertension
Anterior ischemic optic neuropathy
Leukemic infiltration of the optic nerve
Idiopathic
Leber idiopathic stellate neuroretinitis
Recurrent idiopathic neuroretintis

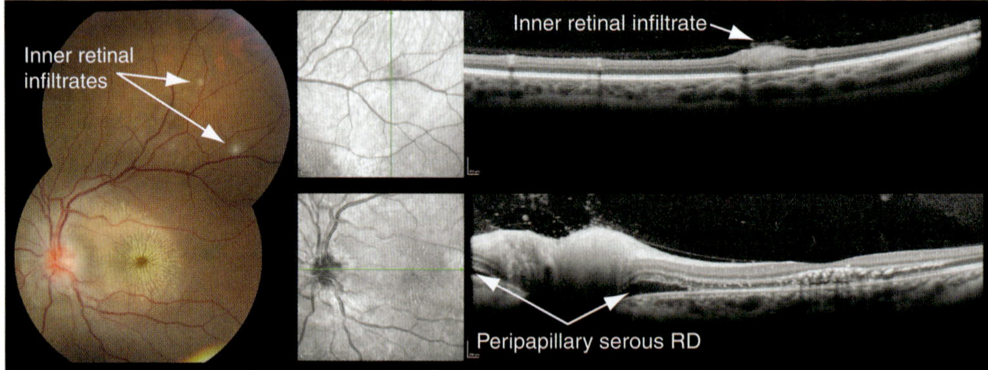

Figure 10-15 *Left,* color fundus photograph of the left eye of a patient with cat-scratch disease shows neuroretinitis with optic disc involvement associated with a macular star. Punctate retinal infiltrates are also visible superiorly *(arrows). Upper right,* spectral-domain optical coherence tomography scan delineates the inner retinal infiltrate *(arrow). Lower right,* scan reveals subretinal fluid *(peripapillary serous retinal detachments, arrows),* intraretinal exudates, vitreous inflammatory infiltration, and optic disc and macular edema. *(Courtesy of Daniel V. Vasconcelos-Santos, MD, PhD.)*

disc swelling, and panuveitis. Immunosuppressed individuals may display a retinal vasoproliferative response, leading to single/multiple angiomatoid lesions involving retina/choroid.

Chi SL, Stinnett S, Eggenberger E, et al. Clinical characteristics in 53 patients with cat scratch optic neuropathy. *Ophthalmology.* 2012;119(1):183–187.

Diagnosis

A diagnosis of CSD is made on the basis of characteristic clinical features together with confirmatory serologic testing. The indirect fluorescent antibody assay for the detection of serum anti–*B henselae* antibodies is 88% sensitive and 94% specific, with titers of greater than 1:64 considered positive. Enzyme immunoassays with a sensitivity for IgG of 86%–95% and a specificity of 96%, together with Western blot analysis, have also been developed. A single positive indirect fluorescent antibody or enzyme immunoassay titer for IgG or IgM is sufficient to confirm the diagnosis of CSD. Other diagnostic approaches include bacterial cultures, which may require several weeks for colonies to become apparent; skin testing, which has a sensitivity of up to 100% and a specificity of up to 98%; and PCR-based techniques that target the bacterial 16S ribosomal RNA gene or *B henselae* DNA.

Suhler ED, Lauer AK, Rosenbaum JT. Prevalence of serologic evidence of cat scratch disease in patients with neuroretinitis. *Ophthalmology.* 2000;107(5):871–876.

Treatment

Definitive treatment guidelines have not emerged for CSD because it is a self-limiting illness in many cases, with an overall excellent systemic prognosis. Visual outcomes may be variable, depending on location/severity of intraocular inflammation. A variety of antibiotics, including doxycycline, ciprofloxacin, erythromycin, rifampin, trimethoprim-sulfamethoxazole, and gentamycin, have been used in the treatment of more severe systemic or ocular manifestations, even though their efficacy has not been demonstrated conclusively. A typical regimen for immunocompetent patients older than 8 years consists of doxycycline, 100 mg orally twice daily for 4–6 weeks. For more severe infections, doxycycline may be given intravenously or used in combination with rifampin, 300 mg orally twice daily; among immunocompromised individuals, this treatment is extended for 4 months. Children with CSD may be treated with azithromycin, as safety of ciprofloxacin in individuals younger than 18 years is of concern. The efficacy of oral corticosteroids on the course of systemic and ocular disease is unknown, even though these are frequently used in cases threatening the optic nerve/macula.

Whipple Disease

Whipple disease is a rare multisystem disease caused by the *Tropheryma whipplei* bacterium. It is most common in middle-aged White men. Migratory arthritis occurs in 80% of cases, and gastrointestinal symptoms, including diarrhea, steatorrhea, and malabsorption, occur in 75%. Intestinal loss of protein results in pitting edema and weight loss. Cardiomyopathy and valvular disease can also occur. Central nervous system involvement occurs in 10% of cases and results in seizures, dementia, and coma. Neuro-ophthalmic signs can include

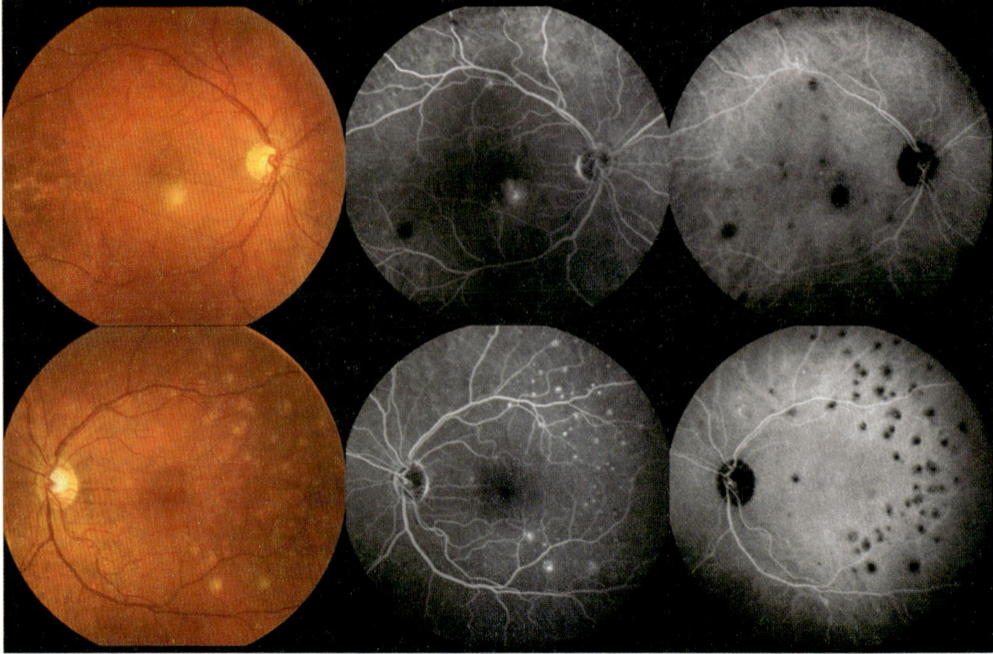

Figure 10-16 Bilateral multifocal chorioretinitis in a patient with Whipple disease, revealed by fundus photography *(left)*, fluorescein angiography *(middle)*, and indocyanine green angiography *(right)*. (Courtesy of Wendy M. Smith, MD.)

cranial nerve palsies, nystagmus, and ophthalmoplegia. Some patients develop a progressive supranuclear palsy–like condition (see also BCSC Section 5, *Neuro-Ophthalmology*, for discussion on neuro-ophthalmologic manifestations of Whipple disease).

Ocular Involvement

Intraocular involvement is rare and occurs in less than 5% of cases. Patients can present with bilateral panuveitis and retinal vasculitis, as well as with multifocal chorioretinitis (Fig 10-16). Both anterior uveitis and moderate vitritis are present. Diffuse chorioretinal inflammation and diffuse retinal vasculitis in the perifoveal and midperipheral regions may occur. Retinal vascular occlusions and retinal hemorrhages may result from the vasculitis. Optic disc edema and, later, optic atrophy may occur. Unusual granular, crystalline deposits on the iris, capsular bag, and intraocular lens have also been reported.

Razonable RR, Pulido JS, Deziel PJ, Dev S, Salomão DR, Walker RC. Chorioretinitis and vitreitis due to *Tropheryma whipplei* after transplantation: case report and review. *Transpl Infect Dis.* 2008;10(6):413–418.

Diagnosis

The gold standard for diagnosis of Whipple disease is a duodenal biopsy that demonstrates a periodic acid–Schiff (PAS)-positive bacillus in macrophages within intestinal villi. A PCR analysis of peripheral blood and vitreous may show *T whipplei* DNA and confirm the diagnosis. Culturing of *T whipplei* is difficult but possible. The differential diagnosis of uveitis associated with Whipple disease includes diseases that can cause retinal vasculitis with multisystem involvement, including sarcoidosis, SLE, polyarteritis nodosa, and Behçet disease. Primary vitreoretinal lymphoma should also be considered in elderly individuals with significant vitreal infiltration.

Chan RY, Yannuzzi LA, Foster CS. Ocular Whipple's disease: earlier definitive diagnosis. *Ophthalmology.* 2001;108(12):2225–2231.

Treatment

Untreated Whipple disease can be fatal. Systemic trimethoprim-sulfamethoxazole is the preferred treatment. Patients allergic to sulfonamides may be treated with ceftriaxone, tetracycline, or chloramphenicol. Treatment duration may vary from 1 to 3 months, but relapses occur in 30% of cases, necessitating prolonged (up to 1 year) treatment. Retinal vasculitis can resolve with treatment, but neurologic deficits become permanent.

Nubourgh I, Vandergheynst F, Lefebvre P, Lemy A, Dumarey N, Decaux G. An atypical case of Whipple's disease: case report and review of the literature. *Acta Clin Belg.* 2008;63(2):107–111.

Touitou V, Fenollar F, Cassoux N, et al. Ocular Whipple's disease: therapeutic strategy and long-term follow-up. *Ophthalmology.* 2012;119(7):1465–1469.

CHAPTER 11

Infectious Uveitis: Nonbacterial Causes

This chapter includes a related video, which can be accessed by scanning the QR code provided in the text or going to www.aao.org/bcscvideo_section09.

Highlights

- The viral necrotizing retinopathies include acute retinal necrosis, cytomegalovirus retinitis, and progressive outer retinal necrosis. Diagnosis is principally clinical; in uncertain cases, polymerase chain reaction testing can be done.
- Human infection by *Toxoplasma gondii* may be either acquired or congenital. Recently acquired disease may present as a focal retinochoroiditis in the absence of a chorioretinal scar.
- Ophthalmic presentations of ocular toxocariasis include a chronic endophthalmitis (25%), a posterior pole granuloma (25%), or a peripheral granuloma (50%).
- Viruses, fungi, protozoa, helminths, and bacteria can all cause infectious uveitis, featuring inflammation in different parts of the uveal tract. This chapter is organized according to the causative organism and subcategorized by the anatomical location of inflammation.

Viral Uveitis

Herpesviridae Family

Herpes simplex virus and varicella-zoster virus

Anterior uveitis Acute anterior uveitis can be associated with herpetic viral disease. BCSC Section 8, *External Disease and Cornea,* extensively discusses herpes simplex virus (HSV) and varicella-zoster virus (VZV) infections. Anterior uveitis in herpetic viral infections may be associated with corneal involvement (keratouveitis) but also occurs without noticeable keratitis. The inflammation may become chronic.

Chickenpox (varicella), which is caused by the same virus that is responsible for secondary VZV reactivation, may be associated with an acute, mild, nongranulomatous, self-limiting, and bilateral anterior uveitis. Cutaneous vesicles at the tip of the nose

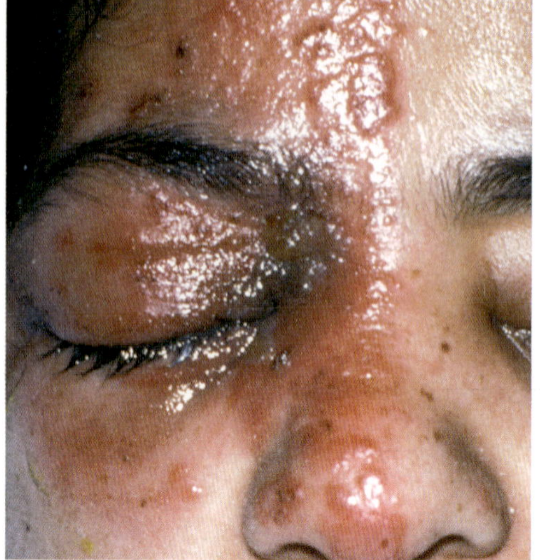

Figure 11-1 Skin lesions in varicella-zoster virus infection. *(Courtesy of Debra A. Goldstein, MD.)*

(Hutchinson sign) indicate nasociliary nerve involvement and a greater likelihood that the eye will be affected (Fig 11-1). Most patients are asymptomatic; however, monitored prospectively, up to 40% of patients with primary VZV infection may develop anterior uveitis.

Herpes zoster (HZ) is defined as varicella zoster emerging from latency, and herpes zoster ophthalmicus (HZO) is defined as HZ within V_1 (ophthalmic division of cranial nerve V). In HZO, the most commonly affected patients are between the ages of 50 and 69, and the eye may or may not be involved. Ophthalmic manifestations of HZO include keratitis, uveitis, conjunctivitis, episcleritis, scleritis, acute retinal necrosis, and cranial nerve palsy. Potential skin manifestations include a painful vesicular eruption within the V_1 dermatome. Infection with VZV can be considered in the differential diagnosis of chronic unilateral anterior uveitis, even if the cutaneous component of the condition occurred in the past or was minimal when present. Patients may develop anterior uveitis without ever having had a cutaneous component (varicella-zoster sine herpete).

Patients with intraocular viral infections, particularly with herpes group viruses, may exhibit granulomatous, nongranulomatous, or stellate (fine and fibrillar) keratic precipitates (KPs). If stellate KPs develop, they are often distributed diffusely, as opposed to a regional distribution in the inferior third of the cornea. Diffuse or stellate KPs are not pathognomonic of any particular condition. For example, Fuchs uveitis syndrome (FUS, historically known as *Fuchs heterochromic uveitis)* may also feature diffuse stellate KPs. Also, notably, patients with herpetic keratouveitis may exhibit diffuse or localized decreased corneal sensation and neurotrophic keratitis.

Ocular hypertension associated with herpetic uveitis may be a helpful diagnostic hallmark. Most other inflammatory syndromes are associated with decreased intraocular pressure (IOP) as a result of ciliary body hyposecretion. However, herpesvirus may cause trabeculitis and thus increase IOP, often to as high as 50–60 mm Hg. In addition, inflammatory cells may contribute to trabecular obstruction and congestion. Cytomegalovirus (CMV)-related anterior uveitis may also present with high IOP (see the section on glaucomatocyclitic crisis in Chapter 8). Other potential findings associated with herpesvirus include hyphema, hypopyon, posterior synechia, KPs, and corneal edema.

Iris atrophy is characteristic of herpetic inflammation and can be present with HSV-, VZV-, or CMV-associated anterior uveitis. The atrophy may be patchy or sectoral (Fig 11-2) and is visualized as transillumination defects upon retroillumination at the slit lamp (Fig 11-3).

Viral retinitis may occur with these entities, particularly in immunocompromised hosts. Vasculitis may occur with HZO, and it may lead to anterior segment ischemia, retinal artery occlusion, and scleritis. Vasculitis in the orbit may cause cranial nerve palsies.

Treatment for viral anterior uveitis includes topical corticosteroids and cycloplegic agents. Topical antiviral drugs are ineffective for intraocular inflammation but may prevent dendritic disease in patients receiving topical steroids. Systemic antiviral drugs such as acyclovir (400–800 mg, 5 times/day), famciclovir (250–500 mg, 3 times/day), or valacyclovir (500 mg to 1 g, 3 times/day) may help treat HSV- or VZV-related intraocular inflammation, with the higher doses used for VZV uveitis. Initiation of oral antiviral therapy at the onset of VZV uveitis is recommended. Patients with herpetic uveitis may require prolonged corticosteroid therapy with very gradual tapering. In fact, some patients with VZV infection require very long-term, albeit extremely low, doses of topical corticosteroids (as infrequent as 1 drop per week) for the condition to remain quiescent. Systemic corticosteroids are sometimes necessary. Long-term, suppressive, low-dose antiviral therapy may be indicated in patients with herpetic uveitis, but controlled studies are lacking. The oral prophylactic dosage for patients with herpes simplex is acyclovir, 400 mg 2 times/day, or valacyclovir,

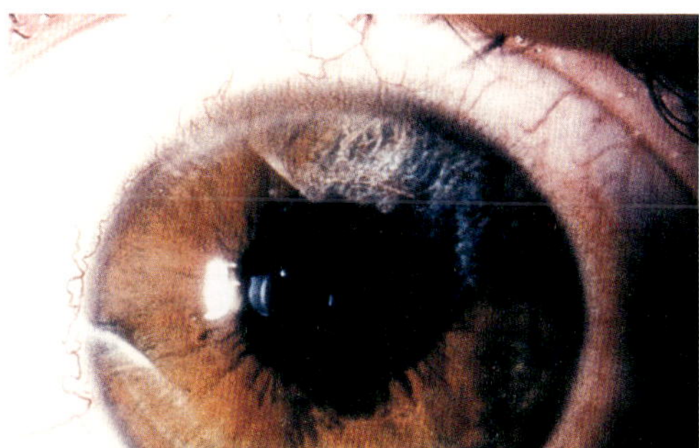

Figure 11-2 Iris stromal atrophy in a patient with varicella-zoster anterior uveitis. *(Courtesy of David Forster, MD.)*

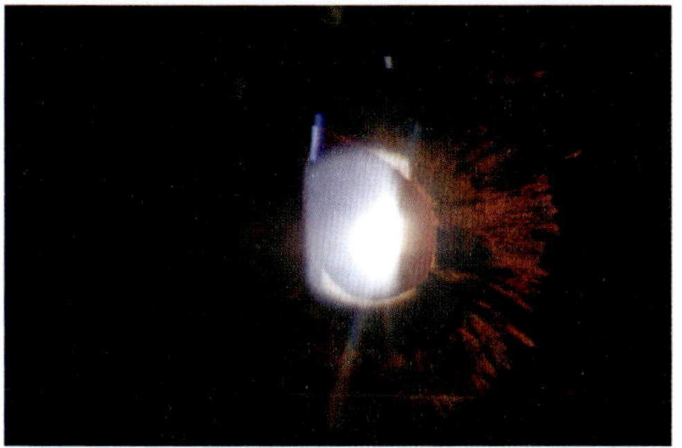

Figure 11-3 Iris transillumination in herpetic anterior uveitis. *(Courtesy of Bryn M. Burkholder, MD.)*

500 mg/day. For VZV disease, dosage is either acyclovir, 800 mg 2 times/day, or valacyclovir, 1 g/day.

A controlled trial of oral acyclovir for iridocyclitis caused by herpes simplex virus. The Herpetic Eye Disease Study Group. *Arch Ophthalmol.* 1996;114(9):1065–1072.

Liesegang TJ. Herpes zoster ophthalmicus natural history, risk factors, clinical presentation, and morbidity. *Ophthalmology.* 2008;115(2 Suppl):S3–12

Siverio Júnior CD, Imai Y, Cunningham ET Jr. Diagnosis and management of herpetic anterior uveitis. *Int Ophthalmol Clin.* 2002;42(1):43–48.

Tran KD, Falcone MM, Choi DS, et al. Epidemiology of herpes zoster ophthalmicus: recurrence and chronicity. *Ophthalmology.* 2016;123(7):1469–1475.

van der Lelij A, Ooijman FM, Kijlstra A, Rothova A. Anterior uveitis with sectoral iris atrophy in the absence of keratitis: a distinct clinical entity among herpetic eye diseases. *Ophthalmology.* 2000;107(6):1164–1170.

Acute retinal necrosis, progressive outer retinal necrosis, and nonnecrotizing herpetic retinitis The necrotizing retinopathies include acute retinal necrosis (ARN), CMV retinitis, and progressive outer retinal necrosis (PORN). Retinal lesions of presumed herpetic etiology that are not consistent with ARN, CMV retinitis, or PORN are grouped under the umbrella designation *nonnecrotizing herpetic retinopathy.*

Acute retinal necrosis may occur in healthy adults or children, but may also occur in immunocompromised patients, including patients with HIV. Acute, fulminant disease may arise without a systemic prodrome, often months or years after primary infection or following cutaneous or systemic herpetic infection such as chickenpox, herpes zoster, or herpetic encephalitis. Patients may have a history of recurrent cutaneous herpetic outbreaks. The prevalence is nearly equal between the sexes, with the majority of cases clustering in patients between the fifth and seventh decades of life. The American Uveitis Society has established criteria for the diagnosis of ARN solely on the basis of clinical findings and disease progression, independent of viral etiology or host immune status (Table 11-1).

Patients with ARN usually present with acute unilateral loss of vision, photophobia, floaters, and pain. Fellow eye involvement occurs in approximately 36% of cases, usually within 6 weeks of disease onset, but sometimes months or years later. Panuveitis develops, beginning with significant anterior segment inflammation, Keratic precipitates, posterior synechiae, and elevated IOP, together with heavy vitreous cellular infiltration and oftentimes vitreous haze. Within 2 weeks, the classic triad of occlusive retinal arteriolitis, vitritis,

Table 11-1 American Uveitis Society Criteria for Diagnosis of Acute Retinal Necrosis

One or more foci of retinal necrosis with discrete borders, located in the peripheral retina[a]
Rapid progression in the absence of antiviral therapy
Circumferential spread
Occlusive vasculopathy with arteriolar involvement
Prominent vitritis, anterior chamber inflammation
Optic neuropathy/atrophy, scleritis, pain supportive but not required

[a]Macular lesions do not exclude diagnosis in the presence of peripheral retinitis.

Data from Holland GN and the Executive Committee of the American Uveitis Society. Standard diagnostic criteria for the acute retinal necrosis syndrome. *Am J Ophthalmol.* 1994;117(5):663–667.

and a multifocal yellow-white peripheral retinitis evolves. Early on, the peripheral retinal lesions may be discontinuous and have scalloped edges that appear to arise in the outer retina. Within days the lesions coalesce to form a confluent 360° creamy retinitis that progresses in a posterior direction, leaving full-thickness retinal necrosis, arteriolitis, phlebitis, and occasional retinal hemorrhage in its wake (Fig 11-4). Widespread necrosis of the peripheral and midzonal retina, multiple posterior retinal breaks, and proliferative vitreoretinopathy may lead to combined tractional–rhegmatogenous retinal detachments in 75% of patients (Figs 11-5, 11-6). Optic nerve swelling and a relative afferent pupillary defect may develop.

In most cases, the diagnosis is made clinically. The differential includes CMV retinitis, atypical toxoplasmic retinochoroiditis, syphilis, lymphoma, leukemia, and autoimmune retinitis with retinal vasculitis such as that of Behçet disease. Acute retinal necrosis may also be present in association with concurrent or antecedent herpetic encephalitis (HSV-1 or -2).

In cases of diagnostic uncertainty, classically intraocular antibody production was assayed from an aqueous humor sample, and a Goldmann-Witmer (GW) coefficient

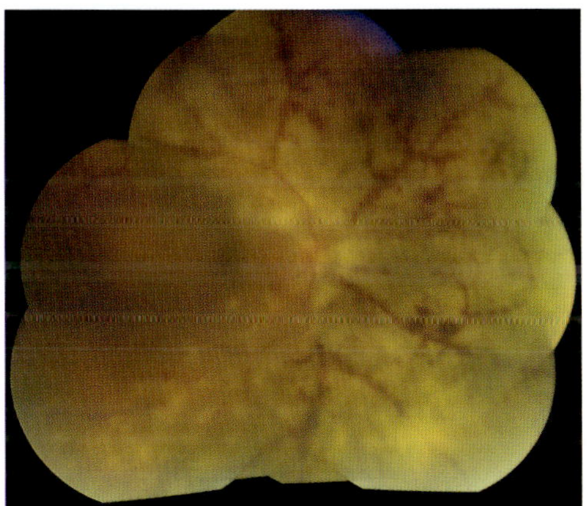

Figure 11-4 Fundus photograph of acute retinal necrosis showing confluent peripheral retinitis. *(Courtesy of H. Nida Sen, MD.)*

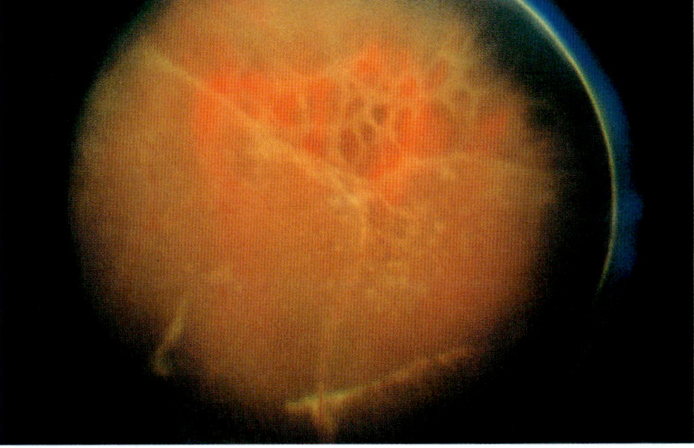

Figure 11-5 Acute retinal necrosis. Retinal detachment with multiple, posterior retinal breaks. *(Courtesy of E. Mitchel Opremcak, MD.)*

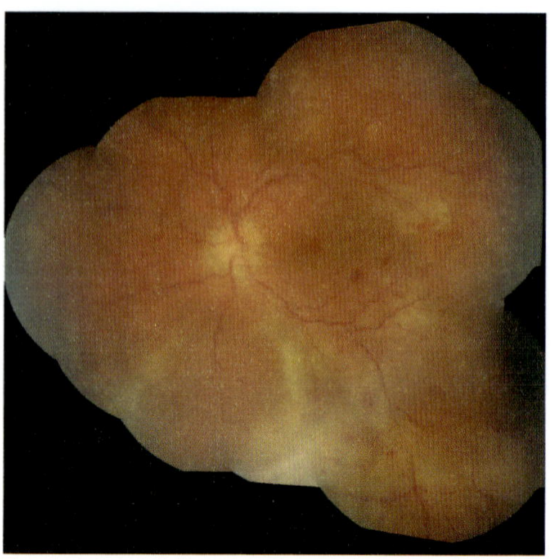

Figure 11-6 Montage fundus photograph of a patient with acute retinal necrosis reveals vitritis, multifocal and confluent areas of retinitis, retinal vasculitis, retinal hemorrhage, optic nerve head edema, and retinal detachment. *(Reprinted with permission from Schoenberger SD, Kim SJ, Thorne JE, et al. Diagnosis and treatment of acute retinal necrosis: a report by the American Academy of Ophthalmology.* Ophthalmology. *2017;124[3]:382–392.)*

calculated. Polymerase chain reaction (PCR) testing of aqueous or vitreous specimens has largely supplanted viral culture, intraocular antibody titers, and serology. For presumed ARN, aqueous sampling is usually sufficient. Quantitative PCR may add information with respect to viral load, disease activity, and response to therapy.

Studies using PCR-based assays suggest that the most common cause of ARN is VZV infection, followed by infections with HSV-1, HSV-2, and, in rare cases, CMV. Patients with ARN caused by HSV-1 or VZV infection tend to be older (mean age, 40 years), whereas those with ARN due to HSV-2 infection tend to be younger (below age 25 years). There is a higher risk of encephalitis and meningitis among patients with ARN caused by HSV-1 infection than by VZV infection. In rare cases in which PCR results are negative but the clinical suspicion for necrotizing herpetic retinitis is high, endoretinal biopsy may be diagnostic.

Timely diagnosis and prompt initiation of antiviral therapy are essential, given the rapidity of disease progression, the frequency of retinal detachment, and the guarded visual prognosis. Intravenous acyclovir, 10 mg/kg every 8 hours for 10–14 days, is effective against HSV and VZV. Reversible elevations in levels of serum creatinine and liver enzymes may occur; in the presence of frank renal insufficiency, the dosage will need to be reduced. After 24–48 hours of antiviral therapy, systemic corticosteroids (prednisone, 1 mg/kg/day) are introduced to treat active inflammation and are subsequently tapered over several weeks. Aspirin and other anticoagulants have been used to treat an associated hypercoagulable state and prevent vascular occlusions, but the results have been inconclusive. Following intravenous antiviral induction for VZV infection, treatment with acyclovir at 800 mg orally 5 times daily, valacyclovir at 1 g orally 3 times daily, or famciclovir at 500 mg orally 3 times daily should be continued for 3 months. For ARN associated with HSV-1 infection, the follow-on oral dose is one-half of that for VZV. Extended antiviral therapy may reduce the incidence of contralateral disease or bilateral ARN by 80% over 1 year.

Oral valacyclovir at doses of up to 2 g 3 times daily has been used successfully as an alternative to intravenous acyclovir as induction therapy. In addition, intravitreal ganciclovir (2.0 mg/0.05 or 0.1 mL) and foscarnet (1.2–2.4 mg/0.1 mL) have been used to achieve a rapid induction in combination with both intravenous and oral antivirals as first-line therapy or for disease that fails to respond to systemic acyclovir (see Chapter 12). High-dose systemic oral therapy, alone or in combination with intravitreal antiviral drugs, has not been demonstrated as superior to the classic intravenous approach. Given the short intravitreal half-life of these drugs, injections may need to be repeated twice weekly until the retinitis is controlled. Effective treatment inhibits the development of new lesions and promotes lesion regression over 4 days.

Retinal detachment may occur within weeks to months of disease onset. The use of prophylactic barrier laser photocoagulation, applied to the areas of healthy retina at the posterior border of the necrotic lesions once the view permits, is controversial and employed by some practitioners. If detachment occurs, vitrectomy techniques are preferred over standard scleral buckling. Optic nerve atrophy may be visually limiting even with a favorable retinal anatomic outcome.

Progressive outer retinal necrosis is a morphologic variant of acute necrotizing herpetic retinitis, occurring in those who are profoundly immunosuppressed, most often in advanced AIDS (CD4$^+$ T lymphocytes ≤50 cells/μL). The most common cause of PORN is VZV infection; HSV has also been isolated. As with ARN, the retinitis begins as patchy areas of outer retinal whitening that coalesce rapidly. In contrast to ARN, the posterior pole may be involved early in the disease course, significant vitreous cell and haze are typically absent, and the retinal vasculature is minimally involved, at least initially (Fig 11-7). Patients with PORN and HIV infection or AIDS frequently have a history of cutaneous zoster (67%) and eventually incur bilateral involvement (71%); they also have a similarly high rate (70%) of retinal detachment as in ARN. The visual prognosis is poor; in the largest series reported to date, 67% of patients had a final visual acuity of no light perception. Although PORN is often resistant to treatment with intravenous acyclovir alone, successful management has been reported with combination systemic and intraocular therapy using foscarnet and ganciclovir. Long-term suppressive antiviral therapy is required in patients with HIV/AIDS who are not able to achieve immune reconstitution through combination antiretroviral treatment. See also BCSC Section 12, *Retina and Vitreous,* for additional discussion of viral retinitis.

Nonnecrotizing herpetic retinitis (nonnecrotizing posterior uveitis) may occur in patients with herpetic infections, including acute retinochoroiditis with diffuse hemorrhages

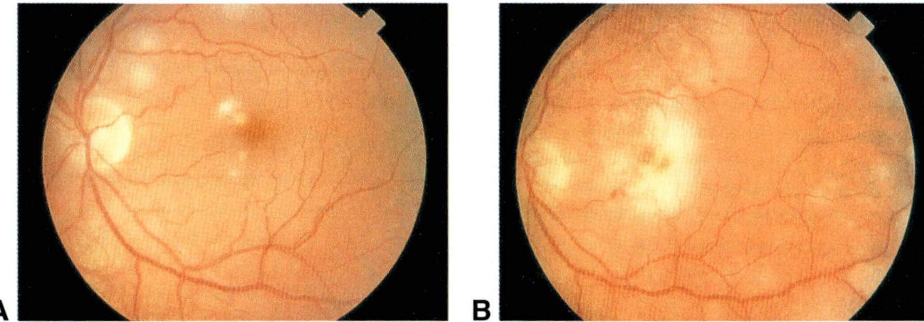

Figure 11-7 **A,** Fundus photograph showing multifocal areas of white retinitis in a patient with progressive outer retinal necrosis. **B,** Fundus photograph taken 5 days later, showing rapid disease progression and confluence of the areas of the viral retinitis. *(Courtesy of E. Mitchel Opremcak, MD.)*

following acute VZV infection in children and chronic choroiditis or retinal vasculitis in adults. Patients may be immune competent or immune compromised. In a study using PCR-based assays and local antibody analysis of aqueous fluid samples for herpesviruses, a viral etiology was confirmed in 13% of cases deemed "idiopathic posterior uveitis." Inflammation is typically bilateral, and the disorder may present with uveitic macular edema, as a birdshot uveitis–like chorioretinopathy, or as an occlusive bilateral retinitis. The disease is initially resistant to conventional therapy with systemic corticosteroids and/or immunomodulatory therapy (IMT), but favorable response is achieved when patients are switched to systemic antiviral medication.

American Academy of Ophthalmology. *Diagnosis and Treatment of Acute Retinal Necrosis.* Ophthalmic Technology Assessment. American Academy of Ophthalmology; 2017.

Chau Tran TH, Cassoux N, Bodaghi B, Lehoang P. Successful treatment with combination of systemic antiviral drugs and intravitreal ganciclovir injections in the management of severe necrotizing herpetic retinitis. *Ocul Immunol Inflamm.* 2003;11(2):141–144.

Engstrom RE Jr, Holland GN, Margolis TP, et al. The progressive outer retinal necrosis syndrome. A variant of necrotizing herpetic retinopathy in patients with AIDS. *Ophthalmology.* 1994;101(9):1488–1502.

Goldstein DA, Pyatetsky D. Necrotizing herpetic retinopathies. *Focal Points: Clinical Modules for Ophthalmologists.* San Francisco, CA: American Academy of Ophthalmology: 2008, module 10.

Wensing B, de Groot-Mijnes JD, Rothova A. Necrotizing and nonnecrotizing variants of herpetic uveitis with posterior segment involvement. *Arch Ophthalmol.* 2011;129(4): 403–408.

Cytomegalovirus

Cytomegalovirus is a double-stranded DNA virus in the Herpesviridae family. It is the most common cause of congenital viral infection and causes clinically relevant disease in neonates. It also causes illness in immunocompromised children and adults (leukemia, lymphoma, or HIV/AIDS), transplant recipients, and patients with conditions requiring systemic IMT. CMV retinitis is the most common ophthalmic manifestation of both congenital CMV infection and CMV as an opportunistic coinfection in patients with HIV/AIDS. The clinical appearance is similar regardless of clinical context, with 3 distinct variants:

- a classic or fulminant retinitis with large areas of retinal hemorrhage against a background of whitened, edematous, or necrotic retina. The retinitis typically appears in the posterior pole, near the vascular arcades, in the distribution of the nerve fiber layer, and associated with blood vessels (Fig 11-8)
- a granular or indolent form found more often in the retinal periphery, characterized by little or no hemorrhage, edema, or vascular sheathing. Active retinitis may progress from the borders of the lesion (Fig 11-9)
- a perivascular form often described as a variant of "frosted-branch" angiitis, an undifferentiated retinal perivasculitis initially described in immunocompetent children (Fig 11-10)

The diagnosis of congenital CMV disease is suggested by the clinical presentation; positive serum antibodies or PCR testing of urine, saliva, or intraocular fluids; and systemic

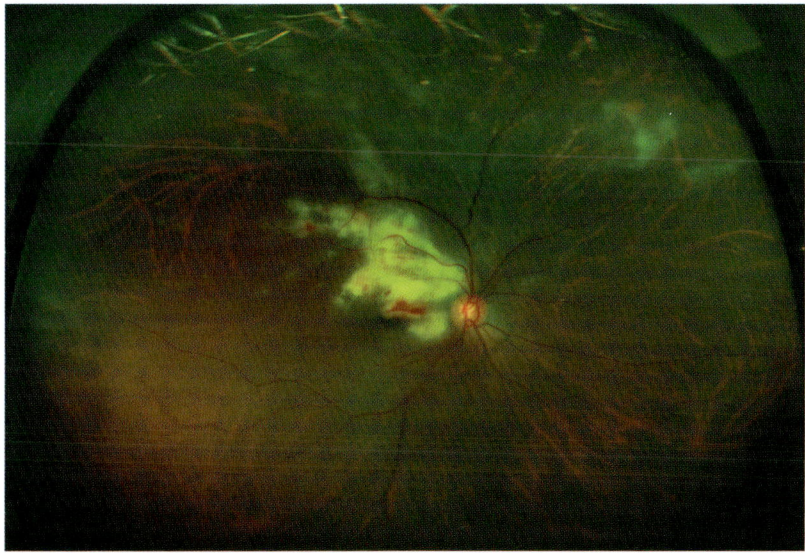

Figure 11-8 Fundus photograph of cytomegalovirus retinitis. *(Courtesy of Bryn M. Burkholder, MD.)*

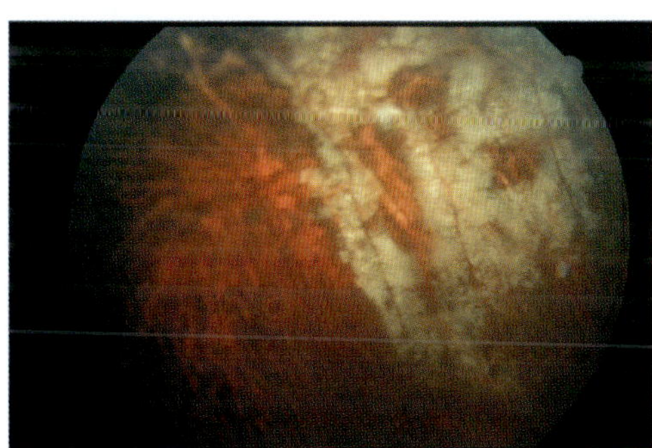

Figure 11-9 Fundus photograph of granular cytomegalovirus retinitis. *(Courtesy of Careen Lowder, MD.)*

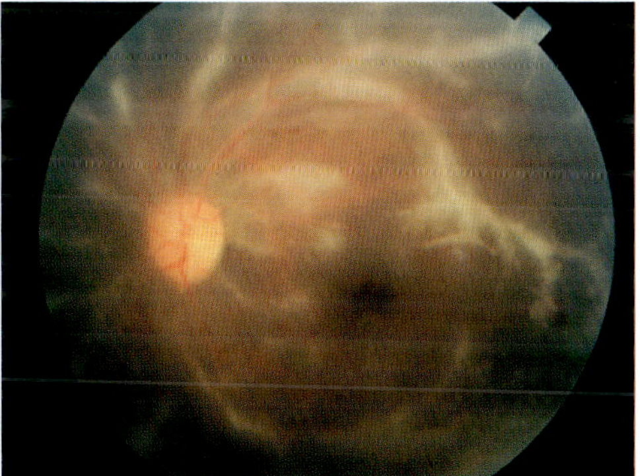

Figure 11-10 Fundus photograph of "frosted-branch" cytomegalovirus perivasculitis. *(Courtesy of Albert T. Vitale, MD.)*

findings. Serum antibody testing may be useful 5–24 months after the loss of maternal antibodies transferred after pregnancy. Congenital CMV retinitis is usually associated with other systemic manifestations of disseminated infection, including fever, thrombocytopenia, anemia, pneumonitis, and hepatosplenomegaly; the reported prevalence in children with congenital CMV infection is between 11% and 22%.

However, CMV retinitis has been reported to occur later in life among children with no discernible lesions ophthalmoscopically and no evidence of systemic disease reactivation. This pattern suggests that even asymptomatic children with evidence of congenital CMV infection should be monitored at regular intervals for potential ocular involvement later into childhood. Resolution of the retinitis leaves both pigmented and atrophic lesions, with retinal detachment occurring in up to one-third of these children. Optic atrophy and cataract formation are not uncommon sequelae.

The diagnosis of CMV retinitis in patients with HIV/AIDS or undergoing IMT is essentially clinical. Early CMV retinitis may present as a small, white retinal infiltrate and look like a cotton-wool spot. Patients may have coincidental HIV-associated retinopathy (dot-blot hemorrhages, cotton-wool spots), and early CMV retinitis is distinguished by its inevitable progression without treatment. In patients with atypical lesions or whose disease is not responding to therapy, early treatment and close follow-up are important. Polymerase chain reaction testing of aqueous or vitreous may help differentiate CMV from necrotizing retinitis secondary to HSV1/2 or VZV and from toxoplasmic retinochoroiditis. Toxoplasmosis may masquerade as a viral retinitis.

Prior to modern antiretroviral therapy, an estimated 30% of patients with HIV/AIDS, usually with $CD4^+$ T lymphocyte counts ≤50 cells/µL, experienced CMV retinitis. Secondary to breaks in areas of peripheral retinal necrosis, rhegmatogenous retinal detachments occurred at a rate of approximately 33% per eye per year. Modern antiretroviral regimens have reduced the incidence of CMV retinitis and its associated complications, such as retinal detachment, by 80%. This decrease has stabilized, and new cases of CMV retinitis can occur in patients where combination antiretroviral treatment fails or in those who abandon treatment or experience immune reconstitution but do not develop CMV-specific immunity.

Cytomegalovirus reaches the eye hematogenously, with passage of the virus across the blood–ocular barrier, infection of retinal vascular endothelial cells, and cell-to-cell transmission of the virus within the retina. The histologic features of both congenital and acquired disease include a primary, full-thickness, coagulative necrotizing retinitis and secondary diffuse choroiditis. Infected retinal cells show pathognomonic cytomegalic changes consisting of large eosinophilic intranuclear inclusions and small basophilic cytoplasmic inclusions. Viral inclusions may also be present in the retinal pigment epithelium (RPE) and vascular endothelium.

Management of CMV retinitis requires antiretroviral regimens and anti-CMV therapy. Anti-CMV therapy is particularly important, since CMV retinitis signifies a twofold-increased mortality risk in patients with a $CD4^+$ T-cell count below 100 cells/µL (an effect not observed with counts ≥100 cells/µL). Resistant CMV infection is further associated with increased mortality in patients with HIV/AIDS and CMV retinitis. Options for systemic coverage include high-dose induction with either intravenous ganciclovir (5 mg/kg twice daily) or foscarnet (90 mg/kg twice daily) for 2 weeks followed by low-dose daily maintenance therapy or oral valganciclovir (900 mg twice daily) for 3 weeks followed by maintenance therapy (900 mg/day).

Intravitreal injection of ganciclovir or foscarnet effectively treats intraocular disease and is a useful alternative in patients who cannot tolerate intravenous therapy because of myelotoxicity. However, intravitreal therapy alone leaves extraocular systemic CMV and the fellow eye untreated. Combination treatment with oral valganciclovir may ameliorate this limitation. This combination is also useful for vision-threatening, posteriorly located retinitis. In patients with CMV retinitis who are on antiretroviral regimens and experience sustained immune recovery ($CD4^+$ T lymphocytes ≥100 cells/µL for 3–6 months), systemic anti-CMV maintenance therapy may be safely discontinued. Antiretroviral therapy–naive patients may require only 6 months of anti-CMV therapy with good immune reconstitution, whereas antiretroviral therapy–experienced patients may require long-term maintenance therapy. Despite immune recovery, patients with a history of CMV retinitis who discontinue maintenance anti-CMV therapy remain at risk for recurrence and should be monitored at 3-month intervals.

Patients with immune recovery may, months or years later, develop intermediate uveitis in the absence of CMV reactivation. Rather, the reconstituted immune system reacts to residual CMV antigens within the eye. Cystoid macular edema may develop. Topical, periocular, and oral steroids are utilized. Initial aggressive anti-CMV therapy initiated at the same time as antiretroviral treatment may ultimately decrease the incidence of immune recovery uveitis.

Among immunocompetent adults, CMV infection may produce a chronic or recurrent unilateral anterior uveitis associated with ocular hypertension, corneal edema, and variable degrees of sectoral iris atrophy. Positive PCR testing of aqueous fluid for CMV DNA combined with negative testing for HSV and VZV is diagnostic. Treatment options for CMV anterior uveitis include systemic anti-CMV treatment (usually valganciclovir), topical ganciclovir gel 0.15%, and intravitreal ganciclovir injections. Relapses are common after discontinuation of therapy.

Chee SP, Bascal K, Jap A, Se-Thoe SY, Cheng CL, Tan BH. Clinical features of cytomegalovirus anterior uveitis in immunocompetent patients. *Am J Ophthalmol.* 2008;145(5):834–840.

Jabs DA, Holbrook JT, Van Natta ML, et al; Studies of Ocular Complications of AIDS Research Group. Risk factors for mortality in patients with AIDS in the era of highly active antiretroviral therapy. *Ophthalmology.* 2005;112(5):771–779.

Jabs DA, Martin BK, Forman MS; Cytomegalovirus Retinitis and Viral Resistance Research Group. Mortality associated with resistant cytomegalovirus among patients with cytomegalovirus retinitis and AIDS. *Ophthalmology.* 2010;117(1):128–132.

Kedhar SR, Jabs DA. Cytomegalovirus retinitis in the era of highly active antiretroviral therapy. *Herpes.* 2007;14(3):66–71.

Kempen JH, Min YI, Freeman WR, et al; Studies of Ocular Complications of AIDS Research Group. Risk of immune recovery uveitis in patients with AIDS and cytomegalovirus retinitis. *Ophthalmology.* 2006;113(4);684–694.

Epstein-Barr virus

Epstein-Barr virus (EBV) is a ubiquitous double-stranded DNA virus with a complex capsid and envelope; it belongs to the subfamily Gammaherpesvirinae. EBV is commonly associated with infectious mononucleosis (IM) and has been implicated in the pathogenesis of Burkitt lymphoma (especially among African children), nasopharyngeal carcinoma, Hodgkin disease, and Sjögren syndrome. EBV has a tropism for B lymphocytes, the only cells known to have surface receptors for the virus.

Ocular manifestations may arise either as a consequence of congenital EBV infection or, more commonly, during primary infection in the context of IM. Cataract may occur with congenital EBV infection. In contrast, a mild, self-limiting follicular conjunctivitis is most common with acquired IM. Other, less frequently reported anterior ocular

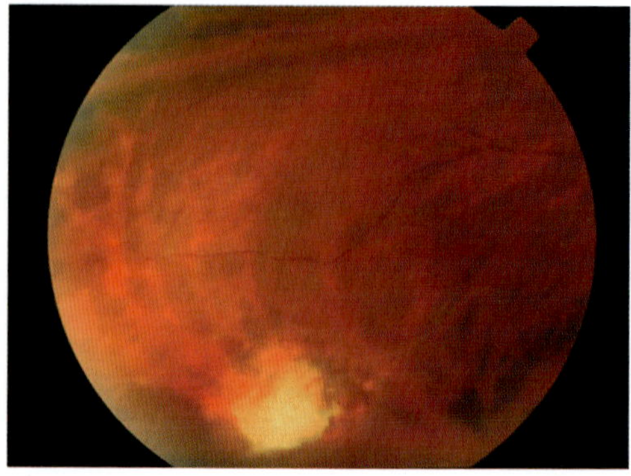

Figure 11-11 Fundus photograph of Epstein-Barr virus–related retinitis and vasculitis. *(Reprinted with permission from Vitale AT, Foster CS. Uveitis affecting infants and children: infectious causes. In: Hartnett ME, Trese M, Capone A, Keats B, Steidl SM, eds.* Pediatric Retina. *Philadelphia, PA: Lippincott Williams & Wilkins; 2004:269; courtesy of Albert T. Vitale, MD.)*

manifestations of acquired IM include epithelial or stromal keratitis; episcleritis; bilateral, granulomatous anterior uveitis; dacryoadenitis; and, less frequently, cranial nerve palsies and Parinaud oculoglandular syndrome.

A variety of posterior segment manifestations have been reported in association with EBV infection, including isolated optic disc edema and optic neuritis, macular edema, retinal hemorrhages, retinitis (Fig 11-11), punctate outer retinitis, choroiditis, multifocal choroiditis and panuveitis (MCP), pars planitis and vitritis, progressive subretinal fibrosis, uveitis, and secondary choroidal neovascularization (CNV). Acute retinal necrosis has also been reported. Epstein-Barr virus is rarely a cause of these findings in the absence of proper systemic context (eg, recent IM). Antibody testing against a variety of EBV-specific capsid antigens is rarely useful given the very high seroprevalence of EBV (90%) in the adult population; PCR assay from intraocular fluid can be helpful.

Most EBV-associated ocular disease is self-limiting. The presence of anterior uveitis may necessitate topical corticosteroids and cycloplegia. Systemic corticosteroids can treat posterior segment inflammation. Systemic antiviral therapy for EBV infection may be considered for the management of necrotizing retinitis/ARN.

Matoba AY. Ocular disease associated with Epstein-Barr virus infection. *Surv Ophthalmol.* 1990;35(2):145–150.

Peponis VG, Chatziralli IP, Parikakis EA, Chaira N, Katzakis MC, Mitropoulos PG. Bilateral multifocal chorioretinitis and optic neuritis due to Epstein-Barr virus: a case report. *Case Rep Ophthalmol.* 2012;3(3):327–332.

Rubella

The rubella virus is the prototypical teratogenic viral agent. It consists of single-stranded RNA surrounded by a lipid envelope, or "toga," hence its inclusion in the Togaviridae family. Although rubella remains an important cause of blindness in resource-limited regions and nations, the epidemic pattern of the disease was interrupted in the United States by introduction of the rubella vaccine in 1969. The peak age incidence shifted from 5–9 years (young children) in the prevaccine era to 15–19 years (older children) and more recently to 20–24 years (young adults). Approximately 5%–25% of women of childbearing age are susceptible to primary infection. Rubella may involve the retina as part of the congenital rubella syndrome (CRS) or during acquired infection (German measles).

The fetus is infected with the rubella virus transplacentally, secondary to maternal viremia during the course of primary infection. The frequency of fetal infection is highest during the first 10 weeks and the final month of pregnancy, with the rate of congenital defects varying inversely with gestational age. Although obvious maternal infection during the first trimester of pregnancy may end in spontaneous abortion, stillbirth, or severe fetal malformations, seropositive asymptomatic maternal rubella may also result in severe fetal disease.

The classic features of CRS include cardiac malformations (patent ductus arteriosus, interventricular septal defects, and pulmonic stenosis), ocular findings (chorioretinitis, cataract, corneal clouding, microphthalmia, strabismus, and glaucoma), and deafness (Fig 11-12). Hearing loss is the most common systemic finding. Individuals with CRS are at greater risk for diabetes mellitus and subsequent diabetic retinopathy later in life.

A unilateral or bilateral pigmentary retinopathy is the most common ocular manifestation of CRS (25%–50%), followed by cataract (15%) and glaucoma (10%). The pigmentary disturbance, often described as "salt-and-pepper" fundus, shows considerable variation, ranging from finely stippled, bone spicule–like, small, black, irregular masses to gross pigmentary irregularities with coarse, blotchy mottling (Fig 11-13). It can be stationary or

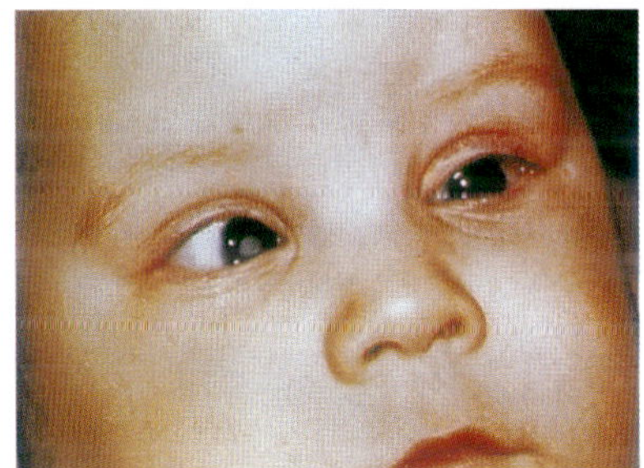

Figure 11-12 Patient with congenital rubella syndrome who exhibited cataract, esotropia, cognitive impairment, congenital heart disease, and deafness. *(Courtesy of John D. Sheppard Jr, MD.)*

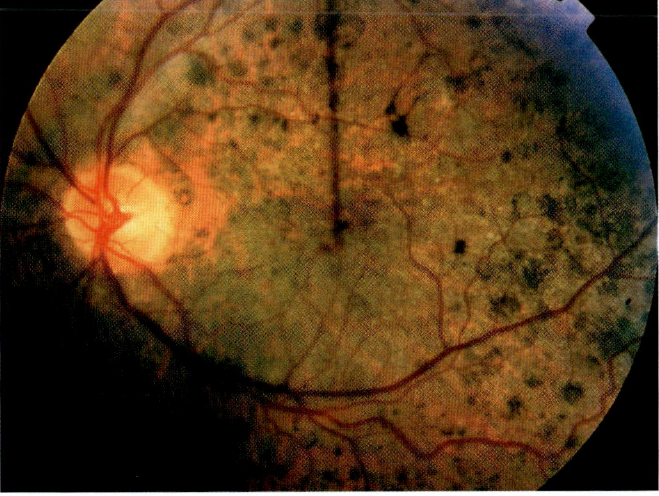

Figure 11-13 Fundus photograph of congenital rubella syndrome with diffuse retinal pigment epithelial mottling showing "salt-and-pepper" appearance. *(Courtesy of Albert T. Vitale, MD.)*

progressive. Despite loss of the foveal light reflex and prominent pigmentary changes, neither vision nor electroretinogram results are typically affected. Congenital (nuclear) cataracts and microphthalmia are the most frequent causes of poor visual acuity and, rarely, CNV. Unless otherwise compromised by glaucoma, the optic nerve and the retinal vessels are typically normal in appearance.

Histologic studies of the lens reveal retained cell nuclei in the embryonic nucleus as well as anterior and posterior cortical degeneration. Poor development of the pupil dilator muscle, necrosis of the iris pigment epithelium, and chronic nongranulomatous inflammation may be present in the iris. The RPE displays alternating areas of atrophy and hypertrophy. The anterior chamber angle appears similar to that of congenital glaucoma. Although the mechanism of rubella embryopathy is not known at the cellular level, it is thought that the virus inhibits cellular multiplication and establishes a chronic, persistent infection during organogenesis. The persistence of viral replication after birth, with ongoing tissue damage, is central to the pathogenesis of CRS and may explain the appearance of hearing and neurologic and/or ocular deficits long after birth.

The pigmentary retinal changes and associated systemic findings, together with a history of maternal exposure to rubella, suggest the diagnosis of CRS. Serologic criteria for rubella infection include a fourfold increase in rubella-specific immunoglobulin G (IgG) in paired sera 1–2 weeks apart or the new appearance of rubella-specific IgM. Because the fetus is capable of mounting an immune response to the rubella virus, specific IgM or IgA antibodies to rubella in the cord blood confirm the diagnosis.

The differential diagnosis of congenital rubella retinitis consists of entities constituting the TORCH (*t*oxoplasmosis, *o*ther agents, *r*ubella, *c*ytomegalovirus, and *h*erpesviruses) syndrome. See also BCSC Section 6, *Pediatric Ophthalmology and Strabismus*, for additional discussion of congenital rubella. Other viral illnesses, such as mumps, roseola subitum, and postvaccination encephalitis, should be considered and ruled out by appropriate serologic tests. There is no specific antiviral therapy for congenital rubella, and treatment is supportive.

Acquired infection (German measles) presents with a prodrome of malaise and fever in adolescents and adults before onset of the rubella exanthem. An erythematous, maculopapular rash appears first on the face, spreads toward the hands and feet, involves the entire body within 24 hours, and disappears by the third day. Although the rash is not always prominent and the occurrence of fever is variable, lymphadenopathy is invariably present.

The most frequent ocular complication of postnatally acquired rubella is conjunctivitis (70%), followed by the infrequent occurrence of epithelial keratitis and retinitis. Acquired rubella retinitis has been described in adults presenting with acute-onset decreased vision and multifocal chorioretinitis, with large areas of bullous neurosensory detachment, underlying pigment epithelial detachment involving the entire posterior pole, anterior chamber and preretinal vitreous cells, dark gray atrophic lesions of the RPE, normal appearance of the retinal vessels and optic nerve, and absence of retinal hemorrhage. The neurosensory detachments resolve spontaneously, and visual acuity returns to normal. Chronic rubella virus infection has been implicated in the pathogenesis of FUS, as evidenced by the presence of rubella-specific intraocular antibody production and the intraocular persistence of the virus (for more detailed discussion of FUS, see Chapter 8).

Uncomplicated acquired rubella does not require specific therapy; however, rubella retinitis and postvaccination optic neuritis may respond well to systemic corticosteroids.

Arnold JJ, McIntosh ED, Martin FJ, Menser MA. A fifty-year follow-up of ocular defects in congenital rubella: late ocular manifestations. *Aust N Z J Ophthalmol.* 1994;22(1):1–6.
Givens KT, Lee DA, Jones T, Ilstrup DM. Congenital rubella syndrome: ophthalmic manifestations and associated systemic disorders. *Br J Ophthalmol.* 1993;77(6):358–363.
Quentin CD, Reiber H. Fuchs heterochromic cyclitis: rubella virus antibodies and genome in aqueous humor. *Am J Ophthalmol.* 2004;138(1):46–54.

Lymphocytic Choriomeningitis Virus

Lymphocytic choriomeningitis virus (LCMV) is an under-recognized fetal teratogen that should probably be listed among the "other agents" in the TORCH group of congenital infections. The microbe is a single-stranded RNA virus of the Arenaviridae family.

Systemic findings include macrocephaly, hydrocephalus, and intracranial calcifications. Neurologic abnormalities, seizures, and mild cognitive impairment may occur. Ocular findings include macular and peripheral chorioretinal scars, similar in morphology and distribution to congenital toxoplasmosis. Serologic testing of the mother and the infant helps differentiate. Other findings include optic atrophy, strabismus, and nystagmus.

Mets MB, Barton LL, Khan AS, Ksiazek TG. Lymphocytic choriomeningitis virus: an underdiagnosed cause of congenital chorioretinitis. *Am J Ophthalmol.* 2000;130(2):209–215.

Mumps

The mumps virus is a member of the Paramyxoviridae family (other members include measles, parainfluenza, and respiratory syncytial virus). A single-stranded RNA virus, mumps is acquired by respiratory droplets and may cause parotitis, aseptic meningitis, and orchitis. Rarely, mumps may cause inflammation involving the cornea, optic nerve, or retina.

Khubchandani R, Rane T, Agarwal P, Nabi F, Patel P, Shetty AK. Bilateral neuroretinitis associated with mumps. *Arch Neurol.* 2002;59(10):1633–1636.

Measles (Rubeola)

Congenital and acquired measles infection is caused by a single-stranded RNA virus of the genus *Morbillivirus* in the Paramyxoviridae family. The virus is highly contagious and is transmitted either directly or via aerosolization of nasopharyngeal secretions to the mucous membranes of the conjunctiva or respiratory tract of susceptible individuals, or transplacentally from a pregnant woman to her fetus.

Despite the existence of an effective vaccine, measles remains a leading cause of mortality worldwide among children. In the United States, however, measles is rare.

Congenital measles infection may cause cataract, optic nerve head drusen, and a bilateral diffuse pigmentary retinopathy involving the posterior pole and retinal periphery. The retinopathy may be associated with normal or attenuated retinal vessels, retinal edema, and macular star formation. Electroretinographic results and visual acuity are usually normal.

The most common ocular manifestations of acquired measles are keratitis and a mild, papillary, nonpurulent conjunctivitis. Corneal scarring in countries with prevalent malnutrition may cause post-measles blindness, a significant problem worldwide.

Measles retinopathy is more common in acquired than in congenital disease, presenting with profound loss of vision 6–12 days after the appearance of the characteristic exanthem; it may be accompanied by encephalitis. Measles retinopathy is characterized by attenuated arterioles, diffuse retinal edema, macular star formation, scattered retinal hemorrhages, blurred disc margins, and clear media. Optic disc pallor and a secondary pigmentary retinopathy with either a bone spicule or salt-and-pepper appearance may subsequently develop.

The differential diagnosis of congenital measles retinopathy includes the TORCH entities, atypical retinitis pigmentosa, and neuroretinitis. For acquired measles retinopathy, considerations include central serous chorioretinopathy, Vogt-Koyanagi-Harada (VKH) syndrome (bullous detachments may resolve, leaving extensive RPE disruption), retinitis pigmentosa, syphilis, and other viral retinopathies.

The diagnosis of measles and its ocular sequelae is made clinically and through serologic testing. Systemic corticosteroids should be considered in cases of acute measles retinopathy.

Foxman SG, Heckenlively JR, Sinclair SH. Rubeola retinopathy and pigmented paravenous retinochoroidal atrophy. *Am J Ophthalmol.* 1985;99(5):605–606.

Lee JH, Agarwal A, Mahendradas P, et al. Viral posterior uveitis. *Surv Ophthalmol.* 2017;62(4):404–445.

Subacute sclerosing panencephalitis

Subacute sclerosing panencephalitis (SSPE) is a rare, late complication of acquired measles infection. It most often affects unvaccinated children 6–8 years after the primary infection. In late childhood or adolescence, visual impairment, behavioral disturbances, and memory impairment may insidiously develop, followed by myoclonus and progression to spastic paresis, dementia, and death within 1–3 years.

Ocular findings are reported in up to 50% of patients with SSPE and may precede the neurologic manifestations by several weeks to 2 years. The most consistent finding is a maculopathy, consisting of focal retinitis and RPE changes, occurring in 36% of patients (Fig 11-14). Retinitis may progress to involve the peripheral retina. Other findings include

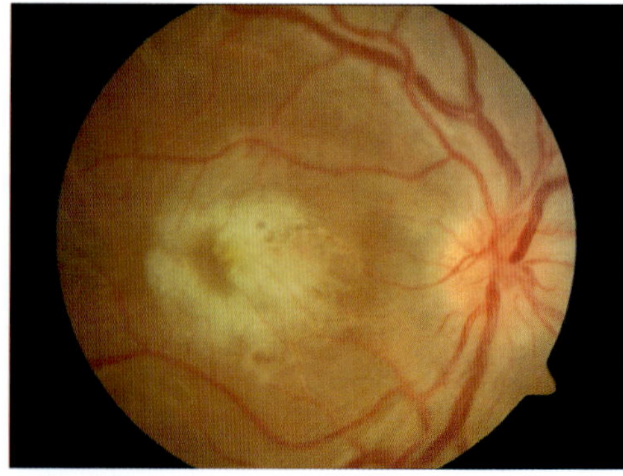

Figure 11-14 Fundus photograph of subacute sclerosing panencephalitis macular retinitis. *(Courtesy of Emad B. Abboud, MD.)*

disc swelling and papilledema, optic atrophy, macular edema, macular pigment epithelial disturbances, small intraretinal hemorrhages, gliotic scar, whitish retinal infiltrates, serous macular detachment, drusen, preretinal membranes, macular hole, cortical blindness, hemianopsia, horizontal nystagmus, and ptosis. Characteristically, there is little, if any, vitritis.

The diagnosis is based on clinical examination, electroencephalographic abnormalities, raised IgG antibody titer against measles in the plasma and cerebrospinal fluid, and/or panencephalitis found on magnetic resonance imaging or brain biopsy.

The differential diagnosis of the ophthalmic findings includes necrotizing viral retinitis caused by HSV, VZV, and CMV infection. Intermediate uveitis and retinal vasculitis associated with multiple sclerosis (MS) may also be considered. Definitive treatment of SSPE remains undetermined.

Garg RK. Subacute sclerosing panencephalitis. *Postgrad Med J.* 2002;78(916):63–70.

Yuksel D, Sonmez PA, Yilmaz D, Senbil N, Gurer Y. Ocular findings in subacute sclerosing panencephalitis. *Ocul Immunol Inflamm.* 2011;19(2):135–138.

West Nile Virus

West Nile virus (WNV) is a single-stranded RNA virus of the family Flaviviridae; it belongs to the Japanese encephalitis virus serocomplex and is endemic to Europe, Australia, Asia, and Africa. The virus is transmitted from birds (the natural host) to humans through the bite of an infected mosquito. The peak onset of the disease occurs in late summer, but it can occur anytime between July and December. The incubation period ranges from 3 to 14 days. Eighty percent of WNV infections are subclinical. Twenty percent of infections present as a febrile illness, often accompanied by myalgia, arthralgia, headache, conjunctivitis, lymphadenopathy, and a maculopapular or roseolar rash. Severe neurologic disease (meningitis or encephalitis) may occur, frequently found in association with diabetes mellitus and advanced age.

Presenting ocular symptoms include pain, photophobia, conjunctival hyperemia, and blurred vision. A characteristic multifocal chorioretinitis is present in most patients, together with nongranulomatous anterior uveitis and vitreous inflammatory cells. Chorioretinal lesions vary in size (200–1000 µm) and number and may affect the midzone and/or posterior pole, often in linear arrays following the course of retinal nerve fibers. Active lesions appear whitish to yellow, are flat and deep, and evolve with varying degrees of pigmentation and atrophy.

Fluorescein angiography reveals central hypofluorescence with late staining of active lesions, and early hyperfluorescence with late staining of inactive lesions. Inactive or partly active lesions may show a target-like appearance with central hypofluorescence caused by blockage from pigment and peripheral hyperfluorescence due to atrophy (Fig 11-15). Indocyanine green angiography reveals hypofluorescent spots, more numerous than those apparent on fluorescein angiography or funduscopy.

Other findings may include intraretinal hemorrhages, disc edema, optic atrophy, and, less commonly, focal retinal vascular sheathing and occlusion, cranial nerve VI palsy, and nystagmus. Congenital WNV infection has been reported in an infant presenting without intraocular inflammation but with chorioretinal scarring.

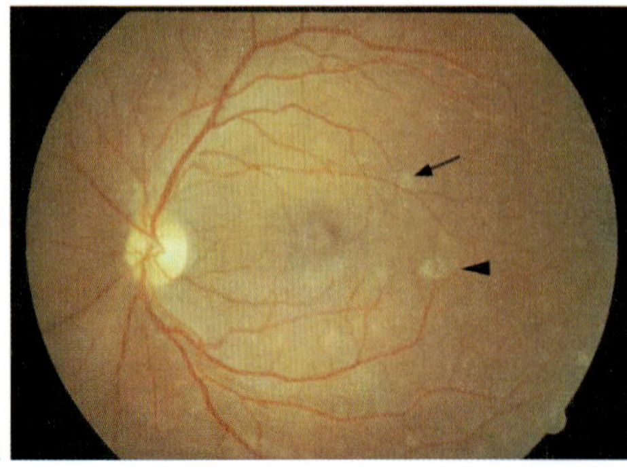

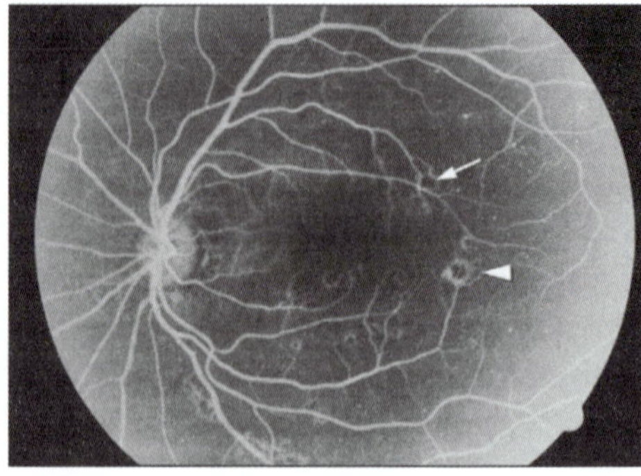

Figure 11-15 West Nile virus chorioretinitis. **A,** Fundus photograph showing multiple active *(arrow)* and partially active *(arrowhead)* discrete cream-colored chorioretinal spots (100–300 μm) in a linear pattern. **B,** The corresponding fluorescein angiogram shows early hypofluorescence *(arrow)* on the active chorioretinal spots (acute stage) and focal hypofluorescence with a surrounding hyperfluorescent ring *(arrowhead)* on the partially active lesions (subacute stage). The late-phase angiogram (not shown) shows subsequent staining. *(Reprinted with permission from Chan CK, Limstrom SA, Tarasewicz DG, Ling SG. Ocular features of West Nile virus infection in North America: a study of 14 eyes.* Ophthalmology. *2006;113[9]:1539–1546.)*

In most patients, intraocular inflammation associated with WNV infection has a self-limiting course, with a return of visual acuity to baseline after several months. Loss of vision may occur because of CNV, foveal scar, ischemic maculopathy, vitreous hemorrhage, tractional retinal detachment, optic nerve pathology, and retrogeniculate damage. Diabetes mellitus has been implicated as a risk factor for WNV-related death and may increase the risk of WNV-associated ocular involvement.

Ocular findings in patients with systemic symptoms suggestive of WNV infection or with meningoencephalitis may suggest the diagnosis and may prompt serologic testing. The differential diagnosis includes syphilis, MCP, histoplasmosis, sarcoidosis, and tuberculosis.

Currently there is no vaccine or specific antiviral treatment for WNV infection. Patients receive supportive therapy. Anterior uveitis may be treated with topical steroids. The efficacy of systemic and periocular corticosteroids for chorioretinal manifestations is unknown. Public health strategies directed at prevention are the mainstays of WNV infection control.

Chan CK, Limstrom SA, Tarasewicz DG, Lin SG. Ocular features of West Nile virus infection in North America: a study of 14 eyes. *Ophthalmology.* 2006;113(9): 1539–1546.

Garg S, Jampol LM. Systemic and intraocular manifestations of West Nile virus infection. *Surv Ophthalmol.* 2005;50(1):3–13.

Khairallah M, Ben Yahia S, Attia S, Zaouali S, Ladjimi A, Messaoud R. Linear pattern of West Nile virus–associated chorioretinitis is related to retinal nerve fibres organization. *Eye (Lond).* 2007;21(7):952–955.

Khairallah M, Ben Yahia S, Letaief M, et al. A prospective evaluation of factors associated with chorioretinitis in patients with West Nile virus infection. *Ocul Immunol Inflamm.* 2007;15(6):435–439.

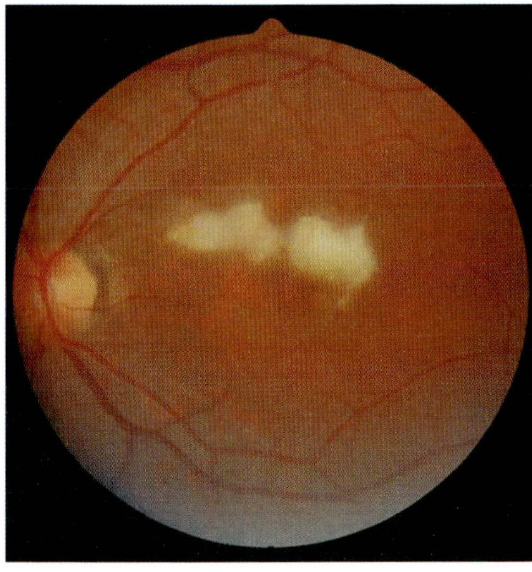

Figure 11-16 Rift Valley fever. Fundus photograph of a 44-year-old male farmer from Saudi Arabia who presented with decreased vision and macular retinitis sparing the fovea; he had a history of fever and contact with animal abortus. *(Courtesy of Albert T. Vitale, MD.)*

Rift Valley Fever

Rift Valley fever (RVF) is a febrile illness caused by the Bunyaviridae family. One of 3 clinical syndromes may develop: (1) an uncomplicated, febrile, influenza-like illness; (2) hemorrhagic fever; or (3) encephalitis. Ophthalmic findings may include anterior uveitis, vitritis, a macular or paramacular retinitis (Fig 11-16), retinal hemorrhage, retinal vasculitis, and optic nerve edema. Anterior uveitis may occur in 31% of patients. Patients may develop macular scarring, vascular attenuation, retinal ischemia, and/or optic atrophy.

The differential diagnosis includes viral entities such as measles, rubella, influenza, dengue fever, and WNV infection as well as bacterial illnesses such as brucellosis, Lyme disease, toxoplasmosis, cat-scratch disease, and rickettsial diseases. The diagnosis of RVF is made clinically and serologically.

Al-Hazmi A, Al-Rajhi AA, Abboud EB, et al. Ocular complications of Rift Valley fever outbreak in Saudi Arabia. *Ophthalmology.* 2005;112(2):313–318.

Human T-Lymphotropic Virus Type 1

Human T-lymphotropic virus type 1 (HTLV-1) is a retrovirus that is endemic in Japan, the Caribbean islands, and parts of Central and South America. It accounts for approximately 1% of uveitis cases in Japan. The diagnosis is made by serologic testing.

The major target cell of HTLV-1 is the $CD4^+$ T cell. HTLV-1 infection is the established cause of adult T-cell leukemia/lymphoma (ATL), HTLV-1–associated myelopathy/tropical spastic paralysis (HAM/TSP), and HTLV-1 uveitis (HU). HU is defined as uveitis of undetermined origin in an HTLV-1 carrier. Additional ocular manifestations of HTLV-1 infection include retinal infiltrates caused by secondary ATL (Fig 11-17), retinal degeneration, optic neuropathy, and keratopathy, as well as keratoconjunctivitis sicca in patients with HAM/TSP.

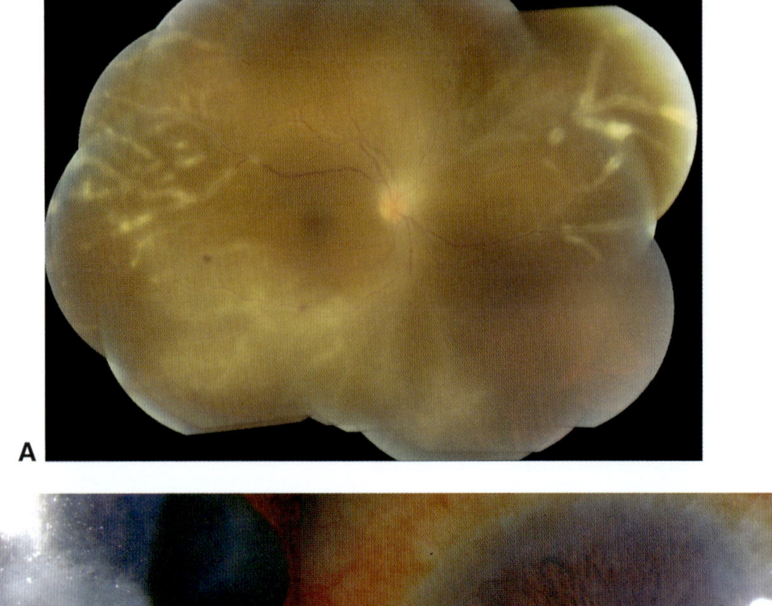

Figure 11-17 Ocular findings in human T-cell lymphotropic virus type 1–associated T-cell leukemia/lymphoma. **A,** Fundus photograph showing HTLV-1– associated retinal and vascular infiltrates. **B,** Anterior segment photograph of HTLV-1–associated keratopathy. *(Courtesy of H. Nida Sen, MD/National Eye Institute.)*

Most cases of HU (75%) are classified as an intermediate uveitis. Patients present with blurred vision and floaters caused by a mild granulomatous anterior uveitis (20%), unilateral vitritis (60%), membranous vitreous opacities, and/or "snowballs." Retinal vasculitis (60%), exudative retinal lesions (25%), optic disc abnormalities (20%), and uveitic macular edema (3%) may also be observed. Retinal vasculitis is responsive to corticosteroids.

For cases that progress despite therapy, the clinician must consider a masquerade syndrome, as retinal infiltration caused by ATL (see Fig 11-17) and retinal degeneration associated with HAM/TSP may mimic HU. HTLV-1–associated keratopathy (previously referred to as *HTLV-1–related chronic interstitial keratitis*) has been described in Brazilian and Caribbean patients but has not been found among Japanese patients. These corneal lesions likely represent lymphoplasmacytic infiltrates and are asymptomatic.

Although HU responds to topical, periocular, or systemic steroids, one-half of patients may experience recurrent disease.

Buggage RR. Ocular manifestations of human T-cell lymphotropic virus type 1 infection. *Curr Opin Ophthalmol.* 2003;14(6):420–425.

Goto H, Mochizuki M, Yamaki K, Kotake S, Usui M, Ohno S. Epidemiological survey of intraocular inflammation in Japan. *Jpn J Ophthalmol.* 2007;51(1):41–44.

Dengue Fever

Dengue fever is the most common mosquito-borne viral disease in humans. A member of the Flaviviridae family and transmitted by the *Aedes aegypti* mosquito, dengue is endemic within more than 100 countries in the tropical and subtropical regions of the globe.

Systemic signs and symptoms include fever, headache, myalgia, purpuric rash, and other bleeding manifestations secondary to thrombocytopenia. For many patients, however, this initial infection may be low grade and escape obvious mention unless specifically elicited upon history. The most common ocular manifestation is petechial subconjunctival hemorrhage. A variable degree of anterior chamber and vitreous cells may occur.

Maculopathy or "foveolitis" may develop in approximately 10% of patients 1 month after the onset of systemic disease, causing a sudden decrease in vision and central scotoma. Fluorescein angiography may show early focal arteriolar knobby hyperfluorescence in the macula with late leakage and/or staining; optical coherence tomography (OCT) angiography may show disruption of the foveal avascular zone (Fig 11-18). Despite no apparent

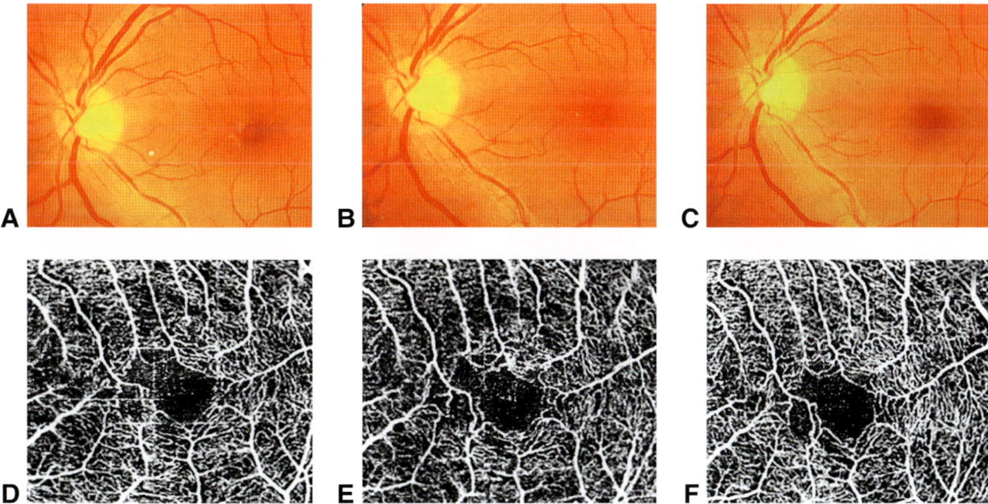

Figure 11-18 A 46-year-old man presented with decreased vision 1 week after an episode of dengue fever. Small, whitish, retinal opacification patches with few superficial hemorrhages are seen **(A)**. The lesions gradually resolve after a course of oral steroids **(B, C)**. Optical coherence tomography angiogram shows broken foveal avascular zone and loss of capillary density in the superficial retina plexus, which remained unchanged on follow-up **(D–F)**. *(Reprinted with permission from Bajgai P, Singh R, Kapil A. Progression of dengue maculopathy on OCT-angiography and fundus photography.* Ophthalmology. *2017;124[12]:1816.)*

lesions on clinical exam, OCT may show macular edema, subretinal fluid, or disruption of the inner segment/outer segment junction.

The diagnosis is based on clinical findings combined with positive serologic testing. While the infection is not endemic to the United States, dengue virus–associated maculopathy should be considered in patients presenting with suggestive findings and a history of recent travel to an endemic area. There is no well-defined treatment algorithm for dengue affecting the posterior segment, but local and systemic steroids may be utilized.

Bacsal KE, Chee SP, Cheng CL, Flores JV. Dengue-associated maculopathy. *Arch Ophthalmol.* 2007;125(4):501–510.

Lim WK, Mathur R, Koh A, Yeoh R, Chee SP. Ocular manifestations of dengue fever. *Ophthalmology.* 2004;111(11):2057–2064.

Ng AW, Teoh SC. Dengue eye disease. *Surv Ophthalmol.* 2015;60(2):106–114.

Chikungunya Fever

Chikungunya fever is a potentially fatal illness resembling dengue fever that is caused by an arthropod-borne *Alphavirus.* Patients present with fever, headache, fatigue, nausea, vomiting, myalgia, arthralgia, and skin rash. Chikungunya translates to "that which bends up," a reference to the polyarthropathy, tenosynovitis, and stooped posture of some affected patients. The virus is typically transmited to humans via mosquito bite. Maternal-fetal transmission has been documented. Recent outbreaks have occurred in Africa, Asia, Europe, and the Americas.

The ocular manifestations in a 2006 epidemic in India included both anterior uveitis and retinitis, and, less frequently, nodular episcleritis. Each had a typically benign course. The anterior uveitis may be granulomatous or nongranulomatous and associated with diffuse pigmented KPs, iris pigment release, and elevated IOP. Chikungunya retinitis may resemble herpetic retinitis. However, chikungunya retinitis features focal, multifocal, or

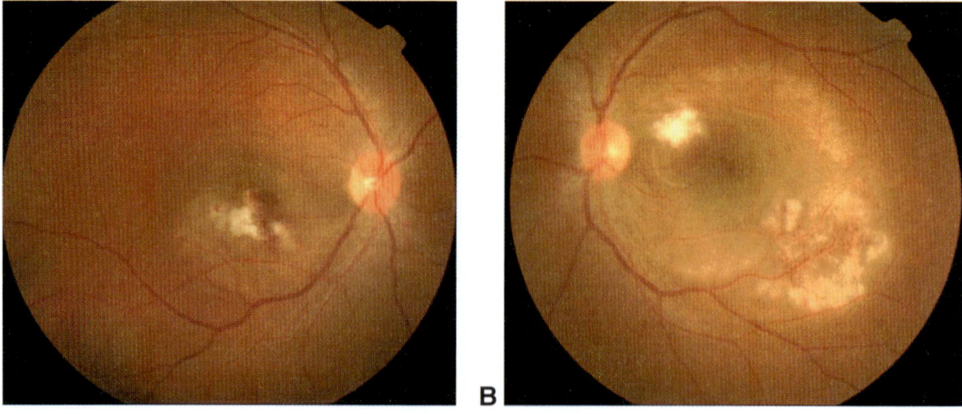

Figure 11-19 Retinitis associated with chikungunya fever. **A,** Retinitis with hemorrhages, right eye. **B,** Multifocal retinitis, left eye. *(Reprinted with permission from Mahendradas P, Ranganna SK, Shetty R, et al. Ocular manifestations associated with chikungunya.* Ophthalmology. *2008;115[2]:287–291.)*

confluent retinochoroiditis in the posterior pole with retinal hemorrhage and minimal vitritis (Fig 11-19), while herpetic retinitis includes the peripheral retina and a more intense vitritis.

Diagnosis may be confirmed serologically by IgM antibodies, virus isolation, or PCR. Although retinitis has been treated with systemic acyclovir and prednisone, there is no evidence to suggest that such therapy improves visual outcome.

Mahendradas P, Avadhani K, Shetty R. Chikungunya and the eye: a review. *J Ophthalmic Inflamm Infect.* 2013;3(1):35.

Zika Virus

Zika virus (ZIKV), an arbovirus and member of the Flaviviridae family, is named after a forest in Uganda. Similar to dengue and chikungunya viruses, mosquitos (often *Aedes aegypti*) transmit ZIKV to humans. Coinfection with any of those 3 distinct viral diseases may occur in endemic areas. Sexual transmission has been reported. A large proportion of patients infected with ZIKV will have no symptoms or minimal symptoms (fever, headache, rash, arthralgia, myalgia, conjunctivitis) that typically resolve within a week.

Acute infection in adults has been reported to cause individual cases of conjunctivitis, anterior uveitis, posterior uveitis with numerous chorioretinal lesions, and unilateral acute maculopathy. There is no defined treatment, but topical, systemic, or local steroids may be considered.

Brazil experienced an epidemic of ZIKV that began in April 2015. A 20-fold spike in newborns with microcephaly was noted in the ensuing months, suggesting ZIKV congenital infection. The United States Centers for Disease Control and Prevention (CDC) has defined congenital Zika syndrome with the following 5 features:

- microcephaly
- structural brain abnormalities
- ocular findings
- congenital contractures such as clubfoot
- hypertonia restricting body movement soon after birth

There have been no reports of uveitis associated with congenital infection. Observed ocular abnormalities include microphthalmia, cataract, glaucoma, iris coloboma, retinal pigment mottling, chorioretinal atrophy, and optic nerve hypoplasia or atrophy (Fig 11-20). No vaccine exists to prevent Zika at this time. Mosquito-borne transmission of ZIKV has been reported in the United States, and current prevention efforts focus on education and mosquito control.

de Paula Freitas B, de Oliveira Dias JR, Prazeres J, et al. Ocular findings in infants with microcephaly associated with presumed Zika virus congenital infection in Salvador, Brazil. *JAMA Ophthalmol.* 2016;134(5):529–535.

de Paula Freitas B, Ventura CV, Maia M, Belfort R Jr. Zika virus and the eye. *Curr Opin Ophthalmol.* 2017;28(6):595–599.

Furtado JM, Espósito DL, Klein TM, Teixeira-Pinto T, da Fonseca BA. Uveitis associated with Zika virus infection. *N Engl J Med.* 2016;375:394–396.

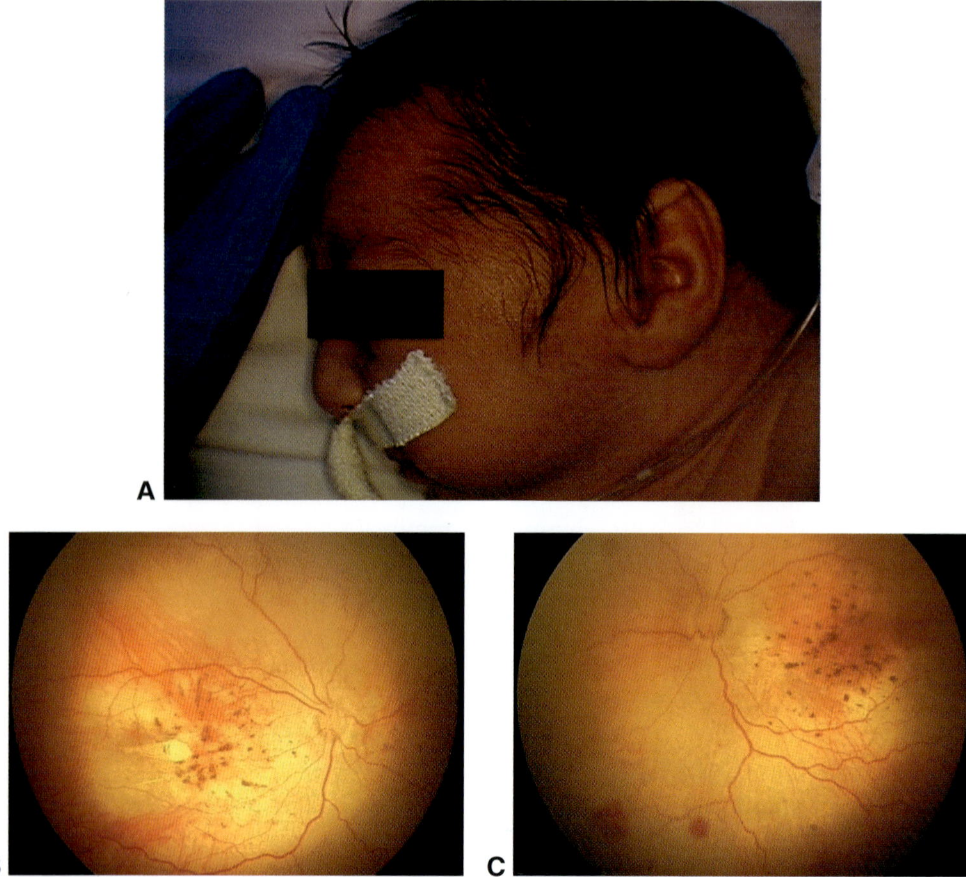

Figure 11-20 Congenital Zika syndrome. **A,** Characteristic features of microcephaly. **B, C,** Fundus photographs showing bilateral pigmentary clumping within the macula. *(Reprinted with permission from Miranda HA 2nd, Costa MC, Frazão MAM, Simão N, Franchischini S, Moshfeghi DM. Expanded spectrum of congenital ocular findings in microcephaly with presumed Zika infection.* Ophthalmology. *2016;123[8]:1788–1794.)*

Kodati S, Palmore TN, Spellman FA, Cunningham D, Weistrop B, Sen HN. Bilateral posterior uveitis associated with Zika virus infection. *Lancet.* 2017;389(10064):125–126.

Parke DW 3rd, Almeida DR, Albini TA, Ventura CV, Berrocal AM, Mittra RA. Serologically confirmed Zika-related unilateral acute maculopathy in an adult. *Ophthalmology.* 2016;123(11):2432–433.

Ebola Virus

Ebola virus disease (EVD) was first discovered in 1976 near the Ebola River in Congo. The virus is transmitted through direct contact with blood or body fluids or needles/syringes from a person who is sick or who has died from Ebola infection. Sexual contact with semen from a man who has recovered from Ebola is debated as a possible mode of transmission. Symptoms are fever, bruising, headache, weakness and fatigue, nausea and vomiting, and abdominal pain. Patients with acute EVD may experience conjunctivitis, conjunctival hemorrhage, and acute vision loss of unclear etiology. Symptoms may appear 2–21 days after initial exposure. There is no vaccine or curative medication for EVD; treatment is aggressive supportive care.

Survivors of EVD may experience "post–Ebola virus disease syndrome," which can include arthralgias, myalgias, fatigue, weight loss, headache, neurocognitive deficits, and psychosocial issues. Uveitis can affect Ebola survivors. In 1 patient, Ebola virus was isolated from aqueous humor 9 weeks after viremia resolved. Iris heterochromia and uveal edema may develop (Fig 11-21). Retinal pigment epithelial cells may be a potential reservoir for the virus. Patients may have episcleritis, interstitial keratitis, anterior uveitis, chorioretinal lesions (Fig 11-22), or optic neuropathy. Uveitis relapses may occur up to 13 months after a negative PCR test on serum.

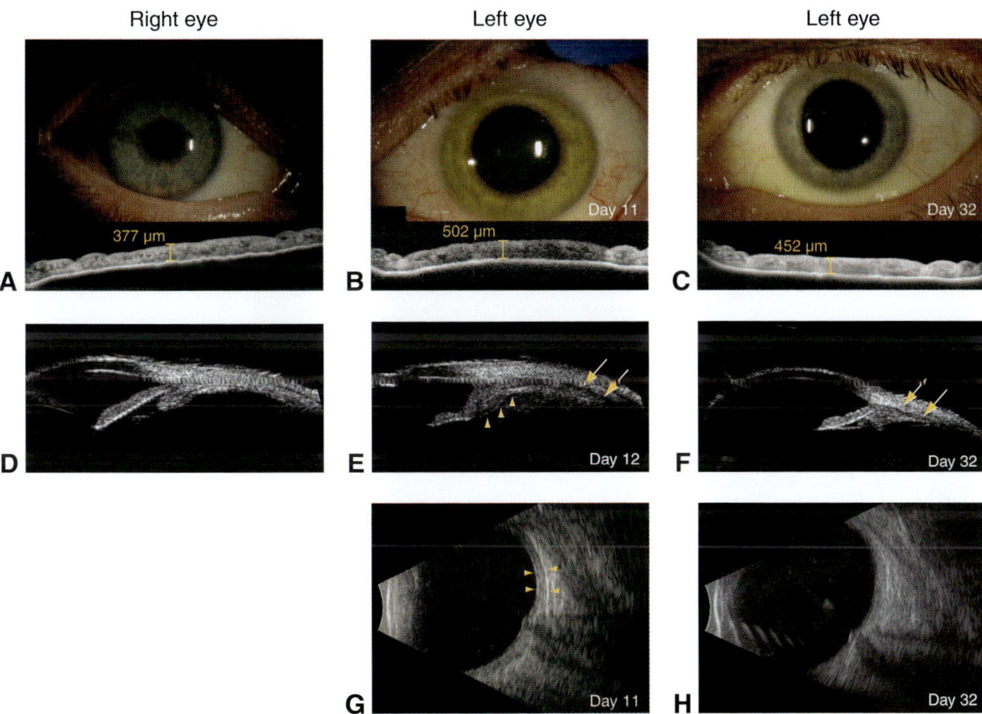

Figure 11-21 Late-onset panuveitis and iris heterochromia in an Ebola survivor. **A,** Slit-lamp photograph of right eye with corresponding anterior segment optical coherence tomography at baseline. **B,** At day 11, the iris of the left eye has turned green and shows edema. **C,** By day 32, the iris has reverted to its original blue color and the iris edema has improved. **D,** Ultrasound biomicroscopy (UBM) image shows normal ciliary body anatomy of the right eye. **E,** At day 12, UBM of the left eye shows ciliary body swelling *(arrowheads)* and supraciliary/choroidal effusion *(arrows)* consistent with progressive panuveitis, choroiditis, and evolving hypotony. **F,** Repeat UBM shows decreased ciliary body swelling and resolution of supraciliary/choroidal effusion *(arrows)* by day 32. **G,** B-scan ultrasound imaging shows choroidal thickening at day 11 *(arrowheads)*. **H,** At day 32, the choroidal thickening has resolved. *(Reprinted with permission from Shantha JG, Crozier I, Varkey JB, et al. Long-term management of panuveitis and iris hetero-chromia in an Ebola survivor.* Ophthalmology. *2016;123[12]:2626–2628.e2.)*

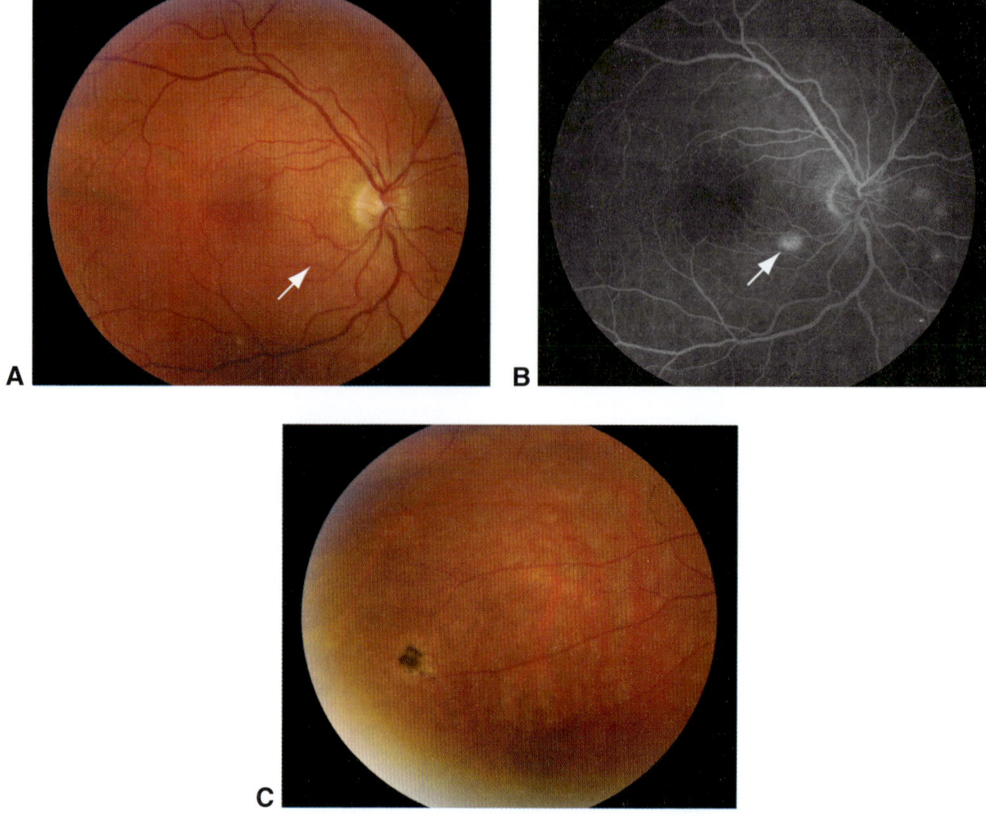

Figure 11-22 Inactive chorioretinitis in a recent Ebola survivor. **A,** Fundus photograph of the right eye shows clear media and a retinal opacity temporal to the optic nerve *(arrow)*. **B,** A corresponding fluorescein angiogram image shows hyperfluorescence with staining of the retinal lesion temporal *(arrow)* and 3 small lesions nasal to the nerve. **C,** Fundus photograph of the inferotemporal retina shows a hyperpigmented scar with a hypopigmented halo. *(Reprinted with permission from Shantha JG, Crozier I, Varkey JB, et al. Long-term management of panuveitis and iris hetero-chromia in an Ebola survivor.* Ophthalmology. *2016;123[12]:2626–2628.e2.)*

Other Viral Diseases

Acute anterior uveitis may also occur with other viral infectious entities. The uveitis observed with influenza, adenovirus infection, and IM is mild and transient. Synechiae and ocular damage seldom occur. Uveitis associated with adenovirus infection is usually secondary to corneal disease (see BCSC Section 8, *External Disease and Cornea)*.

Fungal Uveitis

Ocular Histoplasmosis Syndrome

Ocular histoplasmosis syndrome (OHS) is a multifocal chorioretinitis presumed to be caused by infection with *Histoplasma capsulatum* early in life. Primary infection occurs after inhalation of the fungal spores. Hematogenous dissemination likely results in ocular disease. Initial infection is usually asymptomatic. The initial focal infection of the choroid may subside and leave an atrophic scar and depigmentation of the RPE. The choroiditis may disrupt Bruch membrane, choriocapillaris, and RPE, allowing proliferation of subretinal vessels years later. The syndrome is usually found in endemic areas such as the Ohio and Mississippi River valleys but may occur in nonendemic areas as well. Men and women are affected equally, and the vast majority of patients are of northern European descent.

The diagnosis is suggested by the clinical triad of multiple white, atrophic choroidal scars (so-called *histo spots*); peripapillary pigment changes; and macular CNV in the absence of vitreous cells. Histo spots may appear in the macula or periphery, are discrete and punched out, and are usually asymptomatic (Fig 11-23). Approximately 1.5% of patients from endemic areas exhibit typical peripheral histo spots, first appearing during adolescence. Linear equatorial streaks are present in 5% of patients (Fig 11-24). In contrast, metamorphopsia and a profound reduction in central vision herald macular CNV and bring the patient to the attention of the ophthalmologist. The mean age of patients presenting with maculopathy is 41 years. Funduscopy of active neovascular lesions reveals a yellow-green subretinal membrane typically surrounded by a pigment ring. There may be associated intraretinal or subretinal fluid and subretinal hemorrhage. Subretinal fibrosis may develop.

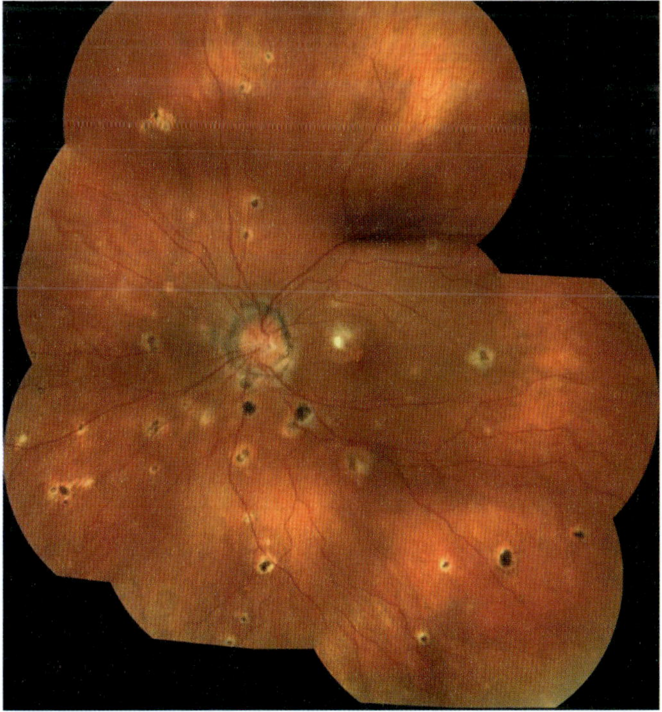

Figure 11-23 Fundus photograph from a patient with ocular histoplasmosis, showing peripapillary pigmentary scarring; midperipheral chorioretinal scars, or "histo spots" (some pigmented and fibrotic); and spontaneously regressed, nasal, juxtafoveal choroidal neovascular membrane in the absence of vitreous cells. Visual acuity, 20/25. *(Courtesy of Ramana S. Moorthy, MD.)*

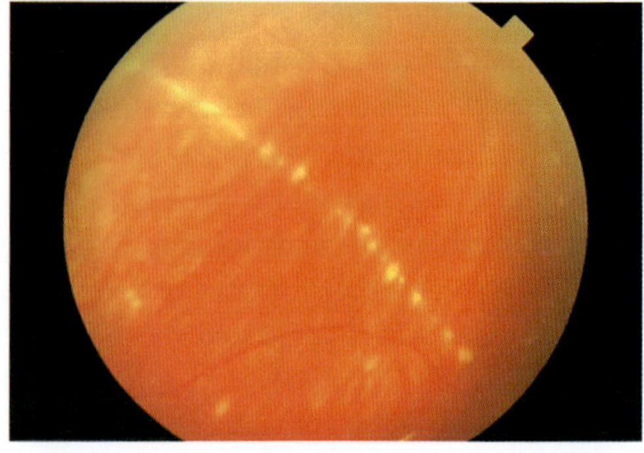

Figure 11-24 Ocular histoplasmosis. Fundus photograph showing linear equatorial streaks. *(Courtesy of E. Mitchel Opremcak, MD.)*

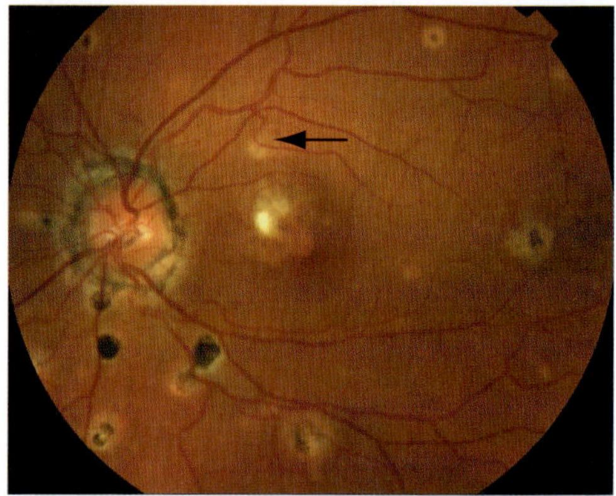

Figure 11-25 Ocular histoplasmosis. Fundus photograph showing macular choroiditis *(arrow)* with multiple yellow elevated lesions. *(Courtesy of Ramana S. Moorthy, MD.)*

The differential diagnosis includes entities associated with CNV, such as age-related macular degeneration, myopic degeneration, angioid streaks, choroidal rupture, undifferentiated CNV, MCP, and punctate inner choroidopathy. Granulomatous fundus lesions (toxoplasmosis, tuberculosis, coccidioidomycosis, syphilis, sarcoidosis, and toxocariasis) may mimic the scarring of OHS.

Over time, new choroidal scars develop in more than 20% of patients; however, only 3.8% of these cases progress to CNV. If histo spots appear in the macular area, the patient has a 15% chance of developing CNV within 5 years; if no spots are observed, the chances fall to 5%. Occasionally massive subretinal exudation and hemorrhagic retinal detachments may occur.

The early, acute granulomatous lesions of OHS are rarely seen but may be treated with oral or regional (periocular) corticosteroids (Fig 11-25). Early in a fluorescein angiography image, foci of active choroiditis hypofluoresce. These lesions hyperfluoresce in a staining pattern late in the imaging.

In contrast, areas of active CNV hyperfluoresce early and then hyperfluoresce in a leak pattern in later fluorescein angiography. Intravitreal vascular endothelial growth factor (VEGF) inhibitors have become mainline therapy for OHS-associated macular CNV. One large retrospective study suggests little benefit to combining VEGF inhibitor therapy with photodynamic therapy. See BCSC Section 12, *Retina and Vitreous*, for further detail about thermal laser photocoagulation, PDT, VEGF inhibitors, intravitreal corticosteroids, and submacular surgery for the treatment of CNV.

For discussions of the ocular manifestations of candidiasis, aspergillosis, cryptococcosis, and coccidioidomycosis, as well as their treatments, see Chapter 12 in this volume.

Cionni DA, Lewis SA, Petersen MR, et al. Analysis of outcomes for intravitreal bevacizumab in the treatment of choroidal neovascularization secondary to ocular histoplasmosis. *Ophthalmology.* 2012;119(2):327–332.

Ehrlich R, Ciulla TA, Maturi R, et al. Intravitreal bevacizumab for choroidal neovascularization secondary to presumed ocular histoplasmosis syndrome. *Retina.* 2009;29(10):1418–1423.

Hawkins BS, Bressler NM, Bressler SB, et al; Submacular Surgery Trials Research Group. Surgical removal vs observation for subfoveal choroidal neovascularization, either associated with the ocular histoplasmosis syndrome or idiopathic: I. Ophthalmic findings from a randomized clinical trial. Submacular Surgery Trials (SST) Group H trial: SST report no. 9. *Arch Ophthalmol.* 2004;122(11):1597–1611.

Macular Photocoagulation Study Group. Five-year follow-up of fellow eyes of individuals with ocular histoplasmosis and unilateral extrafoveal or juxtafoveal choroidal neovascularization. *Arch Ophthalmol.* 1996;114(6):677–688.

Saperstein DA, Rosenfeld PJ, Bressler NM, et al. Verteporfin therapy for CNV secondary to OHS. *Ophthalmology.* 2006;113(12):2371.e1–3.

Spencer WH, Chan CC, Shen DF, Rao NA. Detection of *Histoplasma capsulatum* DNA in lesions of chronic ocular histoplasmosis syndrome. *Arch Ophthalmol.* 2003;121(11): 1551–1555.

Toussaint BW, Kitchens JW, Marcus DM, et al. Intravitreal aflibercept injection for choroidal neovascularization due to presumed ocular histoplasmosis syndrome: The HANDLE Study. *Retina.* 2017;38(1):755 763.

Protozoal Uveitis

Toxoplasmosis

Toxoplasmosis is the most common cause of infectious posterior uveitis in adults and children. It is caused by the parasite *Toxoplasma gondii,* a single-cell obligate intracellular apicomplexan parasite with a worldwide distribution (Fig 11-26). Felines are the definitive hosts of *T gondii,* and humans and a variety of other animals serve as intermediate hosts. *T gondii* has a complex life cycle and exists in 3 major forms:

- the oocyst, or soil form (10–12 μm), which contains sporozoites
- the tachyzoite, or infectious form (4–8 μm)
- the tissue cyst, or latent form (10–200 μm), which contains as many as 3000 bradyzoites

Transmission of *T gondii* to humans and other animals may occur with all 3 forms of the parasite through a variety of vectors. The oocysts reproduce in the cat intestine and are shed in feces, contaminating the environment. After maturation in the soil, these oocysts may then be ingested by intermediate hosts. Tachyzoites, the proliferative form of the parasite, are found in the circulatory system and may invade nearly all host tissue. In an

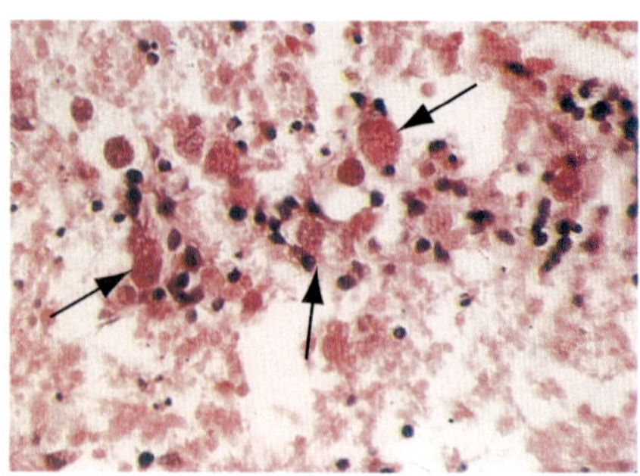

Figure 11-26 Histology of *Toxoplasma gondii* infection of the retina. Note the cysts *(arrows)* in the necrotic retina.

immunocompetent host, tachyzoites proliferation eventually stops. However, some microorganisms may persist as dormant bradyzoites within intercellular tissue cysts.

As of this writing, the CDC estimates that 11% of the United States population age 6 and older has been infected with *T gondii.* Of that group, 2% may develop ocular toxoplasmosis. The reported seropositivity rates among healthy adults vary considerably worldwide. An estimated 80% of the population in southern Brazil is infected with *T gondii,* and up to 18% of these individuals may develop eye disease. Some studies show a greater genotypic heterogeneity of parasites in Brazil than in North America. Such differences may contribute to variance in disease severity and ocular involvement in different regions of the world.

Human infection by *T gondii* may be either acquired or congenital. The principal modes of transmission include

- ingestion of undercooked, infected meat containing tissue cysts
- ingestion of contaminated water, fruit, or vegetables with oocysts
- inadvertent contact with cat feces, cat litter, or soil containing oocysts
- transplacental transmission with primary infection during pregnancy
- blood transfusion or organ transplantation

Five of the epidemics that occurred between 1979 and 2003 have been well studied, and contaminated water supplies or inhaled/ingested sporulated oocysts in dirt were implicated as sources of infection.

Data collected from the 2009–2010 National Health and Nutrition Examination Survey (NHANES) study shows an age-adjusted seroprevalence among women of childbearing age (15–44 years) of 9.1% in the United States population. Thus, most women of childbearing age in the United States are susceptible to *T gondii* infection. The American Academy of Pediatrics estimates that the incidence of primary infection during pregnancy in the United States is approximately 0.2–1.1 per 1000 pregnant women, translating to 800–4400 women per year with acute *T gondi* infection during the 4 million yearly pregnancies in the U.S.

Overall, 40% of primary maternal infections result in congenital infection; transplacental transmission is highest during the third trimester. The risk of severe disease developing in the fetus is inversely proportional to gestational age. Disease acquired early in pregnancy may result in spontaneous abortion, stillbirth, or severe congenital disease. Disease acquired later in gestation may produce an asymptomatic, normal-appearing infant with latent infection. Chronic or recurrent maternal infection during pregnancy is not thought to confer a significant risk of congenital toxoplasmosis because maternal immunity protects against fetal transmission. However, congenital toxoplasmosis may occur in an immune pregnant mother reinfected with a new, more virulent strain.

Pregnant women without serologic evidence of *T gondii* infection should be advised to take the following precautions:

- Avoid ingestion of raw/undercooked meat (freezing at −20°C/−4°F overnight also destroys tissue cysts).
- Drink only well-filtered or boiled water.
- Carefully wash vegetables and fruits before consumption.
- Use gloves and wash hands and kitchen utensils well after handling meat or soil.
- Avoid contact with felines and their feces (including in soil or litter boxes).

The classic presentation of congenital toxoplasmosis, which includes retinochoroiditis, hydrocephalus or microcephaly, intracranial calcifications, and cognitive impairment (Sabin's tetrad), occurs in less than 10% of infected children. Retinochoroidal lesions, found in up to 80% of cases, are the most common abnormality in patients with congenital toxoplasmosis. Lesions are bilateral in approximately 85% of affected individuals and carry a predilection for the posterior pole and macula (Fig 11-27). Posterior segment involvement may be subclinical and chronic. As many as 85% of infected children develop retinochoroiditis after a mean of 3.7 years, and 25% of these become blind in 1 or both eyes. Most experts recommend antiparasitic therapy for newborns with congenital toxoplasmosis during the first year of life to reduce disease burden, regardless of the presence of ocular and/or systemic signs.

Although toxoplasmosis after infancy was previously considered exclusively congenital disease reactivation, it is now recognized that ocular toxoplasmosis in children and adults may represent newly acquired infection in a significant proportion of cases. In one study, acquired postnatal infection was thought to represent up to two-thirds of cases of toxoplasmic ocular disease.

Although dependent on the location of the lesion, presenting symptoms frequently include unilateral blurred or hazy vision and floaters. A mild to moderate granulomatous anterior uveitis is often observed, and up to 20% of patients have acutely elevated IOP at presentation. Classically, ocular toxoplasmosis appears as a focal, white retinochoroiditis, with overlying moderate vitreous inflammation ("headlight in the fog"), often adjacent to

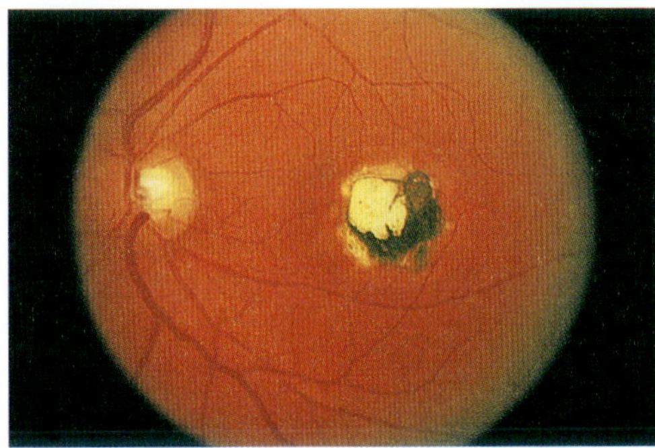

Figure 11-27 Fundus photograph of quiescent, partially pigmented, congenital toxoplasmic macular scar. Patient has 20/400 visual acuity. *(Courtesy of John D. Sheppard Jr, MD.)*

a pigmented retinochoroidal scar (Figs 11-28, 11-29). These lesions occur more commonly in the posterior pole but are occasionally found immediately adjacent to or directly involving the optic nerve; they may be mistaken for optic neuritis. Retinal vessels in the vicinity of an active lesion may show perivasculitis with diffuse venous sheathing and segmental arterial plaques (Kyrieleis arteriolitis). Vascular occlusions may also be present. Additional ocular complications include cataract, persistent vitreous opacities, macular edema, retinal detachment, epiretinal membranes, optic atrophy, and CNV. Recently acquired disease often presents as a focal retinochoroiditis in the absence of a retinochoroidal scarring (Fig 11-30).

Retinochoroiditis developing in immunocompromised and older patients may present with atypical findings, including large, multiple, and/or bilateral lesions, with or without

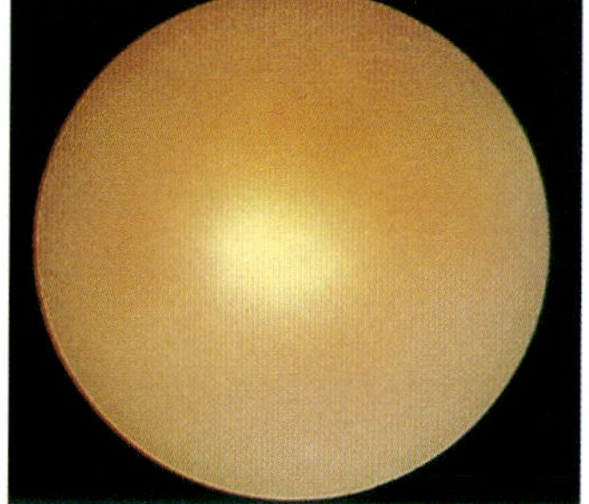

Figure 11-28 Toxoplasmic retinochoroiditis. Fundus photograph showing intense focal retinitis with dense overlying vitritis, producing a "headlight in the fog" appearance.

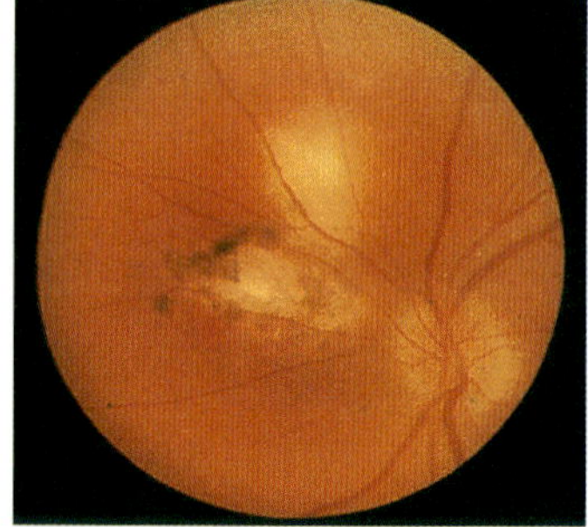

Figure 11-29 Toxoplasmosis. Fundus photograph showing satellite retinochoroiditis around an old scar.

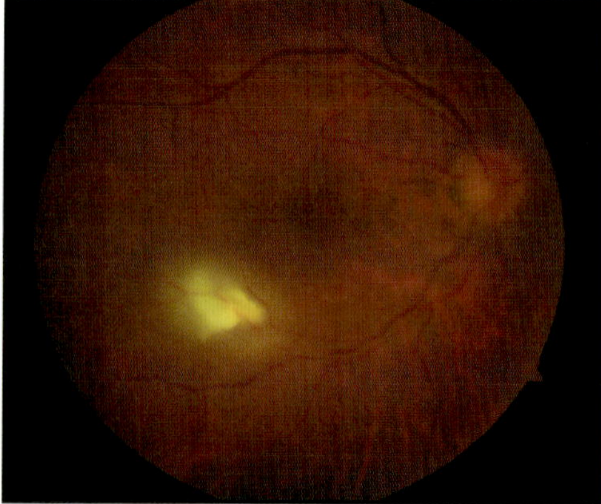

Figure 11-30 Fundus photograph showing *toxoplasmic* retinochoroiditis in the absence of a previous chorioretinal scar. *(Courtesy of Greg Kokame, MD, and the Retina Image Bank, American Society of Retina Specialists.)*

associated retinochoroidal scars. This more severe clinical picture can also occur in patients receiving steroids without concomitant antiparasitic therapy (Fig 11-31). Ocular toxoplasmosis may simulate herpetic ARN. Other atypical presentations include neuroretinitis, punctate outer retinal toxoplasmosis (PORT), unilateral pigmentary retinopathy simulating retinitis pigmentosa, and other forms of intraocular inflammation in the absence of retinochoroiditis. Characteristics of PORT include small, multifocal lesions at the level of the outer retina, with exudation to subretinal space and scant overlying vitreal inflammation (Fig 11-32).

Centers for Disease Control and Prevention; Division of Parasitic Diseases and Malaria. Toxoplasmosis. Available at www.cdc.gov/dpdx/toxoplasmosis/. Accessed November 16, 2020.

Holland GN. Ocular toxoplasmosis: a global reassessment. Part I: epidemiology and course of disease. *Am J Ophthalmol.* 2003;136(6):973–988.

Holland GN. Ocular toxoplasmosis: a global reassessment. Part II: disease manifestations and management. *Am J Ophthalmol.* 2004;137(1):1–17.

Jones JL, Bonetti V, Holland GN, et al. Ocular toxoplasmosis in the United States: recent and remote infections. *Clin Infect Dis.* 201515;60(2):271–273.

Maldonado YA, Read JS; AAP Committee on Infectious Diseases. Diagnosis, treatment, and prevention of congenital toxoplasmosis in the United States. *Pediatrics.* 2017;139(2): e20163860.

Vasconcelos-Santos DV. Ocular manifestations of systemic disease: toxoplasmosis. *Curr Opin Ophthalmol.* 2012;23(6):543–550.

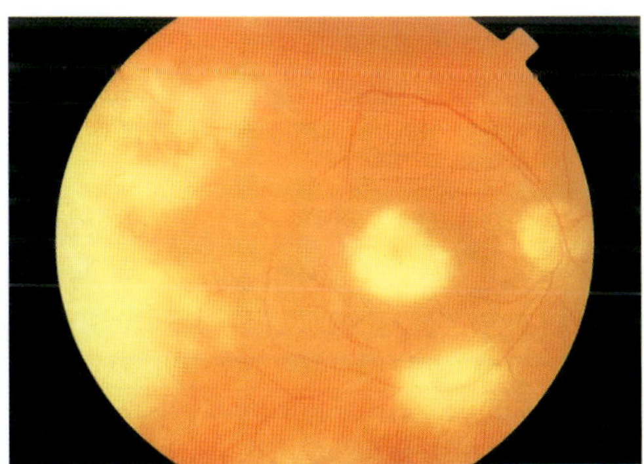

Figure 11-31 Toxoplasmosis. Fundus photograph showing widespread retinal necrosis following periocular corticosteroid injection. *(Courtesy of E. Mitchel Opremcak, MD.)*

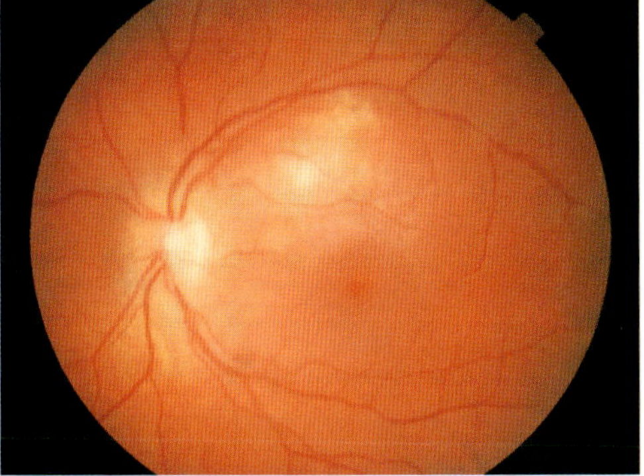

Figure 11-32 Fundus photograph showing punctate outer retinal toxoplasmosis. *(Courtesy of E. Mitchel Opremcak, MD.)*

Diagnosis

In most cases, toxoplasmic retinochoroiditis is clinically diagnosed on the basis of the characteristic fundus lesion. Positive serologic testing for anti–*T gondii* IgG or IgM confirms exposure to the parasite. IgG antibodies appear after the first 2 weeks of infection, typically remain detectable for life at variable levels, and cross the placenta. IgM antibodies, however, increase in number early during the acute phase of the infection, typically remain detectable for less than 1 year, and do not cross the placenta. The presence of anti–*T gondii* IgG antibodies supports the diagnosis of toxoplasmic retinochoroiditis in the appropriate clinical context, whereas a negative antibody titer essentially rules out the diagnosis.

The presence of IgM in newborns confirms congenital infection and indicates acquired disease in adults. In cases of diagnostic uncertainty, PCR testing of aqueous humor and vitreous fluid may be performed.

Montoya JG, Parmley S, Liesenfeld O, Jaffe GJ, Remington JS. Use of the polymerase chain reaction for diagnosis of ocular toxoplasmosis. *Ophthalmology.* 1999;106(8):1554–1563.

Treatment

Ocular toxoplasmosis is a progressive and recurrent disease. New lesions may occur at the margins of old scars as well as elsewhere in the fundus, and toxoplasmic cysts may be present in a normal-appearing retina. In the immunocompetent patient, the disease can have a self-limiting course. The borders of the lesions become sharper and less edematous over a 6–8-week period without treatment, and RPE hyperplasia occurs gradually over a period of months. In the immunocompromised patient, the disease is often more severe and progressive. Treatment can shorten the duration of parasitic replication, leading to more rapid cicatrization and ultimately a smaller retinochoroidal scar. Treatment may also reduce the frequency of inflammatory recurrences and minimize structural complications associated with intraocular inflammation.

Numerous medications may be used to treat toxoplasmosis, and there is no consensus as to the most efficacious regimen. Most antibiotic agents have efficacy against the active tachyzoite, not the tissue-encysted bradyzoite. Little firm evidence exists that antimicrobial therapy alters the natural history of toxoplasmic retinochoroiditis in immunocompetent patients. Some clinicians may elect to observe small lesions in the retinal periphery that are not associated with a significant decrease in vision or vitritis; others treat virtually all patients in an effort to reduce the number of subsequent recurrences. Relative treatment indications include

- lesions threatening the optic nerve or fovea
- decreased visual acuity
- lesions associated with moderate to severe vitreous inflammation
- lesions greater than 1 disc diameter in size
- persistence of disease for more than 1 month
- presence of multiple active lesions

Treatment is indicated in immunocompromised patients (those with HIV/AIDS, with neoplastic disease, or undergoing IMT), patients with congenital toxoplasmosis, and pregnant women with recently acquired disease.

The classic regimen for the treatment of ocular toxoplasmosis consists of 4–8 weeks of pyrimethamine (loading dose, 50–100 mg; treatment dose, 25–50 mg/day) and sulfadiazine (treatment dose, 1 g, 4 times/day). Pyrimethamine has recently become prohibitively expensive. Folinic acid (5–10 mg/day) is added to prevent myelosuppression (leukopenia and/or thrombocytopenia), which may result from pyrimethamine therapy. A complete blood count may be checked approximately every 2 weeks during therapy. Potential adverse effects of sulfa compounds include skin rash, gastrointestinal intolerance, crystalluria, kidney stones, and Stevens-Johnson syndrome. Clindamycin (300 mg, 4 times/day) may be added to the above regimen or substituted for sulfadiazine in the case of sulfa allergy. Clindamycin, either alone or in combination with other drugs, has been effective in managing acute lesions, but pseudomembranous colitis is a potential complication. Azithromycin (500 mg daily) or atovaquone (750 mg, 2–4 times/day) may take the place of sulfadiazine or clindamycin.

Many ophthalmologists utilize trimethoprim-sulfamethoxazole (160 mg/800 mg, 2 times/day) because of its accessibility, simplicity of administration, and cost. Clindamycin (1 mg/0.1 mL) may also be intravitreally injected in an off-label fashion, either in combination with systemic therapy or as monotherapy in patients who do not tolerate systemic therapy.

Systemic corticosteroids (approximately 0.25–0.75 mg/kg, typically not to exceed 60 mg/day) may be considered after 48 hours of antimicrobial therapy in immunocompetent patients. The use of systemic corticosteroids without appropriate antimicrobial coverage or the use of long-acting periocular and intraocular corticosteroid formulations such as triamcinolone acetonide is contraindicated because of the potential for severe panophthalmitis and loss of the eye (see Fig 11-31). Topical corticosteroids, however, are used liberally in the presence of prominent anterior segment inflammation. Systemic corticosteroid treatment may be used for 3–5 weeks, at which time inflammation begins to subside and the retinal lesion shows signs of early cicatrization. Antimicrobial coverage should be continued for the entire period of systemic corticosteroid use.

Newborns with congenital toxoplasmosis are commonly treated with pyrimethamine and sulfonamides (plus folinic acid) for 1 year, in consultation with a specialist in pediatric infectious diseases.

In cases of newly acquired toxoplasmosis during pregnancy, treatment is given to prevent infection of the fetus and limit fetal damage if infection has already occurred, as well as to limit the destructive sequelae of intraocular disease in the mother. Spiramycin (treatment dose, 400 mg 3 times/day) reduces the rate of tachyzoite transmission to the fetus and may be used safely without undue risk of teratogenicity. Because this drug is commonly unavailable in the United States, alternative medications may be needed; options include azithromycin, clindamycin, and atovaquone (treatment dose, 750 mg every 6 hours). Sulfonamides may be used safely in the first 2 trimesters of pregnancy. Alternatively, intravitreal injection of clindamycin and short-acting periocular corticosteroids (eg, dexamethasone) may be utilized in pregnant women to reduce systemic adverse effects.

Patients with HIV/AIDS require extended systemic treatment given the frequent association of ocular disease with cerebral involvement (56%) and the frequency of recurrent ocular disease when antitoxoplasmic medication is discontinued (Fig 11-33). The best

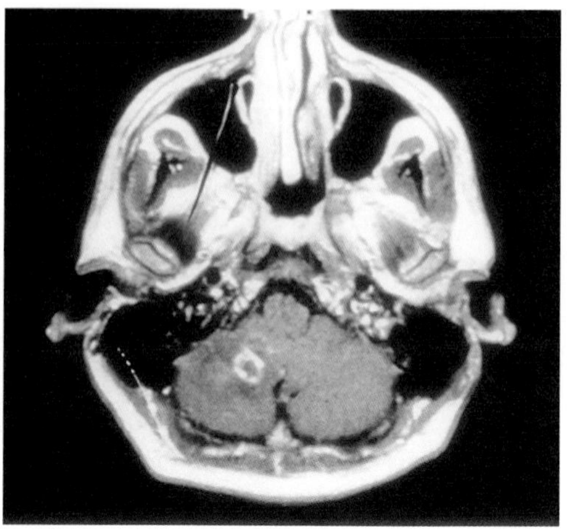

Figure 11-33 Enhanced computed tomography scan revealing a cerebellar lesion caused by central nervous system toxoplasmosis in a patient with AIDS who presented with ataxia. *(Courtesy of John D. Sheppard Jr, MD.)*

regimen for secondary prophylaxis remains to be determined; however, atovaquone acts synergistically with pyrimethamine and sulfadiazine and thus may be useful for reducing the dose and toxicity of these drugs in the treatment of patients with AIDS and toxoplasmosis. The management of ocular toxoplasmosis in association with HIV/AIDS is also covered in Chapter 15.

Long-term intermittent trimethoprim-sulfamethoxazole treatment (160 mg/800 mg 3 times per week) was shown to decrease the risk of reactivation among patients with recurrent toxoplasmic retinochoroiditis observed over a 20-month period. A similar strategy may be useful as prophylaxis in patients with ocular toxoplasmosis and HIV/AIDS.

Similarly, the utility of prophylactic antimicrobial treatment shortly before and after intraocular surgery in patients with inactive toxoplasmic scars—particularly scars that threaten the optic disc or fovea—was raised by a report that describes an association between cataract surgery and an increased risk of reactivation of otherwise inactive toxoplasmic retinochoroiditis. There is, however, no consensus with respect to this treatment approach or to the optimal antibiotic regimen in this clinical situation.

Kim SJ, Scott IU, Brown GC, et al. Interventions for toxoplasma retinochoroiditis: a report by the American Academy of Ophthalmology. *Ophthalmology.* 2013;120(2): 371–378.

Kishore K, Conway MD, Peyman GA. Intravitreal clindamycin and dexamethasone for toxoplasmic retinochoroiditis. *Ophthalmic Surg Lasers.* 2001;32(3):183–192.

Silveira C, Belfort R Jr, Muccioli C, et al. The effect of long-term intermittent trimethoprim/ sulfamethoxazole treatment on recurrences of toxoplasmic retinochoroiditis. *Am J Ophthalmol.* 2002;134(1):41–46.

Helminthic Uveitis

Helminths (derived from the Greek word for *worms*) are multicellular organisms that can be free living or parasitic. Approximately 280 species are recognized.

Toxocariasis

Ocular toxocariasis (OT) is a zoonotic infection caused by *Toxocara canis* and *Toxocara cati.* Dogs and cats, the definitive hosts of the roundworm, pass unembryonated eggs via their feces into the environment (often into the soil). According to the CDC, 30% of dogs younger than 6 months may deposit *Toxocara* eggs in their feces, and 25% of cats are infected with *Toxocara cati.* After 2–4 weeks, those eggs embryonate and become infectious. Transmission to humans occurs through ingestion of soil or contaminated food, or the fecal–oral route. Exposure to playgrounds, sandboxes, kittens, and puppies, as well as the pica eating disorder, are risk factors. Rarely, humans may acquire the infection from undercooked meat. NHANES data from 2011–2014 suggested an overall seroprevalence in the United States of 5.1%. In children, an increased rate of antibody positivity correlated to lack of health insurance. The prevalence was recently estimated to be 1% of a large uveitic population treated at tertiary care centers in northern California.

The organisms grow in the small intestine, enter the portal circulation, and disseminate hematogenously. In humans, the *Toxocara* larvae may migrate to different parts of the body, including the liver, heart, lungs, brains, muscles, or eyes. The larvae do not undergo further development in the human but rather cause a local inflammatory reaction. Because ova are not shed in the gastrointestinal tract, stool analysis for larvae is not useful.

Visceral toxocariasis (VT) may include fever, coughing, enlarged liver, pneumonia, and meningoencephalitis. It more often affects children younger than age 3, and those patients may show peripheral eosinophilia. Ocular toxocariasis is found in older children, typically without significant eosinophilia. These infections rarely present simultaneously.

Ophthalmic presentations include a chronic endophthalmitis (25%), a posterior pole granuloma (25%; Fig 11-34), or a peripheral granuloma, sometimes with fibrous bands in the vitreous that may extend posteriorly (50%; Fig 11-35). Any of these presentations may produce leukocoria. Uncommon variants include unilateral pars planitis with diffuse peripheral inflammatory exudates, granulomas involving the optic nerve, and a diffuse unilateral subacute neuroretinitis. Table 11-2 lists the characteristics of each presentation.

Ocular toxocariasis is principally a clinical diagnosis. Serologic testing may suggest prior exposure. However, patients with OT may have negative serum serology. Antibody testing of ocular fluids may be positive despite negative serum. Polymerase chain reaction

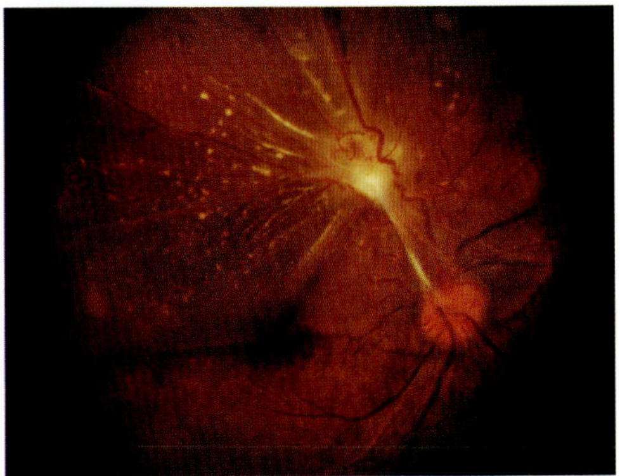

Figure 11-34 Fundus photograph showing *Toxocara* posterior pole granuloma causing macular pucker. *(Courtesy of H. Michael Lambert, MD, and the Retina Image Bank, American Society of Retina Specialists.)*

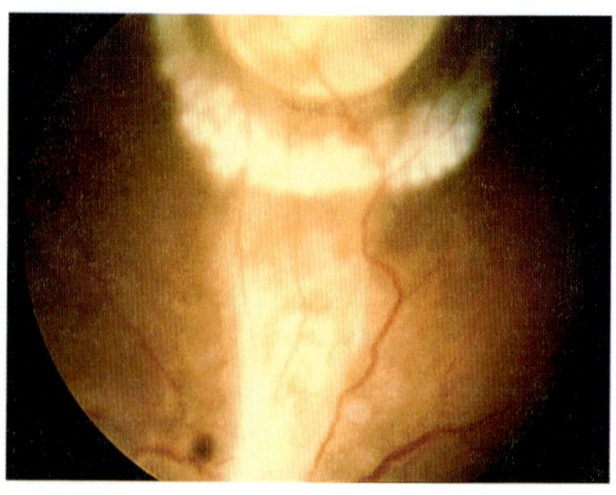

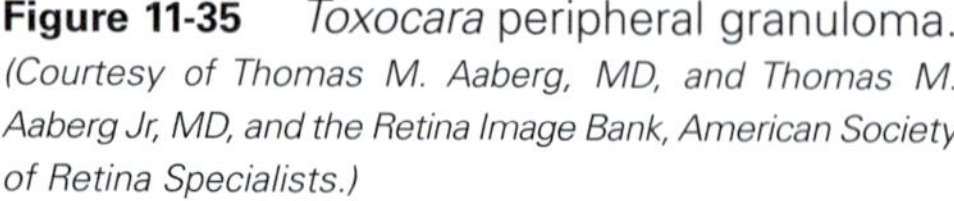

Figure 11-35 *Toxocara* peripheral granuloma. *(Courtesy of Thomas M. Aaberg, MD, and Thomas M. Aaberg Jr, MD, and the Retina Image Bank, American Society of Retina Specialists.)*

Table 11-2 Patterns of Manifestation of Ocular Toxocariasis

Syndrome	Age of Onset, y	Characteristic Lesion
Chronic endophthalmitis	2–9	Chronic unilateral uveitis, cloudy vitreous cyclitic membrane
Localized granuloma	6–14	Present in the macula and peripapillary region Solitary, white, elevated in the retina; minimal reaction; 1–2 disc diameters in size
Peripheral granuloma	6–40	Peripheral hemispheric masses with dense connective tissue strands in the vitreous cavity that may connect to the disc Rarely bilateral

testing is not readily available. Larvae have been recovered from vitrectomy specimens (Fig 11-36). In cases of media opacity, B-scan ultrasonography and/or computed tomography may show vitreous membranes and/or tractional detachment and confirm the absence of calcium, a potential finding in retinoblastoma.

The differential diagnosis includes retinoblastoma, infectious endophthalmitis, Coats disease, familial exudative vitreoretinopathy, persistent fetal vasculature, toxoplasmosis, undifferentiated intermediate uveitis/pars/planitis, retinopathy of prematurity, combined hamartoma of the retina and RPE, and diffuse unilateral subacute neuroretinitis (DUSN). The migrating larvae of other helminths such as *Baylisascaris procyonis* may simulate OT. In contrast to OT, children with retinoblastoma are typically younger, lack significant inflammation, and show lesion growth.

Patients with VT are usually treated with oral albendazole. For OT, the use of antihelminthic therapy is not established but may be considered if the larvae appear active. Typically, local and systemic corticosteroids are used to reduce inflammation and minimize structural complications, which may later be amenable to vitreoretinal surgical techniques.

Centers for Disease Control and Prevention. Ocular toxocariasis—United States, 2009–2010. *MMWR.* 2011;60(22):734–736.

Farmer A, Beltran T, Choi YS. Prevalence of *Toxocara* species infection in the U.S.: Results from the National Health and Nutrition Examination Survey, 2011–2014. *PLoS Negl Trop Dis.* 2017;11(7):e0005818.

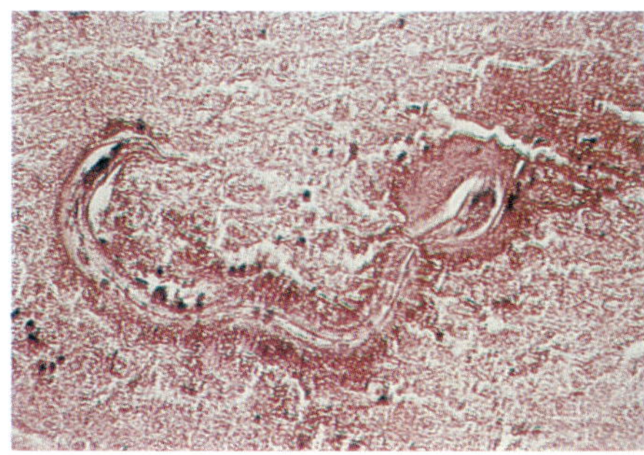

Figure 11-36 Toxocariasis. Histopathology of an eosinophilic vitreous abscess. The organism is in the center of the abscess.

Schneier AJ, Durand ML. Ocular toxocariasis: advances in diagnosis and treatment. *Int Ophthalmol Clin.* 2011;51(4):135–144.

Stewart JM, Cubillan LD, Cunningham ET Jr. Prevalence, clinical features, and causes of vision loss among patients with ocular toxocariasis. *Retina.* 2005;25(8):1005–1013.

Woodhall D, Starr MC, Montgomery SP, et al. Ocular toxocariasis: epidemiologic, anatomic, and therapeutic variations based on a survey of ophthalmic subspecialists. *Ophthalmology.* 2012;119(6):1211–1217.

Cysticercosis

Cysticercosis is the most common ocular tapeworm infection. Human infection is caused by *Cysticercus cellulosae,* the larval stage of the cestode *Taenia solium,* which is endemic to Mexico, Africa, Southeast Asia, eastern Europe, Central and South America, and India. Humans acquire the disease via fecal-oral transmission or consuming undercooked infected pork. The eggs mature into larvae, penetrate the intestinal mucosa, and spread hematogenously to the eye via the posterior ciliary arteries into the subretinal space.

Ocular cysticercosis usually affects individuals between the ages of 10 and 30 years, without sex predilection. Cysticercosis may involve any structure of the eye, orbit, or adnexa, but involves the subretinal space most often (Fig 11-37). Larvae may perforate the retina, gaining access to the vitreous cavity (Fig 11-38). Other presentations include a subconjunctival or eyelid nodule.

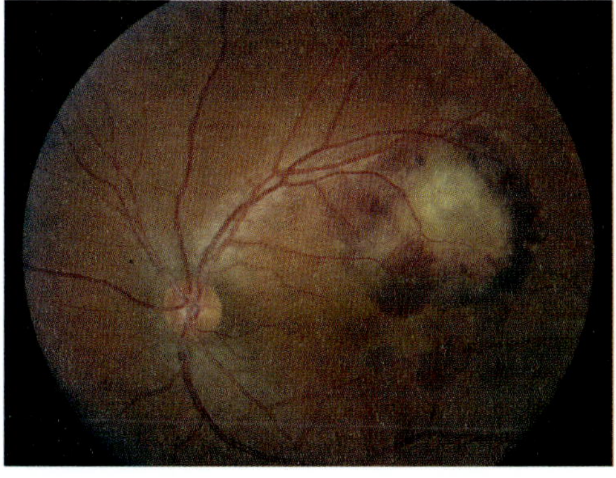

Figure 11-37 Subretinal Fundus photograph of cysticercosis. *(Courtesy of Preema Abraham, MD, and the Retina Image Bank, American Society of Retina Specialists.)*

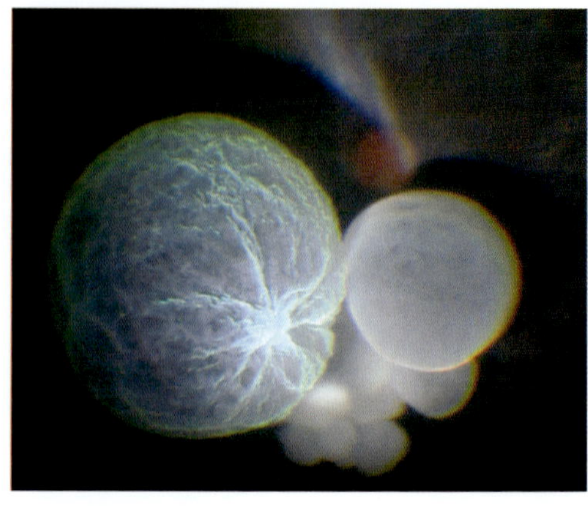

Figure 11-38 Multiple intravitreal cysts associated with cysticercosis. *(Courtesy of Vishal Agrawal, MD, FRCS, and the Retina Image Bank, American Society of Retina Specialists.)*

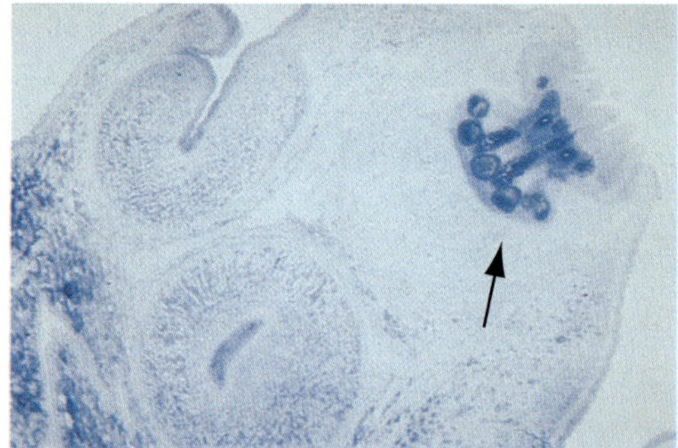

Figure 11-39 Histopathology image of cysticercosis, showing the protoscolex, or head, of the larva *(arrow).*

Patients may be asymptomatic with relatively good vision or may complain of floaters, moving sensations, ocular pain, photophobia, redness, and very poor visual acuity. Larvae may be observed in the vitreous or subretinal space in up to 46% of infected patients. A globular translucent cyst is seen, with an invaginated or evaginated head, or scolex, that undulates in response to the examining light (Figs 11-38, 11-39). Exudative, rhegmatogenous, or tractional retinal detachment may be observed. Computed tomography may reveal intracerebral calcification or hydrocephalus in patients with neural cysticercosis.

The differential diagnosis includes conditions associated with leukocoria (retinoblastoma, Coats disease, retinopathy of prematurity, persistent fetal vasculature, toxocariasis, and retinal detachment) and DUSN.

Larvae death provokes panuveitis. Laser photocoagulation alone may also provoke severe inflammation. Hence, early removal of intraocular larvae, often with vitreoretinal surgical techniques, is advocated. Antihelminthics plus systemic corticosteroids may be utilized for extraocular disease.

Sharma T, Sinha S, Shah N, et al. Intraocular cysticercosis: clinical characteristics and visual outcome after vitreoretinal surgery. *Ophthalmology.* 2003;110(5):996–1004.

Wender JD, Rathinam SR, Shaw RE, Cunningham ET Jr. Intraocular cysticercosis: case series and comprehensive review of the literature. *Ocul Immunol Inflamm.* 2011;19(4):240–245.

Diffuse Unilateral Subacute Neuroretinitis

Diffuse unilateral subacute neuroretinitis is an uncommon but important disease likely caused by nematode infection. It should be considered in the differential diagnosis of posterior uveitis occurring among otherwise healthy, young patients (mean age, 14 years; range, 11–65 years) because early recognition and prompt treatment may preserve vision. Evidence to date suggests that DUSN is caused by solitary nematodes of 2 different sizes, apparently related to geographic region, that migrate through the subretinal space. The smaller worm, measuring 400–1000 µm in length, has been proposed to be either *Ancylostoma caninum* (the dog hookworm) or *Toxocara canis*, though the latter has never been reported to be isolated from an eye with DUSN. The larger worm is believed to be *Baylisascaris procyonis* (the raccoon roundworm), which measures 1500–2000 µm in length and has been found in the northern midwestern United States and Canada. The disease has also been reported outside North America.

The clinical course of DUSN is characterized by the insidious onset of unilateral loss of vision from recurrent episodes of focal, multifocal, or diffuse inflammation of the retina, RPE, and optic nerve. The early stages of the disease are marked by moderate to severe vitritis; optic disc swelling; and multiple, focal, gray-white lesions in the postequatorial fundus that vary in size from 1200 µm to 1500 µm (Fig 11-40). These lesions are transient and may be associated with overlying exudative retinal detachment. The worms may be visualized in the subretinal space, especially in the early stages. Differential diagnosis at this phase of the disease includes sarcoidosis-associated uveitis, MCP, acute posterior multifocal placoid pigment epitheliopathy, multiple evanescent white dot syndrome, serpiginous choroidopathy, Behçet disease, toxocariasis, OHS, nonspecific optic neuritis, and papillitis. The later disease stages are typified by retinal arteriolar narrowing, optic atrophy, diffuse pigment epithelial degeneration, and abnormal electroretinographic results (Fig 11-41). These findings may be confused with posttraumatic chorioretinopathy, occlusive vascular disease, toxic retinopathy, and retinitis pigmentosa. Although highly unusual, bilateral cases have been reported, as have cases of DUSN associated with neurologic disease (neural larvae migrans).

The diagnosis is made according to the aforementioned clinical picture and is most strongly supported by the observation of a worm in the subretinal space (Video 11-1). Results of systemic and laboratory evaluations are typically negative for patients with DUSN.

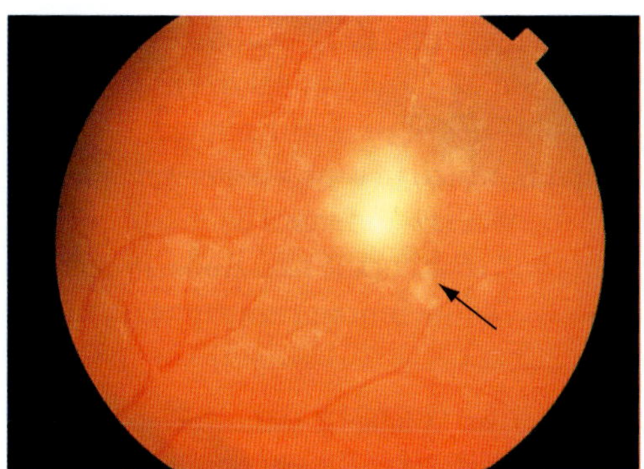

Figure 11-40 Fundus photograph of diffuse unilateral subacute neuroretinitis. Note the multiple white retinal lesions and the nematode in the subretinal space *(arrow)*. *(Courtesy of E. Mitchel Opremcak, MD.)*

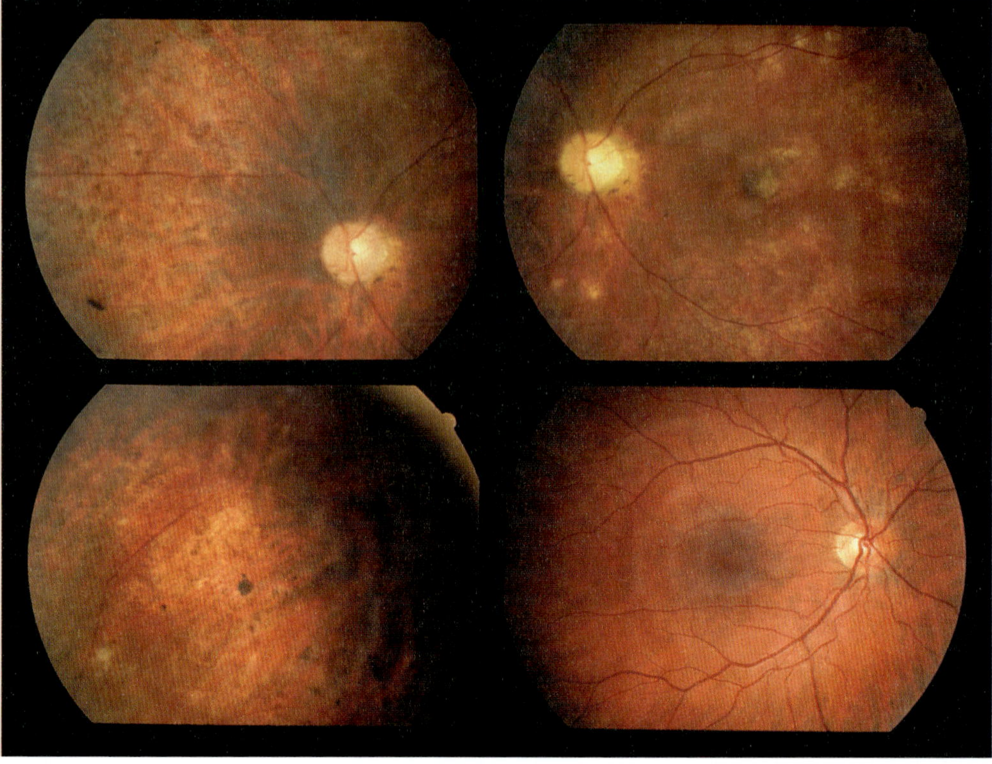

Figure 11-41 Fundus photographs of a 23-year-old male with diffuse unilateral subacute neuroretinitis. *(Courtesy of Howard Schatz, MD, and the Retina Image Bank, American Society of Retina Specialists.)*

Electroretinographic abnormalities may be present even when the test is performed early in the disease course.

VIDEO 11-1 How to find a live worm in diffuse unilateral subacute neuroretinitis.
Courtesy of Carlos A. A. Garcia, MD.
Access the video at www.aao.org/bcscvideo_section09.

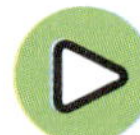

Medical therapy alone with corticosteroids may only transiently control inflammation. Direct laser photocoagulation of the worm in the early phases of the disease does not appear inflammatory and may be highly effective in halting progression of the disease (see Fig 11-38). Successful treatment and immobilization of the subretinal worm have been reported with oral thiabendazole (22 mg/kg twice daily for 2–4 days with a maximum dose of 3 g) and albendazole (200 mg twice daily for 30 days), which may be a better-tolerated alternative. Thus, if the worm cannot be visualized, patients may undergo a course of antihelminthic therapy to increase the chance of identifying and treating the nematode. In patients who undergo laser and inflammation does not improve, antihelminthic therapy may treat a presumed second unvisualized nematode.

Cortez R, Denny JP, Muci-Mendoza R, Ramirez G, Fuenmayor D, Jaffe GJ. Diffuse unilateral subacute neuroretinitis in Venezuela. *Ophthalmology.* 2005;112(12):2110–2114.

de Amorim Garcia Filho CA, Bezerra Gomes AH, de A Garcia Soares AC, de Amorim Garcia CA. Clinical features of 121 patients with diffuse unilateral subacute neuroretinitis. *Am J Ophthalmol.* 2012;153(4):743–749.

Souza EC, Casella AM, Nakashima Y, Monteiro ML. Clinical features and outcomes of patients with diffuse unilateral subacute neuroretinitis treated with oral albendazole. *Am J Ophthalmol.* 2005;140(3):437–445. [Erratum appears in *Am J Ophthalmol.* 2006;141(4):795–796.]

Onchocerciasis (River Blindness)

Humans are the only host for *Onchocerca volvulus* parasite. As the vector, female black flies that breed near rivers bite an infected human and ingest microfilariae. The infective larvae are then transmitted to another human with a future bite. Onchocerciasis is endemic in many areas of sub-Saharan Africa and in isolated foci in Central and South America. Worldwide, at least 25 million people are infected, of whom almost 300,000 are blind and 800,000 are visually impaired. Microfilariae probably reach the eye by various routes:

- direct invasion of the cornea from the conjunctiva
- penetration of the sclera, both directly and through the vascular bundles
- hematogenous spread (possibly)

Microfilariae can be observed swimming freely in the anterior chamber. Live microfilariae can be seen in the cornea; dead microfilariae cause a small stromal punctate keratitis. Anterior uveitis may lead to synechiae, secondary glaucoma, and cataract. In the posterior segment, RPE disruption and focal atrophy may occur. Later, severe chorioretinal atrophy develops. Optic atrophy is common in advanced disease (Fig 11-42).

Diagnosis is based on clinical appearance and a history of pathogen exposure in an endemic area and confirmed by finding microfilariae in small skin biopsies or in the eye. Ivermectin, the treatment of choice, is given every 3–6 months as long as there is evidence of skin or eye infection. Topical corticosteroids can be used to control any anterior uveitis.

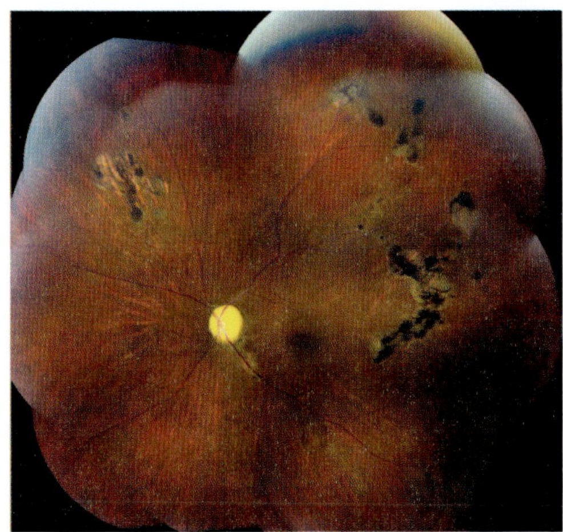

Figure 11-42 Fundus photograph montage showing extensive chorioretinal scars involving both the periphery and the posterior pole as well as optic nerve pallor secondary to onchocerciasis. *(Courtesy of H. Nida Sen, MD.)*

Ivermectin safely kills the microfilariae but does not have a permanent effect on the adult worms. Concomitant doxycycline therapy helps kill the adult worms by eradicating the symbiotic partner—*Wolbachia* bacteria. Lastly, patients coinfected with onchocerciasis and *Loa loa* are at risk of a fatal encephalitic reaction to ivermectin, so infectious disease consultation should be procured for such individuals.

Ejere HO, Schwartz E, Wormald R, Evans JR. Ivermectin for onchocercal eye disease (river blindness). *Cochrane Database Syst Rev.* 2012;8:CD002219.

Winthrop KL, Furtado JM, Silva JC, Resnikoff S, Lansingh VC. River blindness: an old disease on the brink of elimination and control. *J Glob Infect Dis.* 2011;3(2):151–155.

CHAPTER 12

Endophthalmitis

Highlights

- Chronic postoperative endophthalmitis is difficult to diagnose and may require invasive diagnostic testing, antibiotic or antifungal injection, and, in many cases, explantation of an intraocular lens (IOL).
- Suspicion of endogenous endophthalmitis is required in immunosuppressed patients and in patients with a recent history of surgery or hospitalization or of intravenous drug abuse. The diagnosis is often definitively established by cultures and stains from vitreous aspirate obtained by diagnostic vitrectomy.
- Endogenous endophthalmitis requires evaluation for a systemic source of infection, intravitreal antibiotic or antifungal injection, and often systemic antibiotics.

Endophthalmitis is a clinical diagnosis made when intraocular inflammation involving both the posterior and anterior chambers is attributable to bacterial or fungal infection. The retina or the choroid may be involved; occasionally there is concomitant infectious scleritis or keratitis. Acute postoperative and posttraumatic endophthalmitis are covered in BCSC Section 12, *Retina and Vitreous,* and are not discussed here. Chronic postoperative (infectious) endophthalmitis occurs weeks or months after surgery (usually cataract extraction) and can be caused by a myriad of bacteria and fungi. Endogenous endophthalmitis occurs when bacteria or fungi are hematogenously disseminated into the ocular circulation. "Sterile endophthalmitis" describes cases in which infection is suspected but that return negative culture results.

Chronic Postoperative Endophthalmitis

Chronic postoperative endophthalmitis has a distinctive clinical course, with multiple recurrences of chronic indolent inflammation in an eye that had previously undergone surgery, typically cataract extraction. Chronic anterior segment inflammation, hypopyon, keratic precipitates, intracapsular plaques, and/or vitritis may be present. Inflammation may respond to corticosteroid therapy but often recurs after steroids are tapered. This recurrent indolent inflammation may occur at any point during the postoperative course, but it is often delayed by many months to years. Inflammation may cause corneal decompensation or even iris neovascularization in the most severe cases. This course is quite different from the explosive onset of acute postoperative endophthalmitis. The incidence of acute postoperative

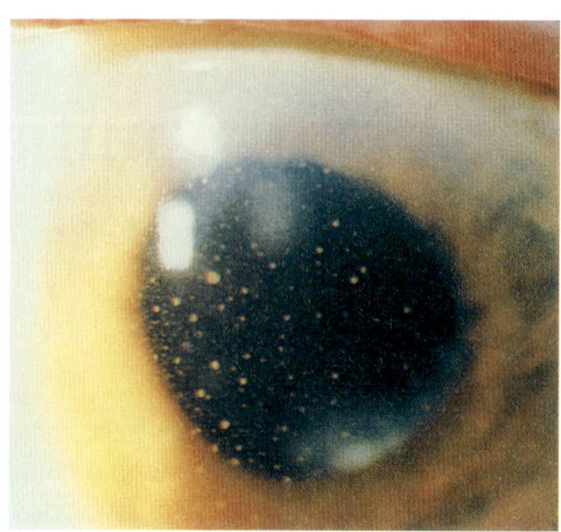

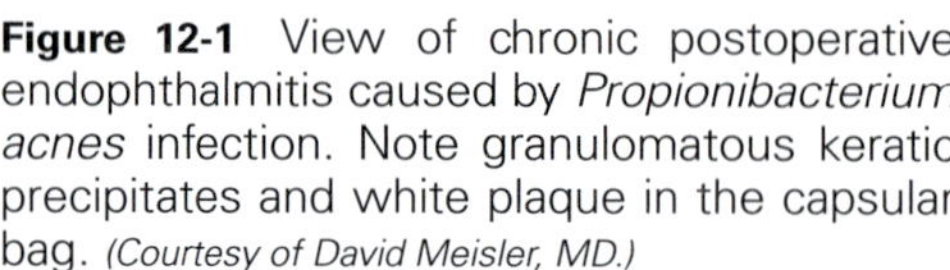

Figure 12-1 View of chronic postoperative endophthalmitis caused by *Propionibacterium acnes* infection. Note granulomatous keratic precipitates and white plaque in the capsular bag. *(Courtesy of David Meisler, MD.)*

endophthalmitis varies between 0.07% and 0.1%. The incidence of chronic endophthalmitis, however, has not been well established, as the condition may often go undiagnosed. Chronic postoperative endophthalmitis can be divided into bacterial and fungal varieties.

Chronic postoperative bacterial endophthalmitis is most commonly caused by *Propionibacterium acnes.* Additionally, gram-positive bacteria with limited virulence (eg, *Staphylococcus epidermidis* and *Corynebacterium* species), gram-negative bacteria, or *Mycobacterium* species may also cause similar chronic infection. *P acnes,* a commensal, anaerobic, gram-positive, pleomorphic rod, is commonly found on the eyelid skin or on the conjunctiva. *P acnes* may sequester itself between an IOL implant and the posterior capsule. In this relatively anaerobic environment, the organism grows and forms colonies, which manifest as whitish plaques between the posterior capsule and the IOL implant (Fig 12-1). A Nd:YAG capsulotomy can trigger chronic endophthalmitis by liberating the organism into the vitreous cavity, resulting in a more severe vitreous inflammation and an exacerbation of the underlying infection.

Shirodkar AR, Pathengay A, Flynn HW Jr, et al. Delayed- versus acute-onset endophthalmitis after cataract surgery. *Am J Ophthalmol.* 2012;53(3):391–398.

Clinical Findings

Chronic postoperative fungal endophthalmitis may present in a very similar fashion to that caused by *P acnes.* Numerous fungal organisms have been implicated in this chronic inflammatory process, including *Candida parapsilosis, Aspergillus flavus, Torulopsis candida,* and *Paecilomyces lilacinus,* as well as *Verticillium* species. Certain clinical signs may be helpful in differentiating a fungal from a bacterial etiology, including the presence of corneal infiltrate or edema, mass in the iris or ciliary body, or development of necrotizing scleritis. The presence of vitreous "snowballs" with a "string-of-pearls" appearance in the vitreous may also be indicative of a fungal infection. The intraocular inflammation may worsen after topical, periocular, or intraocular steroid therapy, which should automatically raise the suspicion of infection.

Diagnosis

The diagnosis of chronic postoperative endophthalmitis is confirmed by obtaining aerobic, anaerobic, and fungal cultures of the aqueous, capsular plaques (if present), and vitreous at the time of pars plana vitrectomy. Gram and fungal stains of undiluted specimens, capsular plaques, and vitreous snowballs should also be obtained. The value of such stains should not be underestimated, especially in cases of fungal endophthalmitis. In addition, polymerase chain reaction (PCR) studies of primers for *P acnes* or pan-fungal and pan-bacterial primers are helpful if available. The bacterial and fungal stains or PCR may yield immediate information, enabling the clinician to tailor therapy and improve clinical prognosis long before the results of the cultures turn positive. Because of the slow-growing and fastidious nature of the organisms that cause chronic endophthalmitis, cultures must be retained by the microbiology laboratory for 2 or more weeks.

The differential diagnosis of chronic postoperative endophthalmitis includes noninfectious causes such as lens-induced uveitis from retained cortical material or retained intravitreal lens fragments, intraocular inflammation from iris chafing resulting from IOL malposition, uveitis-glaucoma-hyphema syndrome, and intraocular lymphoma masquerade syndrome.

Lai JY, Chen KH, Lin YC, Hsu WM, Lee SM. Propionibacterium acnes DNA from an explanted intraocular lens detected by polymerase chain reaction in a case of chronic pseudophakic endophthalmitis. *J Cataract Refract Surg.* 2006;32(3):522–525.

Meisler DM, Mandelbaum S. Propionibacterium-associated endophthalmitis after extracapsular cataract extraction. Review of reported cases. *Ophthalmology.* 1989;96(1):54–61.

Treatment

Pars plana vitrectomy and injection of intravitreal and endocapsular vancomycin are therapeutic in many cases of chronic postoperative bacterial endophthalmitis. However, this treatment may not completely eradicate the infection, especially if equatorial lens capsule sequestrae of bacteria are present. In such cases, IOL explantation, complete capsulectomy, and intravitreal vancomycin injection is curative. The decision to explant the IOL is made on a case-by-case basis and is based on the clinical course, the severity of the intraocular inflammation, and the level of vision loss. There is no preferred method for treating this condition, but existing literature suggests that more than one surgery may be necessary to eradicate this chronic infection.

The treatment of chronic fungal endophthalmitis is more difficult and requires the use of weekly intravitreal antifungal injections (amphotericin or voriconazole) and, possibly, systemic antifungal drugs in the most severe cases. In vitrectomized eyes, antifungals are often injected twice a week. Multiple vitrectomies may be necessary. The role of systemic therapy in this chronic form of fungal endophthalmitis is not well established or proven.

Clark WL, Kaiser PK, Flynn HW Jr, Belfort A, Miller D, Meisler DM. Treatment strategies and visual acuity outcomes in chronic postoperative *Propionibacterium acnes* endophthalmitis. *Ophthalmology.* 1999;106(9):1665–1670.

Endogenous Endophthalmitis

Endogenous Bacterial Endophthalmitis

Endogenous bacterial endophthalmitis is caused by hematogenous dissemination of bacterial organisms, resulting in intraocular infection. This entity is uncommon and accounts for less than 10% of all forms of endophthalmitis. Patients who have compromised immune systems are most at risk for endogenous endophthalmitis. Predisposing conditions include diabetes mellitus, systemic malignancy, sickle cell anemia, systemic lupus erythematosus, and HIV infection. Extensive gastrointestinal surgery, endoscopy, dental procedures, and intravenous drug abuse may increase the risk of endogenous endophthalmitis. Systemic immunomodulatory therapy and chemotherapy may also put patients at risk. Endogenous endophthalmitis can develop in patients with immunosuppression from HIV infection, but it is not clear that this is an independent risk factor. Although the eye may be the only location where the infection can be found, an extraocular focus may exist in as many as 90% of cases. Possible infection sources to be considered are tooth abscess, pneumonia, endocarditis, urinary tract infection, bacterial meningitis, and liver abscess. There may be a history of an indwelling line or port.

A wide variety of bacteria can cause endogenous endophthalmitis. The most common gram-positive organisms are *Streptococcus* species (endocarditis), *Staphylococcus aureus* (cutaneous infections), *Bacillus* species (from intravenous drug use), and *Nocardia* species (in immunocompromised patients; discussed in further detail in Chapter 10). The most common gram-negative organisms are *Neisseria meningitidis, Haemophilus influenzae,* and enteric organisms such as *Escherichia coli* and *Klebsiella* species. In Asia, infection from *Klebsiella* species in liver abscesses is the most common cause of endogenous endophthalmitis.

Jackson TL, Paraskevopoulos T, Georgalas I. Systematic review of 342 cases of endogenous bacterial endophthalmitis. *Surv Ophthalmol.* 2014;59(6):627–635.

Clinical findings and symptoms

The clinical features of endogenous bacterial endophthalmitis are suggestive of an ongoing systemic infection and may include fever greater than 101.5°F, elevated peripheral leukocyte count, and positive bacterial cultures from extraocular sites (blood, urine, sputum). Patients may be ill and undergoing treatment for a primary underlying disease when they present with endogenous endophthalmitis. However, some patients may be ambulatory and afebrile. The underlying disease may include cancer treated with prolonged intravenous chemotherapy as well as other chronic infections, which may subsequently sequester in the eye. A nonocular infection serving as a nidus for bacterial dissemination to the eye may be very difficult to diagnose, especially in cases of osteomyelitis, sinusitis, or pneumonia misdiagnosed as a simple upper respiratory tract infection. In these situations, laboratory tests cannot substitute for a detailed history and review of systems.

Clinical symptoms include acute onset of pain, photophobia, and blurred vision. Examination usually reveals severely reduced visual acuity, and fibrin in the anterior chamber; hypopyon may be present; very rarely there may be periorbital and eyelid edema. There may be significant vitreous inflammation and vitreous cells. Sometimes, both eyes are affected simultaneously. Small microabscesses in the retina or choroid and white-centered retinal hemorrhages (Roth spots) may also be present.

Diagnosis

Diagnosis is based on anterior chamber paracentesis and vitrectomy with vitreous and aqueous cultures and appropriate stains. As for cases of chronic postoperative endophthalmitis, PCR evaluation of ocular fluids with pan-bacterial or pan-fungal primers is extremely useful. Blood and other body fluid cultures should be used along with ocular culture results to confirm the diagnosis and establish therapy.

Treatment

Intravitreal antibiotics are given at the time of vitrectomy. If it is not clear that fungal organisms may be involved, treatment of both fungal and bacterial causes is indicated at the time of vitrectomy. Also, intravenous antibiotic treatment is sometimes needed for several weeks, depending on the organism isolated. Similarly, in patients with endogenous fungal endophthalmitis, systemic antifungal therapy may be warranted for 6 weeks or more. Initial antimicrobial choices may be empiric and subsequently tailored to culture results.

Complications

The complications of endogenous endophthalmitis can be serious. If the diagnosis of systemic infection is missed, the patient may develop sepsis and even die. In severe cases, recurrent or persistent intraocular infection may require numerous surgeries and repeat injections of intravitreal antibiotics. In addition, complications such as cataract development, retinal detachment, suprachoroidal hemorrhage, vitreous hemorrhage, macular scar, hypotony, and phthisis bulbi can occur in the most severe cases. The prognosis is directly related to the offending organism and the systemic status of the patient.

Endogenous Fungal Endophthalmitis

Endogenous fungal endophthalmitis develops slowly as focal or multifocal areas of chorioretinitis. Granulomatous or nongranulomatous inflammation is observed with keratic precipitates, hypopyon, and vitritis with cellular aggregates. The infection usually begins in the choroid, appearing as yellow-white lesions with indistinct borders that range in size from small cotton-wool spots to several disc diameters. It can subsequently break through into the vitreous, producing localized cellular and fungal aggregates overlying the original site(s). Iris nodules and rubeosis may also be noted in severe fungal endophthalmitis.

Endogenous fungal endophthalmitis due to *Candida* (the most common cause; Fig 12-2), *Aspergillus,* and *Coccidioides* species can be mistaken for noninfectious uveitis and treated with corticosteroids alone. This treatment usually worsens the clinical course of the disease, necessitating further investigation to establish the correct diagnosis. There is often a history of indwelling line or intravenous drug abuse. The condition often requires aggressive systemic and local antifungal therapy as well as surgical intervention.

Endogenous fungal endophthalmitis caused by *Histoplasma capsulatum, Cryptococcus neoformans, Sporothrix schenckii,* and *Blastomyces dermatitidis* is less common than that caused by *Candida* and *Aspergillus* species.

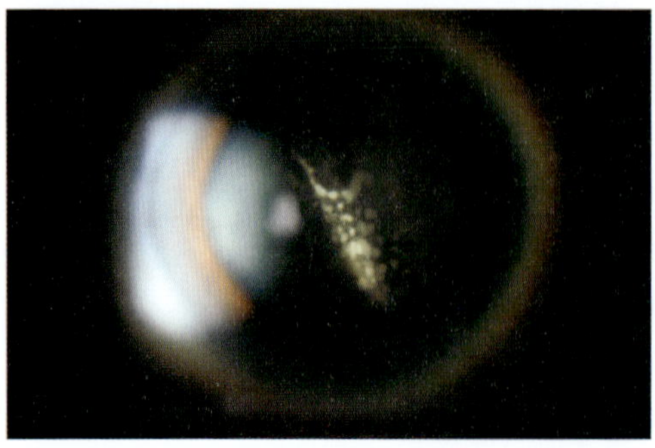

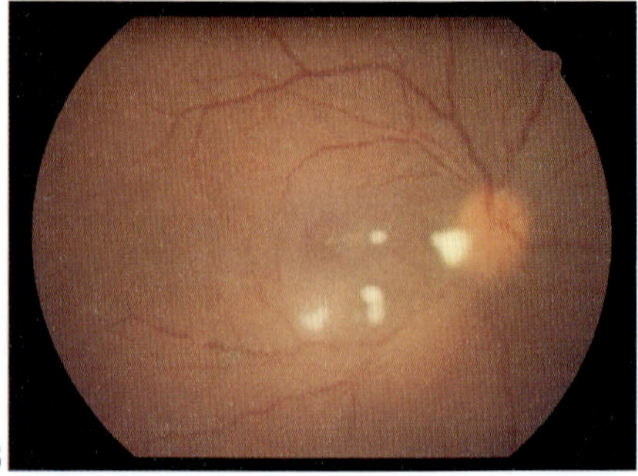

Figure 12-2. Endogenous endophthalmitis. **A,** "String of pearls" seen in the vitreous of a 36-year-old male with endogenous *Candida* endophthalmitis. **B,** Fundus photograph of endogenous endophthalmitis. *(Part A courtesy of H. Nida Sen, MD, and Henry Wiley, MD/National Eye Institute; part B courtesy of Debra A. Goldstein, MD.)*

Sridhar J, Flynn HW Jr, Kuriyan AE, Miller D, Albini T. Endogenous fungal endophthalmitis: risk factors, clinical features, and treatment outcomes in mold and yeast infections. *J Ophthalmic Inflamm Infect.* 2013;3(1):60.

Candida *endophthalmitis*

Candida species are an important cause of nosocomial infections and are the most common fungal organisms, causing endogenous endophthalmitis in both pediatric and adult populations. Although *Candida albicans* remains the most common pathogen, non-*albicans* species (eg, *Candida glabrata*) have also been identified in patients developing ocular disease. In patients with candidemia, the reported prevalence rates of intraocular candidiasis vary widely, ranging between 9% and 78%. However, when strict criteria are applied for the classification of chorioretinitis and endophthalmitis, these numbers drop precipitously. In 1 series, when patients were examined within 72 hours of a positive blood culture result, only 9% had chorioretinitis and none had endophthalmitis. Endogenous *Candida* endophthalmitis occurs in up to 37% of patients with candidemia if they are not receiving antifungal therapy. Ocular involvement drops to 3% in patients who are receiving treatment.

Predisposing conditions associated with candidemia and the development of intraocular infection include

- hospitalization with a history of recent major gastrointestinal surgery
- bacterial sepsis
- systemic antibiotic use
- use of indwelling catheters
- hyperalimentation
- debilitating diseases (eg, diabetes mellitus)
- immunomodulatory therapy
- prolonged neutropenia
- organ transplantation
- a combination of these conditions

Hospitalized neonates and intravenous drug users are also at risk. Immunodeficiency per se does not appear to be a prominent predisposing factor, attested to by the paucity of reported cases of *Candida* chorioretinitis or endophthalmitis among patients with HIV infection or AIDS.

Shah CP, McKey J, Spirn MJ, Maguire J. Ocular candidiasis: a review. *Br J Ophthalmol.* 2008;92(4):466–468.

Manifestations Patients may present with blurred or decreased vision resulting from macular chorioretinal involvement or pain arising from anterior uveitis, which may be severe. Typically, *Candida* chorioretinitis is characterized by multiple, bilateral, white, well-circumscribed lesions less than 1 mm in diameter. These lesions are distributed throughout the postequatorial fundus and associated with overlying vitreous cellular inflammation (Fig 12-3). The chorioretinal lesions may be associated with vascular sheathing and intraretinal hemorrhages. The vitreous exudates may assume a string-of-pearls appearance.

Histologically, *Candida* species are recognized as budding yeast with a characteristic pseudohyphate appearance (Fig 12-4). The organisms reach the eye hematogenously through metastasis to the choroid. Fungi may then break through the Bruch membrane, form subretinal abscesses, and secondarily involve the retina and vitreous.

Rao NA, Hidayat AA. Endogenous mycotic endophthalmitis: variations in clinical and histopathologic changes in candidiasis compared with aspergillosis. *Am J Ophthalmol.* 2001;132(2):244–251.

Diagnosis The diagnosis of ocular candidiasis is suggested by the presence of chorioretinitis or endophthalmitis in the appropriate clinical context and confirmed by positive results on either blood or vitreous cultures. It has been suggested that all patients with candidemia undergo baseline dilated funduscopic examinations and receive monitoring for the development of metastatic ocular candidiasis for at least 2 weeks after an initial eye examination. The reasoning is that earlier treatment of *Candida* endophthalmitis has been associated with better visual outcomes, and patients with ocular lesions are more likely to have infection involving a greater number of organ systems than are patients without eye lesions. The presence of vitreous snowballs and endophthalmitis requires diagnostic and therapeutic vitrectomy. Fungal stains and cultures, and PCR for *Candida* species, should be obtained on undiluted vitreous fluid samples.

The differential diagnosis of *Candida* endophthalmitis includes toxoplasmic retinochoroiditis, which exhibits posterior pole lesions that can appear yellow-white with fluffy borders and range in size from small cotton-wool spots to several disc diameters wide. *Candida* vitreous snowball lesions may also resemble pars planitis.

Hidalgo JA, Alangaden GJ, Eliott D, et al. Fungal endophthalmitis diagnosis by detection of *Candida albicans* DNA in intraocular fluid by use of a species-specific polymerase chain reaction assay. *J Infect Dis.* 2000;181(3):1198–1201.

Krishna R, Amuh D, Lowder CY, Gordon SM, Adal KA, Hall G. Should all patients with candidemia have an ophthalmic examination to rule out ocular candidiasis? *Eye (Lond).* 2000;14(Pt 1):30–34.

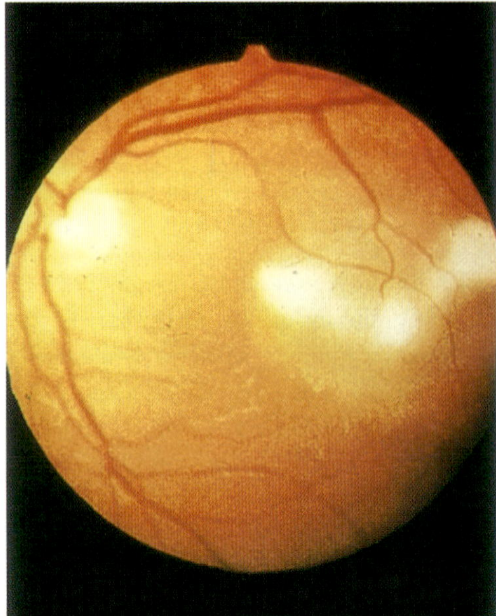

Figure 12-3 Fundus photograph of *Candida* retinitis.

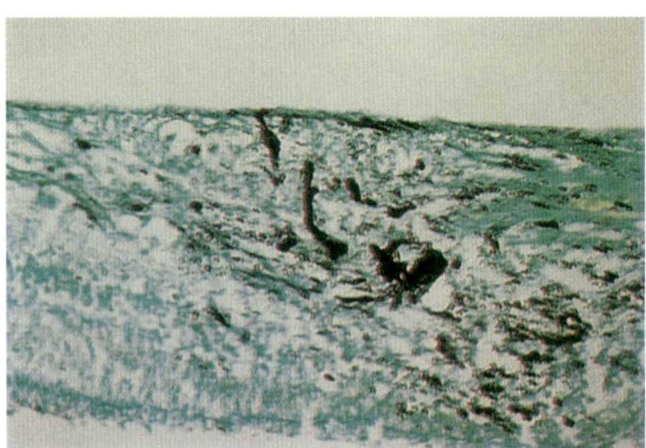

Figure 12-4 Pathology of *Candida* retinitis. Fungi (black) are revealed in a Gomori methenamine silver stain of the retina taken from a patient diagnosed with fungal endophthalmitis.

Treatment The treatment of intraocular candidiasis includes systemic and intravitreal administration of antifungal drugs. Consultation with a specialist in infectious diseases is essential. Chorioretinal lesions not yet involving the vitreous body may be treated effectively with the oral triazole antifungal drugs fluconazole or voriconazole (200 mg, twice daily, for 2–4 weeks), with vigilant monitoring for evidence of progression. Voriconazole has good oral bioavailability, achieving therapeutic intravitreal levels with a broad spectrum of antifungal activity. When the vitreous body is involved, intravitreal injection of antifungal drugs (amphotericin B, 5–10 µg/0.1 mL, or voriconazole, 100 µg/0.1 mL) should be considered, usually in conjunction with pars plana vitrectomy. Long-acting corticosteroid injections should be avoided. Vitrectomy may be useful diagnostically by allowing for the analysis of intraocular fluid by microbiologic and molecular techniques, and therapeutically by debulking the pathogen load.

More severe infections may require intravenous amphotericin B with or without flucytosine. Significant dose-limiting toxicities (renal, cardiac, and neurologic) associated with conventional amphotericin B therapy were greatly reduced by the development of liposomal lipid complex formulations. Finally, intravenously administered caspofungin, an antifungal drug in the echinocandin class (drugs that inhibit synthesis of glucan in the cell wall) with activity against *Candida* and *Aspergillus* species, has been successfully employed in a small number of patients with *Candida* endophthalmitis; some treatment failures have also been reported with this drug, however. Another echinocandin, intravenous micafungin, is also available in the United States and Europe for treatment of candidiasis. Oral voriconazole, flucytosine, fluconazole, or rifampin may be administered in addition to intravenous amphotericin B or caspofungin.

Breit SM, Hariprasad SM, Mieler WF, Shah GK, Mills MD, Grand MG. Management of endogenous fungal endophthalmitis with voriconazole and caspofungin. *Am J Ophthalmol.* 2005;139(1):135–140.

Paulus YM, Cheng S, Karth PA, Leng T. Prospective trial of endogenous fungal endophthalmitis and chorioretinitis rates, clinical course, and outcomes in patients with fungemia. *Retina.* 2016;36(7):1357–1363.

Cryptococcosis

Cryptococcus neoformans is a yeast found in high concentrations worldwide in contaminated soil and pigeon feces. Infection is acquired through inhalation of the aerosolized fungus. It has a predilection for the central nervous system and may produce severe disseminated disease among immunocompromised or debilitated patients. Although overall it remains an uncommon disease, cryptococcosis is the most common cause of fungal meningitis, as well as the most frequent fungal eye infection in patients with HIV infection or AIDS. The fungus probably reaches the eye hematogenously; however, the frequent association of ocular cryptococcosis with meningitis suggests that ocular infection may result from direct extension from the optic nerve. Ocular infections may occur months after the onset of meningitis or, in rare instances, before the onset of clinically apparent central nervous system disease.

Manifestations Ocular findings associated with cryptococcal meningitis include mainly papilledema followed by optic atrophy and cranial nerve palsies. Other manifestations include diplopia, nystagmus, ptosis, and ophthalmoplegia. The most frequent presentation of ocular cryptococcosis that is not directly related to meningoencephalitis is multifocal chorioretinitis. Associated findings include variable degrees of vitritis, vascular sheathing, exudative retinal detachment, papilledema, and granulomatous anterior chamber inflammation. It has been hypothesized that the infection begins as a focus in the choroid, with subsequent extension and secondary involvement of overlying tissues. Severe intraocular infection progressing to endophthalmitis may be observed in the absence of meningitis or clinically apparent systemic disease.

Diagnosis and treatment The clinical diagnosis requires a high degree of suspicion and is supported by demonstration of the organism with India ink stains or by culture of the fungus from cerebrospinal fluid. Intravenous amphotericin B and oral flucytosine are required to halt disease progression. With optic nerve or macular involvement, the prognosis is poor for recovery of vision.

Kestelyn P, Taelman H, Bogaerts J, et al. Ophthalmic manifestations of infections with *Cryptococcus neoformans* in patients with the acquired immunodeficiency syndrome. *Am J Ophthalmol.* 1993;116(6):721–727.

Sheu SJ, Chen YC, Kuo NW, Wang JH, Chen CJ. Endogenous cryptococcal endophthalmitis. *Ophthalmology.* 1998;105(2):377–381.

Wykoff CC, Albini TA, Couvillion SS, Dubovy SR, Davis JL. Intraocular cryptococcoma. *Arch Ophthalmol.* 2009;127(5):700–702.

Aspergillus *endophthalmitis*

Endogenous *Aspergillus* endophthalmitis is a rare disorder associated with disseminated aspergillosis among patients with severe chronic pulmonary diseases, cancer, endocarditis, severe immunocompromise, or intravenous drug abuse. In rare instances, *Aspergillus* endophthalmitis may occur in immunocompetent patients with no apparent predisposing factors. Disseminated infection most commonly involves the lung, with the eye as the second most common site of infection. *Aspergillus fumigatus* and *A flavus* are the species most frequently isolated from patients with intraocular infection.

Aspergillus species are found in soils and decaying vegetation. The spores of these ubiquitous saprophytic molds become airborne and seed the lungs and paranasal sinuses of humans. Human exposure is very common, but infection is rare and depends on the virulence of the fungal pathogen and immunocompetence of the host. Ocular disease occurs via hematogenous dissemination of *Aspergillus* organisms to the choroid.

Manifestations Endogenous *Aspergillus* endophthalmitis results in rapid onset of pain and loss of vision. A confluent yellowish infiltrate is often present in the macula, beginning in the choroid and subretinal space. A hypopyon can develop in the subretinal or subhyaloidal space (Fig 12-5A). Retinal hemorrhages, retinal vascular occlusions, and full-thickness retinal necrosis may occur. The infection can spread to produce a dense vitritis and variable

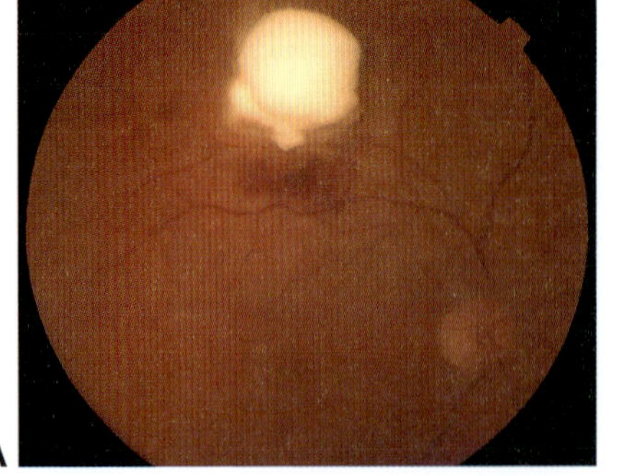

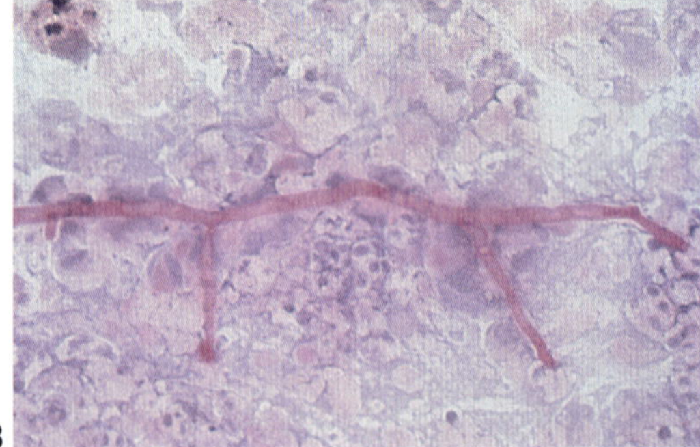

Figure 12-5 Coccidioidal iris granuloma in the pupil. **A,** Fundus photograph. **B,** This granuloma was biopsied and a peripheral iridectomy was performed because it was causing pupillary block and angle-closure glaucoma. *(Courtesy of Ramana S. Moorthy, MD.)*

degrees of cells, flare, and hypopyon in the anterior chamber. The macular lesions form a central atrophic scar when healed. In contrast to the lesions associated with *Candida* chorioretinitis and endophthalmitis, lesions produced by *Aspergillus* species are larger and more likely to be hemorrhagic, and they commonly invade the retinal and choroidal vessels, which may result in broad areas of ischemic infarction.

Diagnosis The diagnosis of endogenous *Aspergillus* endophthalmitis is based on clinical findings combined with positive results from pars plana vitreous biopsy and cultures as well as results from Gram and fungal stains. Coexisting systemic aspergillosis can be a strong clue, especially among high-risk patients. The diagnosis requires a high degree of suspicion within the correct clinical context and is confirmed by the demonstration of septate, dichotomously branching hyphae on analysis of vitreous fluid specimens. *Aspergillus* organisms may be difficult to culture from the blood.

The differential diagnosis of endogenous *Aspergillus* endophthalmitis includes *Candida* endophthalmitis, cytomegalovirus retinitis, *Toxoplasma* retinochoroiditis, coccidioidomycotic choroiditis or endophthalmitis, and bacterial endophthalmitis.

In *Candida* endophthalmitis, the vitreous is the prominent focus of infection, but in *Aspergillus* endophthalmitis, the principal foci are retinal and choroidal vessels and the subretinal or subretinal pigment epithelial space.

Treatment Endogenous *Aspergillus* endophthalmitis usually requires aggressive treatment with diagnostic and therapeutic pars plana vitrectomy combined with intravitreal injection of amphotericin B or voriconazole; intravitreal corticosteroids may be used in conjunction with these drugs. Because most patients with this condition have disseminated aspergillosis, systemic treatment with oral voriconazole, intravenous amphotericin B, or caspofungin is often required. Other systemic antifungal drugs, such as itraconazole, miconazole, fluconazole, and ketoconazole, may also be used. Systemic aspergillosis is best managed by an infectious diseases specialist.

Despite aggressive treatment, the visual prognosis is poor because of frequent macular involvement. Final visual acuity is usually less than 20/200.

Hariprasad SM, Mieler WF, Holz ER, et al. Determination of vitreous, aqueous, and plasma concentration of orally administered voriconazole in humans. *Arch Ophthalmol.* 2004;122(1):42–47.

Coccidioidomycosis

Coccidioidomycosis is a disease produced by the dimorphic soil fungus *Coccidioides immitis,* which is endemic to the San Joaquin Valley of central California, certain parts of the southwestern United States, and parts of Central and South America. Infection follows inhalation of dust-borne arthrospores, most commonly resulting in pulmonary infection and secondary dissemination to the central nervous system, skin, skeleton, and eyes. Approximately 40% of infected patients are symptomatic; the vast majority present with a mild upper respiratory tract infection or pneumonitis approximately 3 weeks after exposure to the organism. Erythema nodosum or multiforme may appear from 3 days to 3 weeks after the onset of symptoms. Disseminated infection is rare, occurring in less than 1% of patients with pulmonary coccidioidomycosis.

Manifestations Ocular coccidioidomycosis is likewise uncommon, even with disseminated disease. Disseminated disease usually causes blepharitis, keratoconjunctivitis, phlyctenular and granulomatous conjunctivitis, episcleritis and scleritis, and extraocular nerve palsies and orbital infection. Uveal involvement is still rarer: fewer than 20 pathologically verified cases have been reported. The anterior and posterior segments are equally involved. Intraocular manifestations include unilateral or bilateral granulomatous anterior uveitis, iris granulomas (Fig 12-5), and a multifocal chorioretinitis characterized by multiple, discrete, yellow-white lesions usually less than 1 disc diameter in size located in the postequatorial fundus. These choroidal granulomas may resolve, leaving punched-out chorioretinal scars. Vitreous cellular infiltration, vascular sheathing, retinal hemorrhage, serous retinal detachment, and involvement of the optic nerve have also been reported.

Diagnosis Positive results of serologic testing for anticoccidioidal antibodies in the serum, cerebrospinal fluid, vitreous, and aqueous, as well as of skin testing for exposure to coccidioidin establish the diagnosis in the correct clinical context.

Treatment The Infectious Diseases Society of America recommends initiating treatment with an oral azole antifungal drug such as fluconazole or itraconazole. Surgical debulking of anterior chamber granulomas, pars plana vitrectomy, and intraocular injections of amphotericin and voriconazole may be required. With systemic disease, much higher doses and a longer duration of intravenous amphotericin therapy or oral voriconazole therapy may be needed. An infectious diseases specialist is essential in the management of coccidioidomycosis.

Despite aggressive treatment, ocular coccidioidomycosis carries a poor visual prognosis, and most eyes require enucleation because of pain and blindness.

Glasgow BJ, Brown HH, Foos RY. Miliary retinitis in coccidioidomycosis. *Am J Ophthalmol.* 1987;104(1):24–27.

Moorthy RS, Rao NA, Sidikaro Y, Foos RY. Coccidioidomycosis iridocyclitis. *Ophthalmology.* 1994;101(12):1923–1928.

Vasconcelos-Santos DV, Lim JI, Rao NA. Chronic coccidioidomycosis endophthalmitis without concomitant systemic involvement: a clinicopathological case report. *Ophthalmology.* 2010;117(9):1839–1842.

CHAPTER 13

Masquerade Syndromes

This chapter includes a related video, which can be accessed by scanning the QR code provided in the text or going to www.aao.org/bcscvideo_section09.

Highlights

- The most common condition to masquerade as uveitis is primary vitreoretinal lymphoma (PVRL), although a number of other neoplastic and nonneoplastic conditions can also masquerade as uveitis.
- Primary vitreoretinal lymphoma can present with vitritis, anterior uveitis, subretinal and/or intraretinal infiltrates. Definitive diagnosis is made by cytology of intraocular fluid.
- Most patients with PVRL will develop central nervous system lymphoma, necessitating evaluation for central nervous system lymphoma even in the absence of central nervous system (CNS) symptoms.
- Masquerade syndromes are a heterogeneous group of disorders noteworthy for mimicking immune-mediated entities and thus are difficult to diagnose. They may be divided into neoplastic and nonneoplastic conditions. Since the underlying diseases often have harmful consequences, early diagnosis and prompt treatment are crucial.

Neoplastic Masquerade Syndromes

Neoplastic masquerade syndromes may account for 2%–3% of all patients evaluated in tertiary uveitis referral clinics. Primary vitreoretinal lymphoma is the most common entity.

Read RW, Zamir E, Rao NA. Neoplastic masquerade syndromes. *Surv Ophthalmol.* 2002;47(2):81–124.

Primary Vitreoretinal Lymphoma

Primary vitreoretinal lymphoma is a subset of primary central nervous system lymphoma (PCNSL). It is an uncommon, but potentially fatal malignancy, which may occur with or without CNS lesions. The usual age of onset is in the 50s and 60s, there is no convincing gender predilection, and immunosuppressed patients are at greater risk. Nearly all (98%) cases of PVRL are non-Hodgkin B-lymphocyte lymphomas. Approximately 2% are T-lymphocyte lymphomas. The incidence of PCNSL appears to be increasing and is projected to occur in 1 of every 100,000 immunocompetent patients.

Chan CC, Rubenstein JL, Coupland SE, et al. Primary vitreoretinal lymphoma: a report from an international primary central nervous system lymphoma collaborative group symposium. *Oncologist.* 2011;16(11):1589–1599.

Clinical features and findings

More than two-thirds of patients with PVRL will develop CNS disease—usually within 29 months of diagnosis. About 25% of patients with intracranial lymphoma will develop intraocular disease. Sites of ocular involvement can include the vitreous, retina, subretinal pigment epithelium (sub-RPE), and any combination thereof. The most common presenting symptoms are decreased vision and floaters.

Examination reveals a variable degree of vitritis and anterior chamber cells. Posterior segment involvement can appear as creamy yellow subretinal infiltrates with overlying RPE detachments (Fig 13-1) and discrete white lesions that may mimic acute retinal necrosis, toxoplasmosis, "frosted-branch" angiitis, or retinal arteriolar obstruction with coexisting multifocal chorioretinal scars (Figs 13-2, 13-3) and retinal vasculitis. The lesions vary in thickness from approximately 1 mm to 2 mm. Because of diagnostic difficulty, often patients

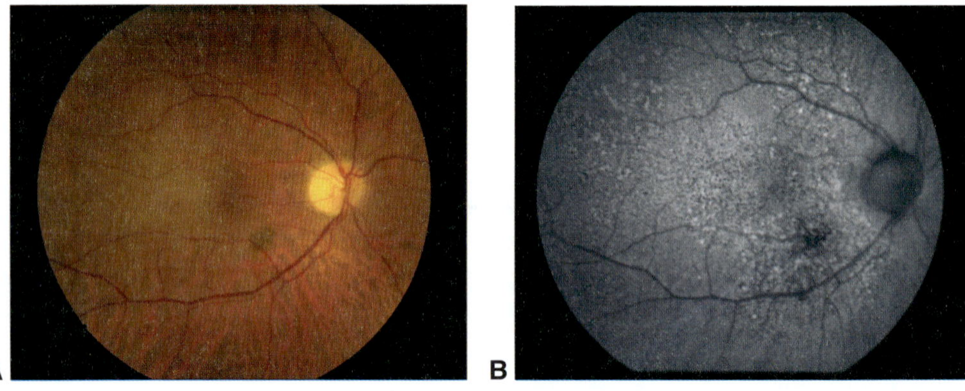

Figure 13-1 Primary central nervous system lymphoma. **A,** Fundus photograph of multifocal, subretinal granular infiltrates. **B,** These infiltrates appear as hyperautofluorescent and hypoautofluorescent granular changes on fundus autofluorescence. *(Courtesy of H. Nida Sen, MD/National Eye Institute.)*

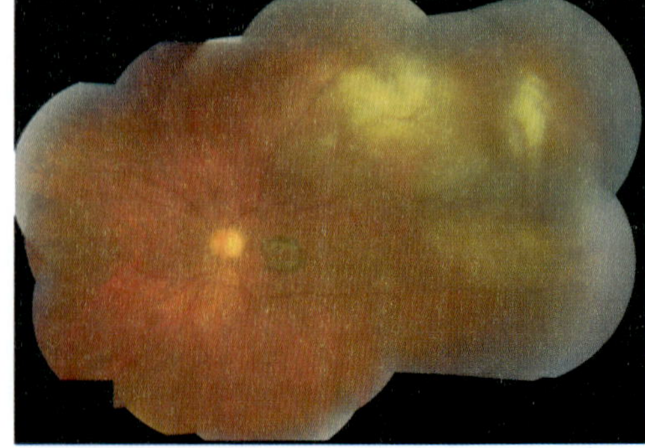

Figure 13-2 Fundus photomontage shows creamy, large, slightly elevated multifocal lesions, some of which are confluent in superotemporal retina in a patient with biopsy-proven primary vitreoretinal lymphoma. The annular atrophic lesion in the macula is less common and is likely secondary to initial corticosteroid treatment for presumed vitritis. *(Courtesy of H. Nida Sen, MD/National Eye Institute.)*

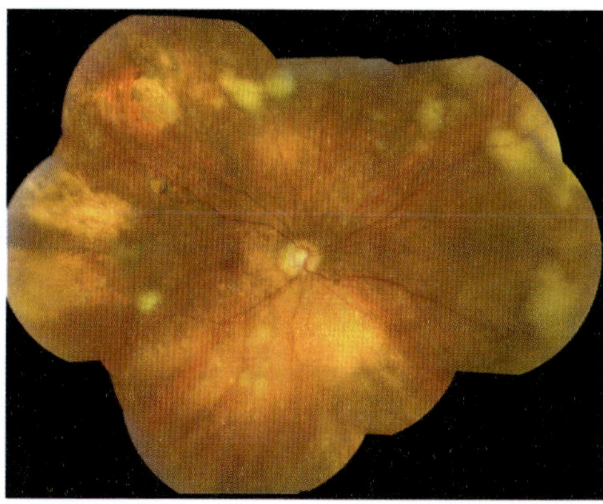

Figure 13-3 Fundus photomontage of a patient with primary vitreoretinal lymphoma shows various lesions. Some are creamy yellowish and elevated; others are more atrophic. There are punctate and granular retinal pigment epithelial changes throughout the fundus. *(Courtesy of H. Nida Sen, MD/National Eye Institute.)*

are already being treated with various anti-inflammatory medications that temporarily can improve the vitreous cellular infiltration, but the effect is not long-lasting. Central nervous system signs may be present and vary in nature from behavioral changes, hemiparesis, and cerebellar signs to epileptic seizures and cranial nerve palsies.

Diagnostic testing

Ultrasonography may indicate vitreous debris, elevated subretinal lesions, and serous retinal detachment. Fluorescein angiography may show hypofluorescent areas due to blockage from a sub-RPE tumor mass or from RPE clumping. Hyperfluorescent window defects may also be caused by RPE atrophy from resolved RPE infiltration. An unusual leopard-spot pattern of alternating hyperfluorescence and hypofluorescence may also be noted. Granular autofluorescence (see Fig 13-1) and nodular elevations at the level of the RPE/sub-RPE corresponding to these areas can also be helpful in the diagnosis. Indocyanine green angiography may show ill-defined hypofluorescent lesions at the late-phase study. Optic coherence tomography (OCT) may reveal mild irregularity of the inner/outer segments of photoreceptors and the RPE/Bruch membrane complex.

All patients with suspected PVRL should be evaluated for CNS lymphoma even in the absence of neurologic symptoms. With CNS involvement, magnetic resonance imaging (MRI) studies of the brain show isointense lesions on T1-weighted images and isointense to hyperintense lesions on T2-weighted images. Computed tomography (CT) without use of contrast shows multiple diffuse periventricular lesions. If intravenous contrast is used with CT, these periventricular lesions may be enhanced. Cerebrospinal fluid analysis reveals lymphoma cells in one-third of patients.

The presence of vitreous cells in cases of uveitis that do not respond to therapy necessitates a vitreous biopsy. Ideally, at least 1 mL of undiluted vitreous sample should be obtained. A retinal biopsy, an aspirate of sub-RPE material, or both may be considered when previous vitreous biopsy results have been negative (Video 13-1). Prior to surgery, communication with an experienced pathologist for instructions on the proper and prompt handling of the specimens is necessary to avoid degeneration of the typically friable cells that may occur with delay. Examination by a pathologist is crucial, as the diagnosis may be difficult to establish because of the frequently sparse cellularity of the specimens. Portions of the specimen are typically prepared for both cytologic examination and cell surface marker determination by flow cytometry. As many as one-third of vitreous biopsies incur a false-negative result; thus, a second biopsy of the vitreous should be performed if the clinical picture warrants.

VIDEO 13-1 Primary vitreoretinal lymphoma.
Courtesy of Emilio M. Dodds, MD.
Access the video at www.aao.org/bcscvideo_section09.

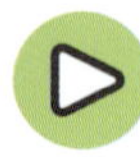

Cytokine analysis of vitreous samples can be helpful in supporting the diagnosis of intraocular lymphoma. Interleukin-10 (IL-10) levels are elevated in the vitreous of patients with lymphoma. In contrast, high levels of IL-6 are found in the vitreous of patients with inflammatory uveitis. Thus, the ratio of IL-10 to IL-6 is often elevated in intraocular lymphoma and supports the diagnosis.

Gene rearrangement studies can provide evidence of monoclonality. Flow cytometry may reveal kappa (κ) or gamma (γ) chain restriction or large B-cell populations, both of which support the diagnosis of B-cell lymphoma. A specific mutation (proline for leucine substitution mutation at position 265) of the myeloid differentiation primary response 88 protein (*MYD88*) is also supportive.

If diagnosis by vitreous aspiration or subretinal aspiration cannot be established, internal or external chorioretinal biopsy techniques may be useful in the diagnosis of PCNSL.

Raparia K, Chang CC, Chévez-Barrios P. Intraocular lymphoma: diagnostic approach and immunophenotypic findings in vitrectomy specimens. *Arch Pathol Lab Med.* 2009;133(8):1233–1237.

Rothova A, Ooijman F, Kerkhoff F, Van der Lelij A, Lokhorst HM. Uveitis masquerade syndromes. *Ophthalmology.* 2001;108(2):386–399.

Sen HN, Bodaghi B, Hoang PL, Nussenblatt R. Primary intraocular lymphoma: diagnosis and differential diagnosis. *Ocul Immunol Inflamm.* 2009;17(3):133–141.

Histology

Cytologic specimens obtained from the vitreous or subretinal space often show pleomorphic cells with scanty cytoplasm, hyperchromatic nuclei with multiple irregular nucleoli, and an elevated nuclear-to-cytoplasm ratio (Fig 13-4). Monoclonality of cells is likely to be present in PCNSL. This can be established through immunophenotyping by immunohistochemistry or flow cytometry to demonstrate the clonality of B lymphocytes by the presence of abnormal immunoglobulin κ or γ light chain predominance, specific B-lymphocyte markers (CD19, CD20, and CD22), and/or gene or oncogene translocations or gene rearrangements. Abnormal lymphocytes may be isolated manually or by laser capture and polymerase chain reaction (PCR)–based assays performed to improve the diagnostic yield of paucicellular samples. See also BCSC Section 4, *Ophthalmic Pathology and Intraocular Tumors*, for discussion of intraocular lymphoma.

Zaldivar RA, Martin DF, Holden JT, Grossniklaus HE. Primary intraocular lymphoma: clinical, cytologic, and flow cytometric analysis. *Ophthalmology.* 2004;111(9): 1762–1767.

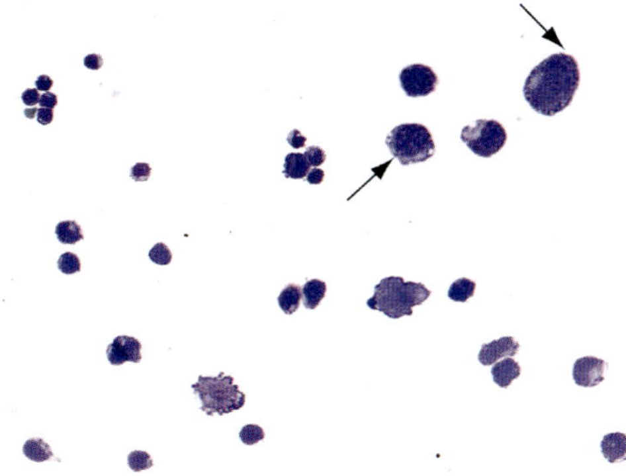

Figure 13-4 Cytology of a vitreous specimen from a patient with primary vitreoretinal lymphoma showing large atypical lymphoid cells *(arrows)*. There are large irregular nuclei and scanty basophilic cytoplasm consistent with large B-cell lymphoma. *(Courtesy of Chi Chao Chan, MD, and H. Nida Sen, MD/National Eye Institute.)*

Treatment

The current treatment of PVRL involves intravitreal chemotherapy (methotrexate and/or rituximab) and local external beam radiation of the eye, with or without systemic chemotherapy depending on CNS involvement. In cases with concomitant PCNSL, systemic high-dose chemotherapy in conjunction with intrathecal therapy, whole-brain radiotherapy, and/or autologous stem cell transplantation are considered. There are various chemotherapy regimens. Among the most commonly used is high-dose systemic methotrexate with rituximab. Some specialists use prophylactic treatment of the CNS even in cases of seemingly isolated ocular disease.

Frenkel S, Hendler K, Siegal T, et al. Intravitreal methotrexate for treating vitreoretinal lymphoma: 10 years of experience. *Br J Ophthalmol.* 2008;92(3):383–388.

Itty S, Pulido JS. Rituximab for intraocular lymphoma. *Retina.* 2009;29(2):129–132.

Prognosis

Primary vitreoretinal lymphoma responds well to initial treatment; however, high rates of relapse and CNS involvement usually lead to poor prognosis and limited survival. The prognosis for survival depends on whether there is CNS involvement. Despite the availability of multiple treatment modalities and regimens, the long-term prognosis for patients with PCNSL remains poor; the median survival with supportive care alone is 2–3 months, and with surgery alone, median survival is in the range of 1–5 months. The longest median survival in various reports approaches 40 months with treatment, and the 5-year overall survival is approximately 60%. Factors that negatively influence outcome include advanced age, worse neurologic functional classification level, multiple rather than single lesions present in the CNS, and deep nuclei/periventricular lesions rather than superficial cerebral and cerebellar hemispheric lesions.

Neoplastic Masquerade Syndromes Secondary to Systemic Lymphoma

Though rare, systemic lymphomas can spread hematogenously to the choroid, subretinal space, vitreous, and anterior chamber. These entities can present with a pseudohypopyon, vitritis, creamy subretinal infiltrates, retinal vasculitis, necrotizing retinitis, and diffuse choroiditis or uveal masses.

Neoplastic Masquerade Syndromes Secondary to Leukemia

Patients with leukemia may have retinal findings, including intraretinal hemorrhages, cotton-wool spots, white-centered hemorrhages, microaneurysms, and peripheral neovascularization. In rare instances, leukemic cells may invade the vitreous cavity. If the choroid is involved, exudative retinal detachment may be present and is angiographically similar to Vogt-Koyanagi-Harada (VKH) syndrome. Leukemia may also present with a hypopyon or hyphema, iris heterochromia, or a pseudohypopyon, which can be gray-yellow.

Neoplastic Masquerade Syndromes Secondary to Uveal Lymphoid Proliferations

The uveal tract may be a site for benign reactive uveal lymphoid hyperplasia that can mimic chronic uveitis. Presenting symptoms may include vision loss that is gradual, painless, and unilateral or bilateral. Early-stage disease shows multifocal creamy choroidal lesions that may mimic sarcoid uveitis or birdshot uveitis. Macular edema may be present. Anterior uveitis with acute symptoms of pain, redness, and photophobia may also be present. Glaucoma and elevated intraocular pressure (IOP) are common. Angle structures may be infiltrated by lymphocytes, resulting in elevation of IOP. There may be overlap in presentation with posterior scleritis and uveal effusion syndrome.

Fleshy episcleral or conjunctival masses that may appear salmon-pink may be present. Unlike subconjunctival lymphomas, these masses are not mobile and are attached firmly to the sclera. Biopsy specimens demonstrate mature lymphocytes and plasma cells, quite different from the appearance of specimens with PCNSL.

Therapy using corticosteroids, radiation, or both has been used with variable results. Systemic and periocular corticosteroid therapy can lead to rapid regression of the lesions, as can external-beam radiation.

Nonlymphoid Malignancies

Uveal melanoma

Approximately 5% of patients with uveal melanoma present with signs of ocular inflammation, including episcleritis, anterior or posterior uveitis, or panuveitis. Most tumors that present in this fashion are epithelioid-cell or mixed-cell choroidal melanomas. Ultrasonography is useful in diagnosing atypical cases because of the characteristically low internal reflectivity of these lesions. Management of uveal melanomas is discussed in BCSC Section 4, *Ophthalmic Pathology and Intraocular Tumors.*

Retinoblastoma

Approximately 1%–3% of retinoblastomas may present with the appearance of inflammation, caused primarily by the relatively rare variant of diffuse infiltrating retinoblastoma. Patients are usually between age 4 and 6 years at presentation. These cases can be diagnostically confusing because of the limited visibility of the fundus and the lack of calcification on radiography or ultrasonography. Patients may have conjunctival chemosis, pseudohypopyon, and vitritis. The pseudohypopyon typically shifts with changes in head position and is usually white as opposed to the yellowish color of inflammatory hypopyon.

Juvenile xanthogranuloma

Juvenile xanthogranuloma is the result of a histiocytic process affecting mainly the skin and eyes, and, in rare instances, viscera. Patients usually present before the age of 1 year with characteristic reddish-yellow skin lesions. Histologic investigation shows large histiocytes with foamy cytoplasm and Touton giant cells. Ocular lesions can involve the iris and result in a spontaneous hyphema. Iris biopsy samples show fewer foamy histiocytes and fewer Touton giant cells than do skin biopsy specimens. Other ocular structures may rarely be involved. If the skin of the eyelids is involved, the globe is usually spared. Intraocular lesions may respond to topical, periocular, or systemic corticosteroid therapy. Resistant cases may require local resection, radiation, or immunomodulatory therapy.

Zamir E, Wang RC, Krishnakumar S, Aiello Leverant A, Dugel PU, Rao NA. Juvenile xanthogranuloma masquerading as pediatric chronic uveitis: a clinicopathologic study. *Surv Ophthalmol.* 2001;46(2):164–171.

Metastatic Tumors

Most intraocular malignancies in adults are metastatic tumors. The most common primary cancers include lung and breast. Choroidal metastasis may be marked by vitritis, serous retinal detachment, and, occasionally, macular edema. These lesions are often bilateral and multifocal.

Anterior uveal metastasis may present with cells in the aqueous humor, iris nodules, neovascularization of the iris, and elevated IOP. Anterior chamber paracentesis may help confirm the diagnosis. Retinal metastases are extremely rare. Primary cancers metastatic to the retina include cutaneous melanoma (the most common), followed by lung, gastrointestinal, and breast cancer. Metastatic melanoma often produces brown spherules in the retina, whereas other metastatic cancers appear white to yellow and may result in perivascular sheathing, simulating a retinal vasculitis or necrotizing retinitis.

Bilateral Diffuse Uveal Melanocytic Proliferation

Bilateral diffuse uveal melanocytic tumors have been associated with systemic malignancy. Such tumors can be accompanied by rapid vision loss, cataracts, multiple pigmented and nonpigmented placoid iris and choroidal nodules, and serous retinal detachments. This condition can mimic VKH syndrome. Histologic investigation shows diffuse infiltration of the uveal tract by benign nevoid or spindle-shaped cells. Necrosis within the tumors may be present, and scleral involvement is common. The cause of this entity is unknown. Treatment should be directed at finding and treating the underlying primary lesion.

Gangaputra S, Kodati S, Kim M, Aranow M, Sen HN. Multimodal imaging in masquerade syndromes. *Ocul Immunol Inflamm.* 2017;25(2):160–168.

Nonneoplastic Masquerade Syndromes

Retinitis Pigmentosa

Patients with retinitis pigmentosa (RP) often have variable numbers of vitreous and anterior chamber cells and can develop macular edema. Features of RP that differentiate it from uveitis include nyctalopia, positive family history, and, on fundus examination, waxy disc pallor, attenuation of arterioles, and a bone-spicule pattern of pigmentary changes in the midperiphery. Electroretinographic responses of patients with RP often appear severely depressed or extinguished, even early in the disease. However, these findings can be found in late posterior uveitis, making differentiation between the entities very difficult in some cases. Late-stage birdshot chorioretinopathy can mimic RP (see BCSC Section 12, *Retina and Vitreous,* for additional information).

Ocular Ischemic Syndrome

Ocular ischemic syndrome results from hypoperfusion of the entire eye and sometimes the orbit, usually because of carotid artery obstruction. Patients with ocular ischemic syndrome are typically men aged 65 years or older. Patients present with decreased vision and mild ocular pain. Examination findings may include corneal edema, anterior chamber cells, and moderate flare, the last often greater than and out of proportion to the number of cells. Anterior segment neovascularization may be present. Intraocular pressure may be low from decreased aqueous production due to ischemia or high due to neovascular glaucoma. A cataract may be more prominent on the involved side. The vitreous is usually clear. Dilated fundus examination may show mild disc edema associated with dilated tortuous retinal venules, narrowed arterioles, and medium to large intraretinal scattered blot hemorrhages in the midperiphery and far periphery of the retina. Neovascularization may be present on the disc or elsewhere in the retina.

Fluorescein angiography shows delayed arteriolar filling, diffuse leakage in the posterior pole as well as from the optic disc, and signs of capillary nonperfusion. Retinal vascular staining may be present in the absence of any physical vascular sheathing on examination.

Diagnostic studies include carotid Doppler ultrasonography; ipsilateral carotid stenosis greater than 90% supports the diagnosis of ocular ischemic syndrome.

Definitive treatment involves carotid endarterectomy. Local treatment consists of topical corticosteroids and cycloplegics, as well as panretinal photocoagulation, especially if rubeosis or retinal neovascularization is present. Intraocular injection of vascular endothelial growth factor (VEGF) inhibitors may also be considered. The 5-year mortality rate of patients with ocular ischemic syndrome is 40%, primarily from cardiovascular disease and myocardial infarction. The visual prognosis is guarded, and many patients improve transiently with treatment but eventually worsen.

Mendrinos E, Machinis TG, Pournaras CJ. Ocular ischemic syndrome. *Surv Ophthalmol.* 2010;55(1):2–34.

Chronic Peripheral Rhegmatogenous Retinal Detachment

Chronic peripheral rhegmatogenous retinal detachment can be associated with anterior segment cell and flare and vitreous inflammatory and pigment cells. Patients often have good vision that can sometimes deteriorate because of macular edema. Careful dilated fundus examination with scleral depression is of paramount importance in establishing the diagnosis. Findings may include peripheral pigment demarcation lines, subretinal fluid, retinal breaks, subretinal fibrosis, and peripheral retinal cysts. Photoreceptor outer segments liberated from the subretinal space may be present in the anterior chamber, simulating inflammatory cells. In such situations, IOP may be elevated, as these photoreceptor outer segments are phagocytosed by the endothelial cells in the trabecular meshwork, resulting in secondary open-angle glaucoma. This condition is called *Schwartz syndrome.*

Schwartz A. Chronic open-angle glaucoma secondary to rhegmatogenous retinal detachment. *Am J Ophthalmol.* 1973;75(2):205–211.

Intraocular Foreign Bodies

Retained intraocular foreign bodies may produce chronic intraocular inflammation as the result of mechanical, chemical, toxic, or inflammatory irritation of uveal tissues (particularly the ciliary body). A high index of suspicion and the following are essential: a careful history; clinical examination; and ancillary testing, including gonioscopy, ultrasonography, and CT of the eye and orbits. If this condition is suspected and recognized quickly, identification and removal of the foreign body are often curative. If the diagnosis is delayed, ocular complications, such as proliferative vitreoretinopathy and endophthalmitis, result in a poorer visual prognosis.

Pigment Dispersion Syndrome

Pigment dispersion syndrome is characterized by pigment granules that have been released from the iris, ciliary body, or both and are floating in the anterior chamber; these granules may be confused with the cells of anterior uveitis. Refer to BCSC Section 10, *Glaucoma,* for a complete discussion.

Other Syndromes

Certain infectious uveitic entities may also be mistaken for immunologic uveitis. Thus, nonneoplastic masquerade syndromes can also include bacterial uveitis caused by infection with *Nocardia* species or *Tropheryma whipplei* (Whipple disease), as well as fungal endophthalmitis due to infection with *Candida* species, *Aspergillus* species, or *Coccidioides immitis.* These entities are discussed in Chapters 10 and 11.

CHAPTER 14

Complications of Uveitis

This chapter includes a related video, which can be accessed by scanning the QR code provided in the text or going to www.aao.org/bcscvideo_section09.

Highlights

- Vision loss in uveitis can result from multiple complications involving the cornea, lens, vitreous, retina, and optic nerve. Consequently, considerations in multiple ophthalmic subspecialties are required for optimal management of difficult cases.
- If surgical interventions are required, optimal perioperative inflammatory control is paramount.
- Uveitic macular edema is a common cause of vision loss in uveitis, can be diagnosed with optical coherence tomography, and is treated usually with optimal inflammatory control and often with adjunctive local steroids.

Calcific Band Keratopathy

Patients with chronic uveitis, especially children, may develop calcium deposition along the epithelial basement membrane and the Bowman layer, a condition termed *band keratopathy.* This complication is most often seen in juvenile idiopathic arthritis (JIA)–associated anterior uveitis and undifferentiated chronic anterior uveitis. It may arise within months of onset of the uveitis. These calcium deposits are usually located in the interpalpebral zone. Calcific band keratopathy may become visually significant when it extends into the visual axis, or it may cause symptoms of foreign-body sensation; in such cases, removal may be required. The calcium deposits are located beneath the corneal epithelium; thus, their removal requires epithelial debridement followed by chelation with disodium ethylenediaminetetraacetic acid (EDTA). Recurrences may require repeat EDTA treatments. Photorefractive keratotomy can also be considered.

Cataracts

Any eye with chronic or recurrent uveitis may develop cataract as a result of the inflammation or the corticosteroids used for treatment. Indications for cataract surgery in uveitic eyes are the same as for all cataracts: when the cataract causes functional impairment that interferes with activities of daily living, when the cataract is responsible for at least a portion of that decrease in vision, and when functional improvement is likely to occur after cataract extraction (a particularly important consideration in children who may develop amblyopia). Additional considerations for cataract surgery in uveitic eyes are whether a cataract precludes the clinician from obtaining an adequate view of the fundus—thereby inhibiting appropriate monitoring of posterior segment disease or health—and the degree to which the uveitis has been controlled.

As mentioned earlier, careful preoperative evaluation is necessary to ascertain whether the cataract is actually contributing to visual dysfunction. Vision loss in uveitis may stem from a variety of other ocular complications of uveitis, including corneal or vitreous opacity, macular edema, macular atrophy or fibrosis, and glaucoma.

Studies have shown that phacoemulsification with posterior chamber (in-the-bag) intraocular lens (IOL) implantation effectively improves vision and is well tolerated in many eyes with uveitis, even over long periods.

Management

Uveitic eyes are at greater risk for postoperative complications than nonuveitic eyes. Thus, careful planning, including preoperative medical management and the timing of the procedure, is critical. The key to a successful visual outcome is meticulous long-term control of inflammation prior to surgery. Common advice is to achieve the best control possible without flare-ups for at least 3 months prior to cataract surgery. The rationale is to ensure the eye is stable on the current medical regimen and the tissues are allowed to recover from prior inflammation before the eye is challenged with a surgical procedure that can lead to a profound postoperative inflammatory response.

The recommendation for maintenance of maximum control for at least 3 months before surgery is based on retrospective clinical case series and clinical experience; no prospective or controlled trials provide definitive data. As such, exceptions may be made when the considered opinion of the treating physician is that a delay in surgery is not indicated. Examples include eyes with mild uveitis lacking sequelae, disorders that have a good surgical prognosis (eg, Fuchs heterochromic uveitis), or special circumstances such as lens-induced uveitis or the need to view the posterior segment (eg, to repair a rhegmatogenous retinal detachment). It should be noted that the "best control possible" is not achieved by incomplete control with corticosteroids alone. The clinician must utilize all appropriate means for control, including immunosuppression if needed. If the clinician is uncomfortable with such means of treatment, then referral to a specialist with that experience is required before proceeding with cataract surgery.

Once appropriate control is achieved, preoperative pulsing with oral corticosteroids (0.5–1.0 mg/kg/day, usually for 3 days, although opinions vary as to dose and duration) and/or intensive topical corticosteroid treatment should be considered. Prospective comparative data regarding optimal perioperative inflammatory control are lacking, and accepted regimens largely rely on the surgeon's preference and experience. Dosages may be tapered over weeks to months after surgery, based on the severity of the underlying uveitis before surgery and the postoperative inflammatory response. Postoperative use of nonsteroidal anti-inflammatory drugs (NSAIDs) has not been studied in eyes with uveitis but is frequently employed in nonuveitic eyes that are undergoing cataract surgery, with the goal of preventing uveitic macular edema (UME). Corneal toxicity from topical NSAIDs used concurrently with topical corticosteroids is a concern. Patients with certain infectious uveitides (eg, uveitis caused by *Toxoplasma gondii* infection and herpetic uveitis) may require perioperative prophylactic antimicrobial therapy to prevent surgically induced recurrence—preoperative oral corticosteroids are usually not given.

Cataract surgery in uveitic eyes is generally more complex than in nonuveitic eyes because of the potential presence of sequelae of uveitis, including posterior synechiae, pupillary membranes, corneal edema or opacity, and hypotony. Entrance into the eye through a clear corneal approach is often used and may be particularly desirable in cases of scleritis that may be prone to postoperative scleral necrosis. Posterior synechiae and pupillary miosis may require mechanical or viscoelastic pupil stretching, sphincterotomies, or the use of flexible iris retractors (Video 14-1).

VIDEO 14-1 Synechiolysis, placement of iris dilator, and capsular staining in a patient with uveitis.
Courtesy of Russell W. Read, MD, PhD.
Access the video at www.aao.org/bcscvideo_section09.

Although a curvilinear capsulorrhexis is preferred, a fibrotic anterior capsule may be more difficult to open with a capsulorrhexis than with a can-opener capsulotomy. Zonular insufficiency may be present, which may make phacoemulsification and lens implantation challenging or impossible. In such cases, there may be few alternatives, and the surgeon's preference may be to perform pars plana lensectomy and vitrectomy and avoid placing an IOL because of the lack of capsular support or zonular dehiscence. Fortunately, this scenario is rare. Meticulous cortical cleanup is important to avoid leaving behind potentially proinflammatory material in the eye. For IOL choice, many surgeons prefer hydrophobic acrylic posterior chamber IOLs placed in the capsular bag. The possibility of future vitreoretinal surgery with silicone oil should be considered when deciding whether to use silicone IOLs. At the conclusion of the surgery, periocular or intravitreal corticosteroids may be administered. Postoperatively, immunomodulation is continued and supplemented with liberal use of topical corticosteroids, which are slowly tapered.

Phacoemulsification with IOL implantation can also be done in conjunction with pars plana vitrectomy if clinical or ultrasonographic findings suggest the presence of substantial vision-limiting vitreous debris or macular pathology such as epiretinal membranes. When there has been significant structural damage from inflammation, or in cases in which the surgical prognosis is more guarded (eg, in JIA-associated uveitis), vitrectomy and aphakia may be the best course. Relative contraindications for IOL implantation include the prior development of rubeosis, a history of extensive membrane formation, and hypotony, although even in these circumstances, an IOL may be used in select cases.

There is controversy regarding IOL placement in children with JIA-associated uveitic cataracts. Avoiding aphakia in children is desirable but may not always be in the best interest of the patient. Choosing the proper IOL power, especially in children under the age of 10 years, is difficult because of normal ocular/orbital growth. (For more information about IOL use in children, see BCSC Section 6, *Pediatric Ophthalmology and Strabismus.*) Regardless, the most important step in the treatment of these children is stringent control of preoperative and postoperative intraocular inflammation using corticosteroids and immunomodulatory therapy (IMT). If IOLs are used, in-the-bag implantation of acrylic IOLs and primary posterior capsulorrhexis are preferred in children. Silicone IOLs are not typically used in uveitic cataracts. These IOLs may lead to suboptimal outcomes and complicate future vitreoretinal surgery. Some surgeons may also perform a core anterior vitrectomy through the posterior capsulorrhexis prior to IOL placement. Administration of intraocular corticosteroids at the end of the procedure is extremely useful for controlling postoperative inflammation and UME. If these methods are used, 75% of patients will obtain a visual acuity of better than 20/40.

Mehta S, Linton MM, Kempen JH. Outcomes of cataract surgery in patients with uveitis: a systematic review and meta-analysis. *Am J Ophthalmol.* 2014;158(4):676–692.

Sen HN, Abreu FM, Louis TA, et al; Multicenter Uveitis Steroid Treatment (MUST) Trial and Follow-up Study Research Group. Cataract surgery outcomes in uveitis: the Multicenter Uveitis Steroid Treatment trial. *Ophthalmology.* 2016;123(1):183–190.

Complications

Close monitoring with immediate attention to any postoperative increase in inflammation or complications is imperative. Visual compromise following phacoemulsification with posterior chamber lens implantation in patients with uveitis is usually attributed to posterior segment abnormalities, most commonly UME. Postoperative UME rates may be reduced through the use of perioperative corticosteroids and with delay of surgery until the uveitis has been controlled for at least 3 months. The postoperative course may also be complicated by the recurrence or exacerbation of uveitis. The incidence of posterior capsule opacification is higher in uveitic than nonuveitic eyes, leading to earlier use of Nd:YAG laser capsulotomy. Furthermore, Nd:YAG capsulotomy may exacerbate uveitis, suggesting that some uveitis patients undergoing capsulotomy may benefit from more careful monitoring after the procedure. In some uveitic conditions, such as pars planitis, inflammatory debris may accumulate, and membranes may form on the surface of the IOL. Strict control of inflammation remains paramount for reducing the chance of these deposits. Long-term administration of topical corticosteroids may be necessary. Despite aggressive use of IMT, inflammatory cocooning of the IOL–lens capsule complex and uncontrolled inflammation may necessitate IOL explantation in 5%–10% of patients. Frequent follow-up, a high index of suspicion, and aggressive IMT can optimize short- and long-term visual results.

AAO PPP Committee, Secretary for Quality of Care, Hoskins Center for Quality Eye Care. Preferred Practice Pattern® Clinical Questions. *Preoperative Control of Uveitis.* San Francisco: American Academy of Ophthalmology; 2013. Available at www.aao.org/ppp

Adán A, Gris O, Pelegrin L, Torras J, Corretger X. Explantation of intraocular lenses in children with juvenile idiopathic arthritis–associated uveitis. *J Cataract Refract Surg.* 2009;35(3):603–605.

Bélair ML, Kim SJ, Thorne JE, et al. Incidence of cystoid macular edema after cataract surgery in patients with and without uveitis using optical coherence tomography. *Am J Ophthalmol.* 2009;148(1):128–135.

Jancevski M, Foster CS. Cataracts and uveitis. *Curr Opin Ophthalmol.* 2010;21(1):10–14.

Nemet AY, Raz J, Sachs D, et al. Primary intraocular lens implantation in pediatric uveitis: a comparison of 2 populations. *Arch Ophthalmol.* 2007;125(3):354–360.

Quiñones K, Cervantes-Castañeda RA, Hynes AY, Daoud YJ, Foster CS. Outcomes of cataract surgery in children with chronic uveitis. *J Cataract Refract Surg.* 2009;35(4):725–731.

Glaucoma

Elevated intraocular pressure (IOP) in uveitic eyes may be acute, chronic, or recurrent. In eyes with long-term ciliary body inflammation, the IOP may fluctuate between abnormally high and low values. Numerous morphologic, cellular, and biochemical alterations occur in the uveitic eye that cause uveitic glaucoma and ocular hypertension. Successful management of uveitic glaucoma and ocular hypertension requires the identification and treatment of each of these contributing factors.

Assessment of patients with uveitis and elevated IOP should include the same measures taken as for any case of ocular hypertension: slit-lamp and dilated fundus examination, gonioscopy, evaluation of the optic nerve head with disc photographs and optical coherence tomography (OCT), and serial automated visual fields.

Moorthy RS, Mermoud A, Baerveldt G, Minckler DS, Lee PP, Rao NA. Glaucoma associated with uveitis. *Surv Ophthalmol.* 1997;41(5):361–394.

Uveitic Ocular Hypertension

Unilateral uveitis of sudden onset with open angles and increased IOP may be of infectious origin, particularly from viral causes but also from *Toxoplasma*. Thus, in the presence of active inflammation early in the course of uveitis, clinicians should resist the urge to prematurely taper corticosteroids because of a fear of corticosteroid-induced ocular hypertension. Corticosteroid-induced ocular hypertension rarely occurs before 3 weeks after the initiation of corticosteroid therapy. Early IOP elevations with active inflammation are almost always caused by inflammation that requires aggressive anti-inflammatory treatment.

Uveitic Glaucoma

Uveitic glaucoma often results from a combination of mechanisms. Glaucoma associated with uveitis is best classified by morphologic changes in angle structure; thus, uveitic glaucoma may be divided into secondary angle-closure and secondary open-angle glaucoma. These entities may be further subdivided into acute and chronic types. In addition, corticosteroid-induced ocular hypertension and glaucoma are other components that must be addressed in cases of chronic uveitic glaucoma. See also BCSC Section 10, *Glaucoma.*

Secondary angle-closure glaucoma

Acute with central shallowing of the anterior chamber Acute secondary angle-closure glaucoma may occur when choroidal inflammation results in forward rotation of the ciliary body and lens–iris diaphragm. It can be the presenting sign of Vogt-Koyanagi-Harada (VKH) syndrome or sympathetic ophthalmia. Patients present with pain, elevated IOP, and no posterior synechiae. Ultrasound biomicroscopy (UBM) or ultrasound evaluation showing choroidal thickening and anterior rotation of the ciliary body is diagnostic. Treatment is with aggressive corticosteroid therapy, aqueous suppressants, and cycloplegia to induce a posterior rotation of the ciliary body. As the inflammation subsides, the chamber deepens and the IOP normalizes. Peripheral iridotomy or iridectomy is not useful in these acute cases because the underlying cause is not pupillary block.

Acute without central shallowing of the anterior chamber Chronic or acute recurrent anterior segment inflammation may result in the formation of circumferential posterior synechiae with pupillary block due to seclusion of the pupil and resultant iris bombé, producing secondary peripheral angle closure. Whereas synechiae formation usually occurs over time, the development of iris bombé may be an acute event. Peripheral laser iridotomy or surgical iridectomy results in resolution of the bombé and angle closure if performed before permanent peripheral anterior synechiae form. Iridotomies should be multiple, created as large as possible. Exacerbation of inflammation can be anticipated after laser iridotomy in these eyes, making the iridotomies prone to close and requiring re-treatment or surgical iridectomy. Intensive topical corticosteroid and cycloplegic therapy is given following the procedure. In patients with brown irides, pretreatment of the iris with an argon laser before using the Nd:YAG laser may lessen the chance of bleeding and facilitate a wider opening. If laser iridotomy is not successful, surgical iridectomy is required. The procedure may be supplemented with goniosynechialysis if peripheral anterior synechiae have started to develop, but this approach is controversial.

Chronic In addition to posterior synechiae, chronic intraocular inflammation may result in peripheral anterior synechiae and chronic secondary angle-closure glaucoma. Eyes with these complications often have chronic secondary open-angle glaucoma and corticosteroid-induced glaucoma superimposed. Topical aqueous suppressants may be inadequate to prevent progression of optic nerve head damage. These eyes may require goniosynechialysis and trabeculectomy with mitomycin C or placement of a glaucoma drainage device. See BCSC Section 10, *Glaucoma,* for a more detailed discussion on surgical treatment of glaucoma.

Secondary open-angle glaucoma

Acute Inflammatory open-angle glaucoma occurs when the trabecular meshwork is inflamed (trabeculitis), as commonly occurs with infectious causes of uveitis such as toxoplasmic retinochoroiditis, necrotizing herpetic retinitis, herpes simplex and varicella-zoster anterior uveitis, cytomegalovirus anterior uveitis (including the Posner-Schlossman type), and sarcoid uveitis or when inflammatory debris clogs the angle. This type of glaucoma usually responds to specific treatment of the infectious agent supplemented by topical cycloplegics and corticosteroids.

Chronic Chronic outflow obstruction is caused by direct damage to the trabecular meshwork. The management of chronic secondary open-angle glaucoma is similar to that of primary open-angle glaucoma (see BCSC Section 10, *Glaucoma*), with the added complexity of maintaining strict control of intraocular inflammation through the use of IMT.

Combined-mechanism uveitic glaucoma

Multiple mechanisms may be responsible for elevated pressure in uveitic eyes. Treatment should be aimed at controlling the inflammation and IOP through a multimodal approach, including both medical and surgical therapy aimed at the responsible mechanisms.

Corticosteroid-Induced Ocular Hypertension and Glaucoma

Elevated IOP in the setting of uveitis should prompt consideration of whether the cause is one of the aforementioned angle issues or is corticosteroid induced. Corticosteroids in any formulation—topical, periocular, intraocular (injection and sustained release), or oral—may induce an elevation of IOP that may be difficult to distinguish from other causes of ocular hypertension in uveitis. Use of the fluocinolone intraocular implant is associated with an eventual need for glaucoma surgery in approximately 40% of eyes. Difluprednate used topically also appears to be associated with significant and sometimes rapid increases in IOP. This IOP rise may be avoided by use of a less-potent topical corticosteroid preparation, a less-frequent administration schedule, or both. Fluorometholone, loteprednol, and rimexolone may be less likely to induce an IOP elevation but are also less effective in controlling intraocular inflammation.

Management

Medical management of uveitic glaucoma requires aggressive control of both intraocular inflammation and IOP as well as prevention of glaucomatous optic nerve damage and visual field loss (see BCSC Section 10, *Glaucoma*). Aqueous suppressants are generally the first-line agents. Prostaglandin analogues may be used to treat uveitic glaucoma and generally do not exacerbate intraocular inflammation, especially when used concomitantly with IMT and corticosteroids. However, caution should be used in eyes with herpetic uveitis. Use of pilocarpine should be avoided in uveitis, as the smaller fixed pupil may be at risk for worsening of posterior synechiae, and pilocarpine causes breakdown of the blood–aqueous barrier.

When medical management fails, glaucoma filtering surgery is indicated. Standard trabeculectomy has a greater risk of failure in these eyes. Results may be improved by using mitomycin C with intensive topical corticosteroids. However, intense and recurrent postoperative inflammation can often lead to failure of filtering surgery in uveitic eyes. Up to 90% of patients 1 year after surgery and approximately 62% 5 years after surgery achieve IOP control with 1 or 0 medications. Surgical complications include cataract formation, bleb leakage (early and late) that could lead to endophthalmitis, and choroidal effusions.

Alternatives to classic trabeculectomy are numerous and have been used with some short-term success in uveitic glaucoma. Nonpenetrating deep sclerectomy with or without a drainage implant has been shown effective in controlling IOP in up to 90% of uveitic eyes for 1 year after surgery. Viscocanalostomy has shown higher success rates in a limited number of studies. Among pediatric uveitis patients, goniotomy has up to a 75% chance of reducing IOP to 21 mm Hg or less after 2 surgeries. This procedure may be complicated by transient hyphema and worsening of the preexisting cataract. Trabeculodialysis and laser sclerostomy have high rates of failure because of recurrent postoperative inflammation. The role of minimally invasive glaucoma surgery remains unclear in uveitis.

Most cases of uveitic glaucoma, especially in pseudophakic or aphakic eyes, require aqueous drainage devices. These devices may be tunneled into the anterior chamber or placed through the pars plana directly into the vitreous cavity after vitrectomy. A unidirectional valve design (valve implant) can prevent postoperative hypotony. These implants are more likely than trabeculectomy to successfully control IOP in the long term; results indicate up to a 75% reduction of IOP from preoperative levels and that nearly 75% of patients achieve target IOP levels with use of 0 or 1 topical antiglaucoma medication after 4 years. Complications of glaucoma-drainage-device surgery (10%/patient-year) include shallow anterior chamber, hypotony, suprachoroidal hemorrhage, and blockage of the drainage device by blood, fibrin, or iris. Long-term complications include device erosion through the conjunctiva, valve migration, corneal decompensation, drainage device–cornea touch, and retinal detachment. Unlike trabeculectomy, these drainage devices have proven to be robust and continue to function despite chronic, recurrent inflammation; they provide excellent long-term IOP control in eyes with uveitic glaucoma.

Cyclodestructive procedures may worsen ocular inflammation and lead to hypotony and phthisis bulbi. Laser trabeculoplasty is generally considered ineffective in eyes with uveitis.

As with all surgeries in uveitic eyes, tight and meticulous control of perioperative inflammation—including the use of preoperative regimens similar to those used before cataract surgery as well as of immunomodulators and corticosteroids—not only improves the success of glaucoma surgery but also improves visual acuity outcomes by limiting sight-threatening complications such as UME and hypotony. Additional details and information on surgical procedures for uveitic glaucoma are described in BCSC Section 10, *Glaucoma.*

Bohnsack BL, Freedman SF. Surgical outcomes in childhood uveitic glaucoma. *Am J Ophthalmol.* 2013;155(1):134–142.

Fortuna E, Cervantes-Castañeda RA, Bhat P, Doctor P, Foster CS. Flare-up rates with bimatoprost therapy in uveitic glaucoma. *Am J Ophthalmol.* 2008;146(6):876–882.

Heinz C, Koch JM, Heiligenhaus A. Transscleral diode laser cyclophotocoagulation as primary surgical treatment for secondary glaucoma in juvenile idiopathic arthritis: high failure rate after short term follow up. *Br J Ophthalmol.* 2006;90(6):737–740.

Kafkala C, Hynes A, Choi J, Topalkara A, Foster CS. Ahmed valve implantation for uncontrolled pediatric uveitic glaucoma. *J AAPOS.* 2005;9(4):336–340.

Markomichelakis NN, Kostakou A, Halkiadakis I, Chalkidou S, Papakonstantinou D, Georgopoulos G. Efficacy and safety of latanoprost in eyes with uveitic glaucoma. *Graefes Arch Clin Exp Ophthalmol.* 2009;247(6):775–780.

Noble J, Derzko-Dzulynsky L, Rabinovitch T, Birt C. Outcome of trabeculectomy with intraoperative mitomycin C for uveitic glaucoma. *Can J Ophthalmol.* 2007;42(1):89–94.

Papadaki TG, Zacharopoulos IP, Pasquale LR, Christen WB, Netland PA, Foster CS. Long-term results of Ahmed glaucoma valve implantation for uveitic glaucoma. *Am J Ophthalmol.* 2007;144(1):62–69.

William A, Spitzer MS, Doycheva D, Dimopoulos S, Leitritz MA, Voykov B. Comparison of ab externo trabeculotomy in primary open-angle glaucoma and uveitic glaucoma: long-term outcomes. *Clin Ophthalmol.* 2016:10;929–934.

Hypotony

Acute inflammation of the ciliary body may cause aqueous hyposecretion and low IOP. This reduction in IOP is reversible with control of intraocular inflammation. In contrast, chronic inflammation may lead to ciliary body damage and atrophy of the ciliary processes, resulting in permanent hypotony. Hypotony may result in hypotony maculopathy, vision loss, and/or phthisis. Serous choroidal detachment often accompanies hypotony and complicates management. Prolonged choroidal effusions may require surgical drainage. Chronic hypotony can be treated with long-term local steroid administration in some cases. Surgery is indicated if there is ciliary body traction from a cyclitic membrane that can be released and if the ciliary processes are preserved (as shown on UBM). If ciliary processes are atrophic, vitrectomy with intraocular silicone oil or viscoelastic may help maintain ocular anatomy and increase IOP. In some of these cases, vision improvement after surgery can be significant; these gains may, however, be transient.

Daniel E, Pistilli M, Kothari S, et al; Systemic Immunosuppressive Therapy for Eye Diseases Research Group. Risk of ocular hypertension in adults with noninfectious uveitis. *Ophthalmology.* 2017;124(8):1196–1208.

Kapur R, Birnbaum AD, Goldstein DA, et al. Treating uveitis-associated hypotony with pars plana vitrectomy and silicone oil injection. *Retina.* 2010;30(1):140–145.

Sen HN, Drye LT, Goldstein DA, et al; Multicenter Uveitis Steroid Treatment (MUST) Trial Research Group. Hypotony in patients with uveitis: The Multicenter Uveitis Steroid Treatment (MUST) Trial. *Ocul Immunol Inflamm.* 2012;20(2):104–112.

Uveitic Macular Edema

Uveitic macular edema is a common cause of vision loss in eyes with uveitis. The edema is usually caused by active intraocular inflammation and appears to be mediated by the proinflammatory cytokines vascular endothelial growth factor (VEGF) and interleukin-6, which cause retinal vascular leakage and retinal pigment endothelium dysfunction. Less commonly, UME may be caused by mechanical vitreomacular traction; the distinction can be differentiated by OCT. It can also be quantitatively evaluated and monitored by serial spectral-domain OCT and fluorescein angiography studies. The severity of UME does not necessarily correspond to the level of inflammatory disease activity; UME is often slow to respond and clear and frequently remains even after visible, active inflammation has resolved. Smoking appears to be associated with a greater prevalence of UME, especially in patients with intermediate uveitis and panuveitis.

Lin P, Loh AR, Margolis TP, Acharya NR. Cigarette smoking as a risk factor for uveitis. *Ophthalmology.* 2010;117(3):585–590.

Rothova A. Inflammatory cystoid macular edema. *Curr Opin Ophthalmol.* 2007;18(6):487–492.

Treatment

Treatment of UME must first be directed toward control of intraocular inflammation. If UME persists despite control of inflammation, therapy directed specifically toward the UME is required. This treatment may be regional or systemic. Periocular injections of corticosteroid may be used; a superotemporal posterior sub-Tenon injection of 20–40 mg of triamcinolone acetonide is preferred. Theoretically, this technique delivers juxtascleral corticosteroid closest to the macula. The injections may be repeated monthly. If UME persists, then 2–4 mg of intravitreal preservative-free triamcinolone may be considered. Intravitreal triamcinolone can be highly effective in reducing UME, particularly in non-vitrectomized eyes, but its effect is time limited; the drug is eliminated more quickly from the vitreous cavity of vitrectomized eyes. Visual improvement and reduction of UME after intravitreal triamcinolone injection typically occur within 4 weeks. Eyes with a longer duration of UME and worse vision on presentation tend to show the least amount of vision improvement after treatment with intravitreal triamcinolone. Corticosteroid-induced elevation of IOP may occur in up to 40% of patients, especially in those younger than 40 years.

Sustained delivery of corticosteroid to the vitreous cavity through the use of implants is also effective. Currently available implants in the United States include Retisert (Bausch + Lomb), Ozurdex (Allergan), and Yutiq (EyePoint Pharmaceuticals). The risk of ocular hypertension is lower for the dexamethasone delivery system than for the fluocinolone implant. The VEGF inhibitors can also reduce inflammatory UME, but the action is of short duration and repeat injections are required. Intravitreal methotrexate (400 μg/0.1 mL) has been shown to be effective in reducing UME in a limited number of patients and is under active investigation. See Chapter 5 for additional information on the use of corticosteroids in the treatment of uveitis including UME.

Topical NSAIDs can be beneficial in treating pseudophakic UME, but their effectiveness in the treatment of UME has not been established. Oral acetazolamide, 500 mg once or twice daily, has also been effective in reducing UME, particularly in patients whose inflammation is well controlled. Systemic interferon therapy has shown efficacy in resolving recalcitrant UME, with complete control in 62.5% of patients in one study. Common adverse effects include flulike symptoms.

Surgical therapy for UME is still controversial. Pars plana vitrectomy for UME in the presence of hyaloidal traction on the macula (as demonstrated on OCT imaging) may be visually and anatomically beneficial. In the absence of vitreomacular traction, however, the efficacy of pars plana vitrectomy in treating UME is not well understood. There is some suggestion that vitrectomy may be beneficial in managing recalcitrant UME, but this application requires further investigation.

Becker M, Davis J. Vitrectomy in the treatment of uveitis. *Am J Ophthalmol.* 2005;140(6): 1096–1105.

Deuter CM, Kötter I, Günaydin I, Stübiger N, Doycheva DG, Zierhut M. Efficacy and tolerability of interferon alpha treatment in patients with chronic cystoid macular oedema due to non-infectious uveitis. *Br J Ophthalmol.* 2009;93(7):906–913.

Jennings T, Rusin MM, Tessler HH, Cunha-Vaz JG. Posterior sub-Tenon's injections of corticosteroids in uveitis patients with cystoid macular edema. *Jpn J Ophthalmol.* 1988;32(4): 385–391.
Kok H, Lau C, Maycock N, McCluskey P, Lightman S. Outcome of intravitreal triamcinolone in uveitis. *Ophthalmology.* 2005;112(11):1916.e1–e7.
Schilling H, Heiligenhaus A, Laube T, Bornfeld N, Jurklies B. Long-term effect of acetazolamide treatment of patients with uveitic chronic cystoid macular edema is limited by persisting inflammation. *Retina.* 2005;25(2):182–188.
Taylor SR, Habot-Wilner Z, Pacheco P, Lightman SL. Intraocular methotrexate in the treatment of uveitis and uveitic cystoid macular edema. *Ophthalmology.* 2009;116(4): 797–801.
Tran TH, de Smet MD, Bodaghi B, Fardeau C, Cassoux N, Lehoang P. Uveitic macular oedema: correlation between optical coherence tomography patterns with visual acuity and fluorescein angiography. *Br J Ophthalmol.* 2008;92(7):922–927.

Epiretinal Membrane and Macular Hole

Epiretinal membranes, both with and without traction, and macular holes can occur in patients with active or inactive uveitis. They often are associated with significant vision loss. Although it makes intuitive sense to apply standard surgical therapy with pars plana vitrectomy, membrane peel, internal-limiting membrane peel, and/or gas tamponade, there is a lack of consensus on the optimal techniques, timing, and case selection for surgical therapy. Isolated cases of both conditions that have improved with maximal medical management alone have been described. It is clear that optimal control of inflammation is essential in optimizing visual results. If surgery is performed, aggressive perioperative inflammatory control is paramount. This is typically achieved with perioperative oral or local steroids. Standard vitreoretinal techniques are described in in BCSC Section 12, *Retina and Vitreous.* These techniques have been reported to produce favorable results in multiple case series in the treatment of epiretinal membranes and macular holes in uveitic eyes,

Branson SV, McClafferty BR, Kurup SK. Vitrectomy for epiretinal membranes and macular holes in uveitis patients. *J Ocul Pharmacol Ther.* 2017;33(4):298–303.
Callaway NF, Gonzalez MA, Yonekawa Y, et al. Outcomes of pars plana vitrectomy for macular hole in patients with uveitis. *Retina.* 2018;38(Suppl 1):S41–S48.

Vitreous Opacification and Vitritis

Vitreous membranes in chronic cases not responding to steroid treatment to a degree that vision is affected may occur in uveitis. Vitrectomy in eyes with quiet inflammation may improve visual acuity in these cases, with 1 review of studies on pars plana vitrectomy in uveitis showing visual acuity improved in 68%. A standard small (25- or 23-gauge) 3-port pars plana vitrectomy is the preferred technique, with a few minor variations (see BCSC Section 12, *Retina and Vitreous*).

Davis JL, Miller DM, Ruiz P. Diagnostic testing of vitrectomy specimens. *Am J Ophthalmol.* 2005;140(5):822–829.
Manku H, McCluskey P. Diagnostic vitreous biopsy in patients with uveitis: a useful investigation? *Clin Exp Ophthalmol.* 2005;33(6):604–610.

Rhegmatogenous Retinal Detachment

Rhegmatogenous retinal detachment (RRD) occurs in 3% of patients with uveitis. Panuveitis and infectious uveitis are the entities most frequently associated with RRD, although pars planitis and posterior uveitis can also be associated with rhegmatogenous or tractional retinal detachments. Uveitis is often still active in eyes that present with RRD. Up to 30% of patients with uveitis and RRD may have proliferative vitreoretinopathy (PVR) at presentation; this percentage is significantly higher than in primary RRD in patients without uveitis. Repair is often complicated by preexisting PVR, vitreous membranes, and poor visualization. Repair of retinal detachment in uveitis is challenging and may require the full armamentarium of surgical strategies employed in complex retinal detachment repair. Additionally, it is essential to control inflammation aggressively in the perioperative period.

Acute retinal necrosis and cytomegalovirus retinitis frequently lead to retinal detachments that are difficult to repair because of multiple, often occult, posterior retinal breaks. The benefit of prophylactic laser treatment applied as soon as adequate visualization can be achieved is controversial. Pars plana vitrectomy and endolaser treatment with internal silicone oil tamponade are most often required to repair these detachments.

Kerkhoff FT, Lamberts QJ, van den Biesen PR, Rothova A. Rhegmatogenous retinal detachment and uveitis. *Ophthalmology.* 2003;110(2):427–431.
Nussenblatt RB, Whitcup SM. *Uveitis: Fundamentals and Clinical Practice.* 4th ed. Philadelphia, PA: Mosby; 2010.

Retinal and Choroidal Neovascularization

Retinal neovascularization is most often associated with posterior uveitis. Some diseases are more prone to be complicated by CNV (eg, as multifocal choroiditis, punctate inner choroiditis, or serpiginous choroiditis), whereas some are more likely to be complicated by retinal neovascularization (eg, retinal vasculitis of various causes, including Eales disease). Retinal neovascularization results from chronic inflammation or capillary nonperfusion. Treatment is directed toward the underlying etiology. The presence of uveitic retinal neovascularization does not always require panretinal photocoagulation. Some cases of sarcoid panuveitis, for example, may present with neovascularization of the disc that resolves completely with immunomodulatory and corticosteroid therapy alone. Thus, treatment must first be directed toward reduction of inflammation. If ischemia is angiographically extensive, as in retinal vasculitis or Eales disease, scatter laser photocoagulation in the ischemic areas is therapeutic. Dramatic regression of neovascularization of the disc and elsewhere in various inflammatory disorders typically occurs after 1 or 2 intravitreal injections of a VEGF inhibitor. This treatment may be used as an adjunct to IMT and scatter laser photocoagulation.

Choroidal neovascularization (CNV) can develop in uveitis as a result of a disruption of the Bruch membrane from choroidal inflammation and the presence of inflammatory cytokines that promote angiogenesis. The prevalence of CNV varies among different entities; for example, it can occur in up to 10% of patients with VKH syndrome. Patients present with metamorphopsia and scotoma, and diagnosis is based on clinical and angiographic findings. Treatment should be directed toward reducing inflammation as well as anatomical ablation of the CNV. Treatment of subfoveal CNV is accomplished with VEGF inhibitors; results of one study showed that 2–3 intravitreal injections improved vision and reduced the size of subfoveal CNV in nearly all patients. Control of inflammation in these cases may reduce the risk of recurrence of CNV and the need for repeated intravitreal injections.

Baxter SL, Pistilli M, Pujari SS, et al. Risk of choroidal neovascularization among the uveitides. *Am J Ophthalmol.* 2013;156(3):468–477.e2.

Doctor PP, Bhat P, Sayed R, Foster CS. Intravitreal bevacizumab for uveitic choroidal neovascularization. *Ocul Immunol Inflamm.* 2009;17(2):118–126.

Lott MN, Schiffman JC, Davis JL. Bevacizumab in inflammatory eye disease. *Am J Ophthalmol.* 2009;148(5):711–717.

O'Toole L, Tufail A, Pavesio C. Management of choroidal neovascularization in uveitis. *Int Ophthalmol Clin.* 2005;45(2).157–177.

Vision Rehabilitation

Despite optimal treatment, inflammatory disorders of the eye can lead to decreased vision. Worldwide, inflammatory disease is a significant cause of blindness and low vision. In the United States, 10% of all blindness is attributed to inadequately treated uveitis. Clinicians can assist their patients by inquiring if vision loss secondary to inflammation is affecting day-to-day functions, such as reading or enjoying leisure activities, and by advising patients about vision rehabilitation resources. Referral to vision rehabilitation is recommended for patients with visual acuity less than 20/40 in the better eye, reduced contrast sensitivity, disabling glare, or central or peripheral visual field loss (see BCSC Section 3, *Clinical Optics*). The low vision section of the American Academy of Ophthalmology website (www.aao.org/low-vision-and-vision-rehab) defines low vision and discusses low vision symptoms, diagnosis, treatment, rehabilitation, vision aids, and how patients can identify vision rehabilitation resources in their community.

It is particularly important for clinicians to provide parents of children with uveitis information about rehabilitation to optimize functioning at school and in other activities. A useful guide for teachers and parents can be found at www.uveitis.org/patients/education/patient-guides.

American Academy of Ophthalmology Vision Rehabilitation Committee. Preferred Practice Pattern® Guidelines. *Vision Rehabilitation.* San Francisco: American Academy of Ophthalmology; 2017. Available at www.aao.org/ppp

CHAPTER 15

Ocular Involvement in AIDS

Highlights

- Acquired immunodeficiency syndrome (AIDS) causes a microangiopathy known as *human immunodeficiency virus (HIV) retinopathy.*
- Opportunistic infections—such as cytomegalovirus (CMV) retinitis, *Pneumocystis jirovecii* choroiditis, and *Cryptococcus neoformans* choroiditis—have become less common since the introduction of highly active antiretroviral therapy.
- Immune recovery uveitis is intraocular sterile inflammation that occurs following CMV retinitis as the T-cell count improves with successful HIV therapy.
- Malignancies such as vitreoretinal lymphoma and Kaposi sarcoma are associated with AIDS.

Acquired immunodeficiency syndrome is caused by HIV, which infects and results in the depletion of $CD4^+$ helper T lymphocytes. This loss of $CD4^+$ T lymphocytes causes profound immune deficiency with subsequent opportunistic infections. Refer to BCSC Section 1, *Update on General Medicine,* for a full discussion of HIV infection and AIDS.

Ophthalmic Manifestations

Ophthalmic manifestations may be the first sign of disseminated systemic HIV infection and have been reported in up to 70% of infected people. These manifestations include

- HIV-related microangiopathy of the retina
- opportunistic viral, bacterial, parasitic, and fungal infections
- Kaposi sarcoma of the eyelid and conjunctiva
- lymphomas primarily involving the retina/vitreous (primary vitreoretinal lymphoma), adnexal structures, and orbit
- squamous cell carcinoma of the conjunctiva

Reports also suggest that HIV infection itself may cause anterior or intermediate uveitis that is not responsive to corticosteroids but improves with antiretroviral therapy.

The most common ocular finding in patients infected with HIV is HIV retinopathy. It is a microangiopathy, characterized mainly by cotton-wool spots (Fig 15-1) but also by microaneurysms and retinal hemorrhages. HIV has been isolated from the human retina, and its antigen has been detected in retinal endothelial cells. The HIV endothelial infection

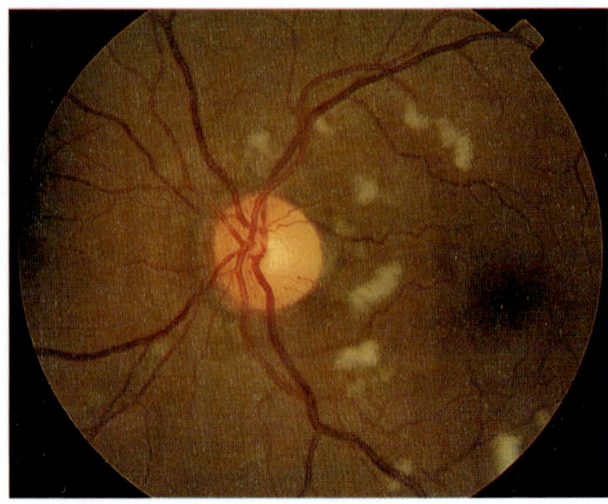

Figure 15-1 Fundus photograph of human immunodeficiency virus (HIV) retinopathy with numerous cotton-wool spots. *(Reprinted with permission from Cunningham ET Jr, Belfort R Jr.* HIV/AIDS and the Eye: A Global Perspective. Ophthalmology Monograph 15. *San Francisco, CA: American Academy of Ophthalmology; 2002:55.)*

and/or rheologic abnormalities may play a role in the development of cotton-wool spots and other vascular alterations. In addition, accelerated aging may be a part of HIV-associated eye disease, with earlier onset of macular degeneration and cataracts.

Other infectious agents that can affect the eye in HIV-infected patients include cytomegalovirus (CMV), herpes simplex and zoster viruses, *Toxoplasma gondii, Treponema pallidum, Mycobacterium tuberculosis, Mycobacterium avium-intracellulare, Cryptococcus neoformans, Pneumocystis jirovecii, Histoplasma capsulatum, Candida* species, molluscum contagiosum virus, microsporidia, and others. These pathogens can infect the ocular adnexa, anterior segment, or posterior segment. Visual morbidity, however, occurs primarily with posterior segment involvement, particularly retinitis caused by CMV, herpes simplex or zoster virus, *T pallidum*, or *T gondii*.

Dadgostar H, Holland GN, Huang X, et al. Hemorheologic abnormalities associated with HIV infection: in vivo assessment of retinal microvascular blood flow. *Invest Ophthalmol Vis Sci.* 2006;47(9):3933–3938.

Kalyani PS, Fawzi AA, Gangaputra S, et al; Studies of the Ocular Complications of AIDS Research Group. Retinal vessel caliber among people with acquired immunodeficiency syndrome: relationships with visual function. *Am J Ophthalmol.* 2012;153(3):428–433.

Cytomegalovirus Retinitis

Before the availability of potent antiretroviral treatment regimens, disseminated CMV infection was the most common opportunistic infection in people with AIDS, and retinal infection was its most clinically important manifestation, occurring in up to 40% of patients with AIDS. CMV retinitis is found mostly in the eyes of individuals with $CD4^+$ counts of 50 cells/μL or less. It is now uncommon in areas where potent combination antiretroviral therapy is available and is an increasing problem in the resource-limited world, particularly in Southeast Asia. Even so, it remains the most common opportunistic ocular infection in patients with AIDS and occasionally is the first AIDS-defining infection found in an individual. See Chapter 11 for a full discussion of CMV retinitis.

Ford N, Shubber Z, Saranchuk P, et al. Burden of HIV-related cytomegalovirus retinitis in resource-limited settings: a systematic review. *Clin Infect Dis.* 2013;57(9):1351–1361.

Holland GN, Vaudaux JD, Shiramizu KM, et al; Southern California HIV/Eye Consortium. Characteristics of untreated AIDS-related cytomegalovirus retinitis. II. Findings in the era of highly active antiretroviral therapy (1997 to 2000). *Am J Ophthalmol.* 2008;145(1):12–22.

Jabs DA, Van Natta ML, Thorne JE, et al; Studies of Ocular Complications of AIDS Research Group. Course of cytomegalovirus retinitis in the era of highly active antiretroviral therapy: 1. Retinitis progression. *Ophthalmology.* 2004;111(12):2224–2231.

Immune recovery uveitis

Immune recovery uveitis (IRU) is an inflammatory process that affects patients with AIDS who previously had CMV retinitis and whose immune status improves with combination antiretroviral therapy. Immune recovery uveitis was defined as an increase in $CD4^+$ T-lymphocyte count of at least 50 cells/µL to the level of 100 cells/µL. The risk factors for developing inflammation depend on the extent of CMV retinitis (CMV retinitis surface area of 25% or more), amount of intraocular CMV antigen, degree of immune constitution, and previous treatment (higher in patients treated with cidofovir). Manifestations of IRU include anterior uveitis, vitritis, uveitic macular edema, epiretinal membrane formation, papillitis, neovascularization of the optic disc or retina and others. Vitreous inflammation may be transient, but some patients may need short courses of systemic or periocular corticosteroids. The risk of recurrent CMV retinitis should be weighed against the benefit of local steroid injections.

El-Bradey MH, Cheng L, Song MK, Torriani FJ, Freeman WR. Long-term results of treatment of macular complications in eyes with immune recovery uveitis using a graded treatment approach. *Retina.* 2004;24(3):376–382.

Kempen JH, Min YI, Freeman WR, et al; Studies of Ocular Complications of AIDS Research Group. Risk of immune recovery uveitis in patients with AIDS and cytomegalovirus retinitis. *Ophthalmology.* 2006;113(4):684–694.

Urban B, Bakunowicz-Łazarczyk A, Michalczuk M. Immune recovery uveitis: pathogenesis, clinical symptoms, and treatment. *Mediators Inflamm.* 2014;2014:971417.

Retinal detachment

Retinal detachment occurs in up to 50% of patients with CMV retinitis. It may occur during active disease or after successful treatment. With potent antiretroviral regimens available, the rate of retinal detachment has been reduced to 0.06 per patient-year. Risk factors for developing retinal detachment include involvement of all 3 retinal zones, lower $CD4^+$ T-lymphocyte count, and more extensive retinitis. Since there is extensive retinal necrosis and multiple posterior holes, most of these detachments require pars plana vitrectomy with long-term silicone oil tamponade. Anatomical reattachment can be achieved in 90% of patients.

Jabs DA, Van Natta ML, Thorne JE, et al; Studies of Ocular Complications of AIDS Research Group. Course of cytomegalovirus retinitis in the era of highly active antiretroviral therapy: 2. Second eye involvement and retinal detachment. *Ophthalmology.* 2004;111(12):2232–2239.

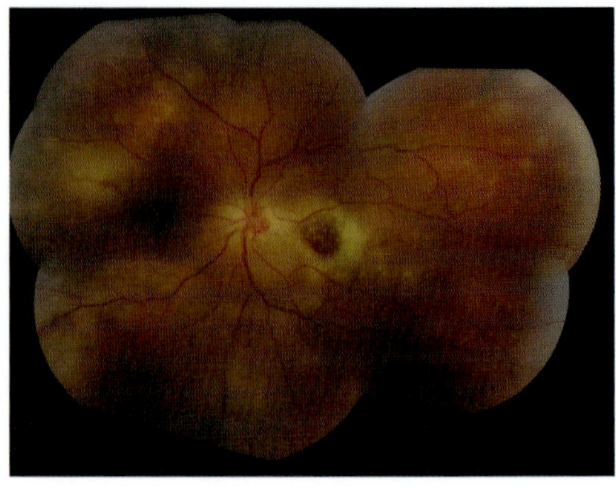

Figure 15-2 Fundus photomontage of progressive outer retinal necrosis with relative preservation of vessels and early involvement of posterior pole in a patient with acquired immune deficiency syndrome. *(Courtesy of H. Nida Sen, MD/National Eye Institute.)*

Necrotizing Herpetic Retinitis

Patients with AIDS may develop necrotizing herpetic retinitis, which appears to manifest as a spectrum of disease; the severity is directly proportional to the level of immunologic compromise. Patients may develop typical acute retinal necrosis or progressive outer retinal necrosis (PORN; see Chapter 11). In its early stages, PORN may be difficult to differentiate from peripheral CMV retinitis (Fig 15-2).

Kim SJ, Equi R, Belair ML, Fine HF, Dunn JP. Long-term preservation of vision in progressive outer retinal necrosis treated with combination antiviral drugs and highly active antiretroviral therapy. *Ocul Immunol Inflamm.* 2007;15(6):425–427.

Toxoplasmic Retinochoroiditis

Toxoplasmosis in patients with AIDS differs from toxoplasmosis in immunocompetent patients. In general, the lesions are larger in people with AIDS, and up to 40% of cases have bilateral disease. Solitary or multifocal patterns of retinitis have been observed (Fig 15-3). A vitreous inflammatory reaction usually appears overlying the area of active retinochoroiditis, but the degree of vitreous reaction may be less than that observed in immunocompetent patients (see also Chapter 11).

A
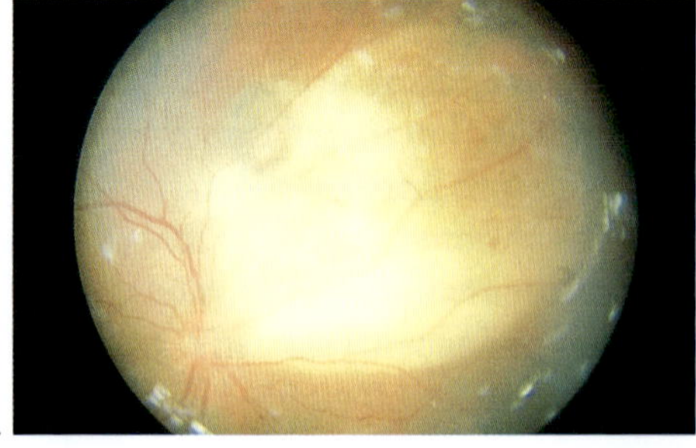

B
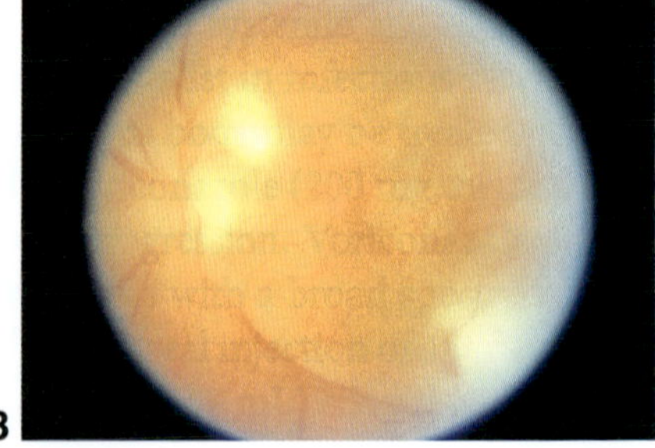

Figure 15-3 Toxoplasmic retinochoroditis. **A,** Fundus photograph showing a large area of macular toxoplasmic retinochoroiditis in a patient infected with human immunodeficiency virus (HIV). **B,** Fundus photograph of multifocal toxoplasmic retinochoroiditis in another HIV-infected patient. *(Courtesy of Emmett T. Cunningham Jr, MD.)*

The diagnosis of ocular toxoplasmosis may also be more difficult in patients with AIDS. Ocular toxoplasmosis may result from newly acquired *T gondii* infection or from reactivation of chronic infection within the retina and even in nonocular sites. Preexisting retinochoroidal scars may be absent. Newly acquired *T gondii* infections or dissemination from nonocular sites are the most likely causes among patients with AIDS, although reactivation of quiescent toxoplasmosis also occurs. Ocular toxoplasmosis in patients with AIDS may be difficult to distinguish from acute retinal necrosis, necrotizing herpetic retinitis, or syphilitic retinitis. Definitive diagnosis may require aqueous and vitreous samples for culture and polymerase chain reaction techniques.

In general, the inflammatory reaction in the choroid, retina, and vitreous is less prominent than in patients with an intact immune system. Trophozoites and cysts can be observed in greater numbers within areas of retinitis, and *T gondii* organisms can occasionally be noted invading the choroid, a finding not present in immunocompetent patients.

The prompt diagnosis of ocular toxoplasmosis is especially important in patients who are immunocompromised because the condition inevitably progresses if left untreated, in contrast to the self-limiting disease in immunocompetent patients. In addition, ocular toxoplasmosis in immunocompromised patients may be associated with cerebral or disseminated toxoplasmosis, an important cause of morbidity and mortality in patients with AIDS. For HIV-infected patients with active ocular toxoplasmosis, computer-assisted tomography (CT) and/or magnetic resonance imaging (MRI) of the head and consultation with specialists in infectious diseases should be pursued to rule out central nervous system (CNS) involvement.

Antitoxoplasmic therapy with synergic combination of pyrimethamine, sulfadiazine, sulfamethoxazole and trimethoprim, azithromycin, atovaquone, and/or clindamycin is required. Corticosteroids should be used with caution and only in the presence of appropriate antimicrobial cover because of the risk of further immunosuppression in this population. In selecting the therapeutic regimen, the physician should consider the possibility of coexisting cerebral or disseminated toxoplasmosis as well as the toxic effects of pyrimethamine and sulfadiazine on bone marrow. Continued maintenance therapy may be necessary for patients with poor immune status that is not improving.

Moshfeghi DM, Dodds EM, Couto CA, et al. Diagnostic approaches to severe, atypical toxoplasmosis mimicking acute retinal necrosis. *Ophthalmology.* 2004;111(4):716–725.

Ocular Syphilis

Syphilis is reemerging globally, particularly in association with HIV coinfection. The clinical presentations of ocular syphilis include scleritis; anterior, intermediate or posterior uveitis; and even optic neuritis. Patients may also experience mucocutaneous and CNS symptoms A classic manifestation of syphilis in patients with AIDS is unilateral or bilateral, pale-yellow, placoid retinal lesions that preferentially involve the macula (syphilitic posterior placoid chorioretinitis). Patients with AIDS may also present with discrete creamy yellow superficial retinal precipitates overlying areas of syphilitic retinitis as a very suggestive finding, although they can occur regardless of HIV status. In patients with AIDS, vitritis without chorioretinitis can be the first manifestation of syphilis. For discussion of other manifestations, refer to Chapter 10.

The course of syphilis may be more aggressive in HIV-infected patients. These patients require treatment with 18–24 million units of intravenous penicillin G administered daily for 10–14 days, followed by 2.4 million units of intramuscular benzathine penicillin G administered weekly for 3 weeks. Monitoring of results from the quantitative rapid plasma reagin (RPR) test is recommended, as symptomatic disease can recur.

Browning DJ. Posterior segment manifestations of active ocular syphilis, their response to a neurosyphilis regimen of penicillin therapy, and the influence of human immunodeficiency virus status on response. *Ophthalmology.* 2000;107(11):2015–2023.

Multifocal Choroiditis and Systemic Dissemination

Multifocal choroidal lesions from a variety of infectious agents are found in up to 10% of patients with AIDS. Most of these lesions are caused by *C neoformans, P jirovecii, M tuberculosis,* or atypical mycobacteria. Because of the profound immunosuppression, multiple infectious agents may cause simultaneous infectious multifocal choroiditis.

The choroid is often a site of opportunistic disseminated infections and thus needs to be carefully examined in patients with AIDS. Multifocal choroiditis should prompt an exhaustive workup because it frequently is a sign of disseminated infection.

Pneumocystis jirovecii Choroiditis

Patients with AIDS are at greater risk for *P jirovecii* pneumonia. In rare cases, this infection can result in choroidal infiltrates that contain the microorganisms.

P jirovecii can present as choroiditis that consists of slightly elevated, plaquelike, yellow-white lesions located in the choroid, with minimal vitritis (Fig 15-4). On fluorescein angiography, these lesions tend to be hypofluorescent in the early phase and hyperfluorescent in the later phases. If disseminated *P jirovecii* infection is suspected, an extensive examination is required by an infectious disease specialist.

Treatment of *P jirovecii* choroiditis involves a 3-week regimen of intravenous trimethoprim (20 mg/kg/day) and sulfamethoxazole (100 mg/kg/day) or pentamidine (4 mg/kg/day). Within 3–12 weeks, most of the yellow-white lesions disappear, leaving mild overlying pigmentary changes. Vision is usually not affected.

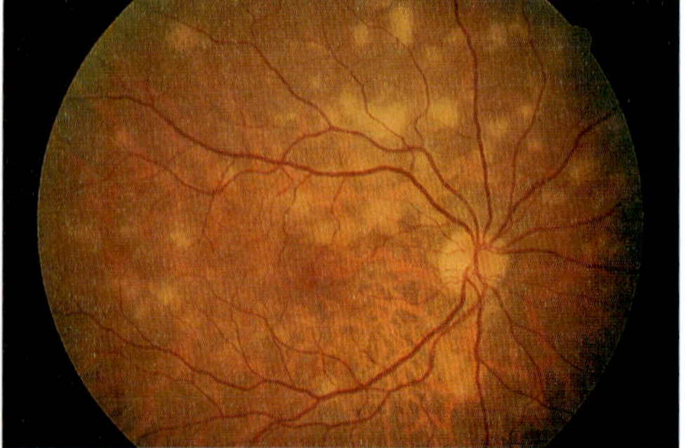

Figure 15-4 Fundus photograph of *Pneumocystis jirovecii* choroiditis. The fellow eye revealed similar findings. *(Reprinted with permission from Cunningham ET Jr, Belfort R Jr.* HIV/AIDS and the Eye: A Global Perspective. Ophthalmology Monograph 15. *San Francisco, CA: American Academy of Ophthalmology; 2002:67.)*

Cryptococcus neoformans Choroiditis

The dissemination of *C neoformans* in patients with AIDS may result in a multifocal choroiditis. Some patients with *C neoformans* choroiditis show choroidal lesions before clinical evidence of dissemination develops. More typically, *C neoformans* infection involves the cerebrospinal fluid, and there is secondary optic nerve edema as a result of increased intracranial pressure that can slowly lead to optic atrophy. Direct invasion of the optic nerve by organisms is also possible and can lead to more rapid vision loss. Treatment may include amphotericin and flucytosine.

Kestelyn P, Taelman H, Bogaerts J, et al. Ophthalmic manifestations of infections with *Cryptococcus neoformans* in patients with the acquired immunodeficiency syndrome. *Am J Ophthalmol.* 1993;116(6):721–727.

External Eye Manifestations

Other ophthalmic manifestations of AIDS include Kaposi sarcoma; molluscum contagiosum; herpes zoster ophthalmicus; and keratitis caused by various viruses, protozoa, conjunctival infections, and microvascular abnormalities. All of these conditions affect mainly the anterior segment of the globe and the ocular adnexa. These conditions are also discussed in BCSC Section 8, *External Disease and Cornea.*

Ocular Adnexal Kaposi Sarcoma

Human herpesvirus 8 is associated with Kaposi sarcoma. Two aggressive variants of this tumor have been described: an endemic variety especially prevalent in Kenya and Nigeria and a second variant, epidemic Kaposi sarcoma, which was first noted in renal transplant recipients and in patients with AIDS. AIDS-associated Kaposi sarcoma may be found in visceral organs (the gastrointestinal tract, lung, and liver) in up to 50% of patients. Before the availability of potent antiretroviral therapy, ocular adnexal involvement occurred in approximately 20% of patients with AIDS-associated systemic Kaposi sarcoma (Fig 15-5). Histologic investigation shows spindle cells mixed with vascular structures. Treatment of Kaposi sarcoma consists of excision, cryotherapy, radiation, or a combination of these methods and is based on the clinical stage of the tumor as well as its location and the presence or absence of disseminated lesions.

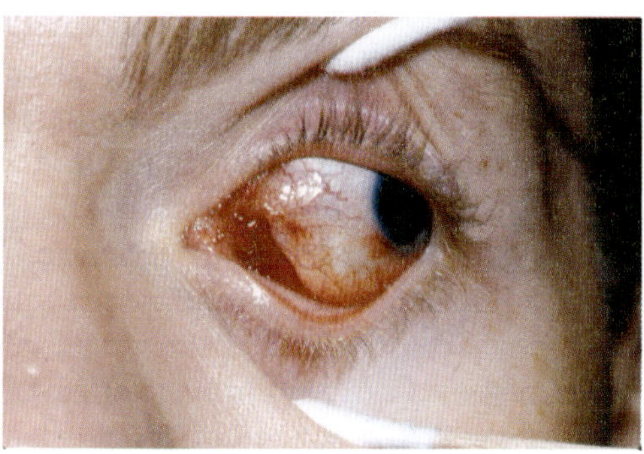

Figure 15-5 Conjunctival involvement in Kaposi sarcoma; hemorrhagic conjunctival tumor. *(Courtesy of Elaine Chuang, MD.)*

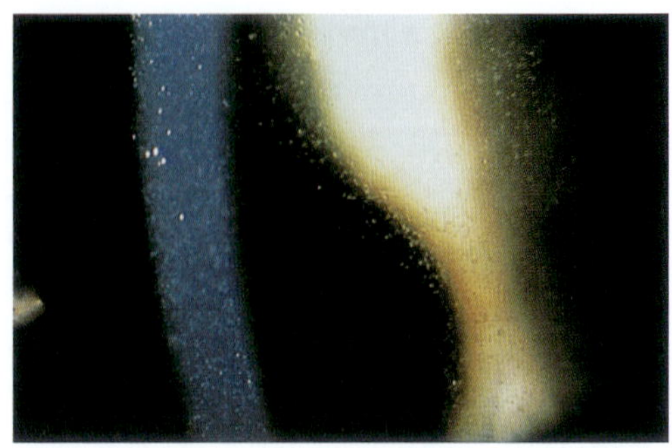

Figure 15-6 Slit-lamp photograph of cornea showing punctate epithelial keratitis caused by microsporidia.

Molluscum Contagiosum

Molluscum contagiosum is caused by a DNA virus of the poxvirus family. The characteristic skin lesions show a small elevation with central umbilication. Molluscum contagiosum lesions in immunocompetent individuals are few, unilateral, and involve the eyelids. In patients with AIDS, however, these lesions may be numerous and bilateral. If molluscum contagiosum lesions in patients with AIDS are symptomatic or cause conjunctivitis, surgical excision may be necessary.

Herpes Zoster

People younger than 50 years of age who present with herpes zoster lesions of the face or eyelids should be considered for HIV testing. Corneal involvement can cause a persistent, chronic epithelial keratitis. Treatment consists of systemic and topical acyclovir. These patients should receive periodic monitoring with retinal examinations to ensure that posterior segment involvement does not occur.

Other Infections

Infection with HIV does not appear to predispose patients to bacterial keratitis, although bacterial and fungal keratitis can occur in patients with AIDS who have no obvious predisposing factors such as trauma or topical corticosteroid use. Infections appear to be more severe and are more likely to cause corneal perforation in patients with AIDS than in immunocompetent patients. Similarly, herpes simplex keratitis does not appear to have a higher incidence in patients with AIDS, but it may have a prolonged course or multiple recurrences and involve the limbus. Microsporidia have been shown to cause a coarse, punctate epithelial keratitis with minimal conjunctival reaction in patients with AIDS (Fig 15-6). Electron microscopy of epithelial scrapings has revealed the organism, which is an obligate, intracellular, protozoal parasite.

Solitary granulomatous conjunctivitis caused by cryptococcal or mycotic infections or by tuberculosis can occur in HIV-infected persons. The possibility of dissemination must be aggressively investigated and, if present, treated. Both orbital and intraocular lymphomas have been described in patients with AIDS.

APPENDIX

Diagnostic Survey for Uveitis

FAMILY HISTORY

These questions refer to your grandparents, parents, aunts, uncles, brothers and sisters, children, or grandchildren.

To your knowledge, has anyone in your family ever had any of the following?

Arthritis or rheumatism	Yes	No
Syphilis	Yes	No
Tuberculosis	Yes	No
Sickle cell disease or trait	Yes	No
Lyme disease	Yes	No
Uveitis, or inflammation in the eye?	Yes	No

SOCIAL HISTORY

Your age (years):		
Your current job:		
Have you ever traveled outside of the United States?	Yes	No
If yes, where and when?		
Have you ever owned a dog or cat?	Yes	No
Have you ever eaten raw meat or uncooked sausage?	Yes	No
Have you ever had unpasteurized milk or cheese?	Yes	No
Have you ever been exposed to sick animals?	Yes	No
Do you drink untreated stream, well, or lake water, or have you gone hunting or camping?	Yes	No
Do you smoke cigarettes?	Yes	No
Have you ever used recreational intravenous drugs?	Yes	No
Have you ever had sexual relations with a person of the same sex or with a person who engages in same-sex relations?	Yes	No

PERSONAL MEDICAL HISTORY

Are you allergic to any medications?	Yes	No
If yes, which medications?		

Please list the medications that you are currently taking, including nonprescription or over-the-counter drugs, nutritional supplements, and herbal or other alternative remedies:

Please list all the eye surgeries you have had (including laser surgery) and the dates of the surgeries:

Please list all the operations besides on the eye you have had and the dates of the surgeries:

____

____

____

____

Have you ever been told by a medical doctor that you have the following conditions?

Anemia (low blood count)	Yes	No
Cancer	Yes	No
Diabetes mellitus	Yes	No
Hepatitis	Yes	No
High blood pressure	Yes	No
Pleurisy	Yes	No
Pneumonia	Yes	No
Ulcers	Yes	No
Herpes (sores in or on the mouth or genitals)	Yes	No
Chickenpox	Yes	No
Shingles (zoster)	Yes	No
German measles (rubella)	Yes	No
Measles (rubeola)	Yes	No
Mumps	Yes	No
Chlamydia or trachoma	Yes	No
Syphilis	Yes	No
Gonorrhea	Yes	No
Any other sexually transmitted disease	Yes	No
Tuberculosis	Yes	No
Leprosy	Yes	No
Leptospirosis	Yes	No
Lyme disease	Yes	No
Histoplasmosis	Yes	No
Candida infection or moniliasis	Yes	No
Coccidioidomycosis	Yes	No
Sporotrichosis	Yes	No
Toxoplasmosis	Yes	No
Toxocariasis	Yes	No
Cysticercosis	Yes	No
Trichinosis	Yes	No
Whipple disease	Yes	No
HIV infection or AIDS	Yes	No
Hay fever	Yes	No
Allergies	Yes	No
Vasculitis	Yes	No
Arthritis	Yes	No
Rheumatoid arthritis	Yes	No
Lupus (systemic lupus erythematosus)	Yes	No
Scleroderma	Yes	No
Reactive arthritis	Yes	No
Colitis (Crohn disease, ulcerative colitis)	Yes	No
Behçet disease	Yes	No

Sarcoidosis	Yes	No
Ankylosing spondylitis	Yes	No
Erythema nodosa	Yes	No
Temporal arteritis	Yes	No
Multiple sclerosis	Yes	No

Have you ever had any of the following symptoms?

GENERAL HEALTH

Chills	Yes	No
Fever (persistent or recurrent)	Yes	No
Painful or swollen glands	Yes	No
Night sweats	Yes	No
Fatigue (tire easily)	Yes	No
Poor appetite	Yes	No
Unexplained weight loss	Yes	No
Do you feel sick?	Yes	No

HEAD

Headaches	Yes	No
Fainting	Yes	No
Numbness or tingling in your body	Yes	No
Paralysis in parts of your body	Yes	No
Seizures or convulsions	Yes	No

EARS

Hard of hearing or deafness	Yes	No
Ringing or noise in your ears	Yes	No
Frequent or severe ear infections	Yes	No
Painful or swollen ear lobes	Yes	No

NOSE AND THROAT

Sores in your nose or mouth	Yes	No
Severe or recurrent nosebleeds	Yes	No
Frequent sneezing	Yes	No
Sinus trouble	Yes	No
Persistent hoarseness	Yes	No
Tooth or gum infections	Yes	No

SKIN

Rashes	Yes	No
Skin sores	Yes	No
Sunburn easily (photosensitivity)	Yes	No
White patches of skin or hair	Yes	No
Loss of hair	Yes	No
Tick or insect bites	Yes	No
Painfully cold fingers	Yes	No
Severe itching	Yes	No

RESPIRATORY

Severe or frequent colds	Yes	No
Constant coughing	Yes	No

Coughing up blood	Yes	No
Recent flu or viral infection	Yes	No
Wheezing or asthma attacks	Yes	No
Difficulty breathing	Yes	No
CARDIOVASCULAR		
Chest pain	Yes	No
Shortness of breath	Yes	No
Swelling of your legs	Yes	No
BLOOD		
Frequent or easy bruising	Yes	No
Frequent or easy bleeding	Yes	No
Have you received blood transfusions?	Yes	No
GASTROINTESTINAL		
Trouble swallowing	Yes	No
Diarrhea	Yes	No
Bloody stools	Yes	No
Stomach ulcers	Yes	No
Jaundice or yellow skin	Yes	No
BONES AND JOINTS		
Stiff joints	Yes	No
Stiff lower back	Yes	No
Back pain while sleeping or awakening	Yes	No
Muscle aches	Yes	No
GENITOURINARY		
Kidney problems	Yes	No
Bladder trouble	Yes	No
Blood in your urine	Yes	No
Urinary discharge	Yes	No
Genital sores or ulcers	Yes	No
Prostatitis	Yes	No
Testicular pain	Yes	No
Are you pregnant?	Yes	No
Do you plan to be pregnant in the future?	Yes	No

Adapted with permission from Foster CS, Vitale AT. *Diagnosis and Treatment of Uveitis.* 2nd ed. Jaypee Brothers Medical Publishers, New Delhi, India; 2012:123–128.

Basic Texts

Uveitis and Ocular Inflammation

Albert DM, Miller JW, Azar DT, Blodi BA, eds. *Albert & Jakobiec's Principles and Practice of Ophthalmology.* 3rd ed. Philadelphia: Saunders; 2008.

Delves PJ, Martin SJ, Burton DR, Roitt IM. *Roitt's Essential Immunology.* 13th ed. Hoboken, NJ: Wiley-Blackwell; 2017.

Dick AD, Okada AA, Forrester JV. *Practical Manual of Intraocular Inflammation.* New York: Informa Healthcare USA; 2008.

Foster CS, Vitale AT, eds. *Diagnosis & Treatment of Uveitis.* 2nd ed. New Dehli, India: Jaypee Brothers Medical Publishers; 2013.

Giles CL. Uveitis in childhood. In: Tasman W, Jaeger EA, eds. *Duane's Clinical Ophthalmology.* Philadelphia: Lippincott Williams & Wilkins; 2005.

Bowling B. *Clinical Ophthalmology: A Systematic Approach.* 8th ed. London: Elsevier; 2016.

Michelson JB. *Color Atlas of Uveitis.* 2nd ed. St Louis: Mosby; 1992.

Nussenblatt RB, Whitcup SM. *Uveitis: Fundamentals and Clinical Practice.* 4th ed. St Louis: Mosby; 2010.

Pepose JS, Holland GN, Wilhelmus KR, eds. *Ocular Infection and Immunity.* St Louis: Mosby; 1996.

Rao NA, section ed. Part 7: Uveitis and other intraocular inflammations. In: Yanoff M, Duker JS, eds. *Ophthalmology.* 5th ed. St Louis: Mosby; 2019.

Related Academy Materials

The American Academy of Ophthalmology is dedicated to providing a wealth of high-quality clinical education resources for ophthalmologists.

Print Publications and Electronic Products

For a complete listing of Academy products related to topics covered in this BCSC Section, visit our online store at https://store.aao.org/clinical-education/topic/uveitis.html. Or call Customer Service at 866-561-8558 (toll free, US only) or +1 415-561-8540, Monday through Friday, between 8:00 AM and 5:00 PM (PST).

Online Resources

Visit the Ophthalmic News and Education (ONE®) Network at aao.org/onenetwork to find relevant videos, online courses, journal articles, practice guidelines, self-assessment quizzes, images and more. The ONE Network is a free Academy-member benefit.

Access free, trusted articles and content with the Academy's collaborative online encyclopedia, EyeWiki, at aao.org/eyewiki.

Get mobile access to the *Wills Eye Manual*, watch the latest 1-minute videos, and set up alerts for clinical updates relevant to you with the AAO Ophthalmic Education App. Download today: Search for "AAO Ophthalmic Education" in the Apple app store or in Google Play.

Requesting Continuing Medical Education Credit

The American Academy of Ophthalmology is accredited by the Accreditation Council for Continuing Medical Education (ACCME) to provide continuing medical education for physicians.

The American Academy of Ophthalmology designates this enduring material for a maximum of 10 *AMA PRA Category 1 Credits*™. Physicians should claim only the credit commensurate with the extent of their participation in the activity.

To claim *AMA PRA Category 1 Credits*™ upon completion of this activity, learners must demonstrate appropriate knowledge and participation in the activity by taking the posttest for Section 9 and achieving a score of 80% or higher.

This activity meets the Self-Assessment CME requirements defined by the American Board of Ophthalmology (ABO). Please be advised that the ABO is not an accrediting body for purposes of any CME program. ABO does not sponsor this or any outside activity, and ABO does not endorse any particular CME activity. Complete information regarding the ABO Self-Assessment CME Maintenance of Certification requirements is available at https://abop.org/maintain-certification/cme-self-assessment/.

To take the posttest and request CME credit online:

1. Go to www.aao.org/cme-central and log in.
2. Click on "Claim CME Credit and View My CME Transcript" and then "Report AAO Credits."
3. Select the appropriate media type and then the Academy activity. You will be directed to the posttest.
4. Once you have passed the test with a score of 80% or higher, you will be directed to your transcript. *If you are not an Academy member, you will be able to print out a certificate of participation once you have passed the test.*

CME expiration date: June 1, 2022. *AMA PRA Category 1 Credits*™ may be claimed only once between June 1, 2019, and the expiration date.

For assistance, contact the Academy's Customer Service department at 866-561-8558 (US only) or +1 415-561-8540 between 8:00 AM and 5:00 PM (PST), Monday through Friday, or send an e-mail to customer_service@aao.org.

Study Questions

Please note that these questions are *not* part of your CME reporting process. They are provided here for your own educational use and identification of any professional practice gaps. The required CME posttest is available online (see "Requesting CME Credit"). Following the questions are a blank answer sheet and answers with discussions. Although a concerted effort has been made to avoid ambiguity and redundancy in these questions, the authors recognize that differences of opinion may occur regarding the "best" answer. The discussions are provided to demonstrate the rationale used to derive the answer. They may also be helpful in confirming that your approach to the problem was correct or, if necessary, in fixing the principle in your memory. The Section 9 faculty thanks the Self-Assessment Committee for developing the study questions and answers.

1. What is a mechanism of the innate immune response?
   a. production of reactive oxygen species
   b. induction of plasma cells
   c. production of antibodies
   d. formation of memory B cells

2. What are the blood and tissue-equivalent cells of the immune system?
   a. basophil (blood) and mast cell (tissue)
   b. dendritic cell (blood) and macrophage (tissue)
   c. eosinophil (blood) and mast cell (tissue)
   d. monocyte (blood) and Langerhans cell (tissue)

3. A 78-year-old man presents for an eye examination. He reports no symptoms and has a history of bilateral cataract extraction. On examination, there is low-grade cell and flare in the anterior chamber of the right eye, an intraocular pressure of 6, and an otherwise normal fundus examination in that eye. Examination of the left eye is normal and a review of systems is notable for a history of smoking, but is otherwise unremarkable. The patient is not on any eye drops. What would be next step in management of this patient's condition?
   a. extensive uveitic workup, including assessing for sarcoidosis, syphilis, and tuberculosis, and starting the patient on topical corticosteroids
   b. vitreous biopsy with flow cytometry to look for primary intraocular lymphoma
   c. carotid Doppler ultrasonography to assess for significant stenosis of the right carotid artery
   d. reassurance and observation, as this is a common finding after intraocular surgery, presumably due to breakdown of the blood–aqueous barrier

4. A 52-year-old White man from North Dakota presents with bilateral panuveitis and retinal vasculitis. He also has complaints of arthralgia, diplopia, diarrhea, and poor performance at work. What test may help with the diagnosis?
   a. duodenal biopsy
   b. HLA-B51
   c. angiotensin-converting enzyme
   d. HLA-A29

5. Peripheral necrotizing retinochoroiditis resembling acute retinal necrosis can be seen in patients infected with what pathogen?
   a. *Pneumocystis jirovecii*
   b. *Nocardia asteroides*
   c. *Treponema pallidum*
   d. *Mycobacterium tuberculosis*

6. What risk factor in a patient with West Nile virus (WNV)-associated uveitis is associated with an increased risk of WNV-associated mortality?
   a. young age
   b. cardiomyopathy
   c. presence of fever
   d. diabetes mellitus

7. When stellate keratic precipitates are present in herpes simplex type 1 intraocular infections, what typically characterizes their distribution on the corneal endothelium?
   a. diffuse, often extending above the corneal equator
   b. inferiorly, specifically only in the Arlt triangle
   c. in coin-shaped, or circinate, lesions
   d. keratic precipitates are not found in herpes simplex type 1 intraocular infections

8. What is the best induction treatment option for a patient with varicella-zoster virus–associated acute retinal necrosis?
   a. oral acyclovir 800 mg 5 times/day
   b. oral valacyclovir 2 g 3 times/day
   c. oral valganciclovir 900 mg twice/day
   d. oral valacyclovir 1 g 3 times/day

9. A patient with candidemia reports a rapid decrease in vision unilaterally and is found to have creamy yellowish chorioretinal lesions in the posterior pole but clear vitreous. What is the best initial treatment option?

   a. oral fluconazole and pars plana vitrectomy

   b. oral voriconazole

   c. posterior sub-Tenon triamcinolone injection followed by oral voriconazole

   d. intravitreal injection of amphotericin B, 5 μg/0.1 mL

10. A patient is referred with a history of disseminated coccidioidomycosis. What is the most common ocular manifestation of the disease?

    a. phlyctenular and granulomatous conjunctivitis

    b. hypertensive anterior uveitis

    c. intermediate uveitis

    d. multifocal choroidal granulomas

11. A 65-year-old White woman with vitritis and negative treponemal antibody and interferon-gamma release assay test results initially responds well to systemic corticosteroids; however, as the steroids are tapered, her vitritis becomes robust. A diagnostic and therapeutic pars plana vitrectomy is performed, and cytopathology discloses large, atypical lymphocytes with a large nucleus-to-cytoplasm ratio. What is the approximate chance that she has or will develop intracranial lesions characterized by the same cells?

    a. 15%–30%

    b. 30%–45%

    c. 45%–60%

    d. 60%–75%

12. A child with juvenile idiopathic arthritis–associated chronic bilateral nongranulomatous uveitis has developed band keratopathy. What material makes up band keratopathy, and at what level of the cornea is it found?

    a. calcium carbonate deposition at the level of the Descemet membrane

    b. calcium hydroxyapatite at the level of the Descemet membrane

    c. calcium carbonate deposition at the level of the Bowman membrane

    d. calcium hydroxyapatite at the level of the Bowman membrane

13. A patient with bilateral pars planitis who is being treated with mycophenolate mofetil exhibits recurrent uveitic macular edema in the right eye. The anterior chamber and vitreous are inactive with respect to inflammation in both eyes, yet the macular edema persists. Optical coherence tomography (OCT) of the macula demonstrates uveitic macular edema in the right eye, but the OCT image is otherwise unremarkable. What is the best initial choice in managing the macular edema in this patient?
    a. discontinuation of mycophenolate mofetil and advancement of systemic therapy to cyclophosphamide for better control of the underlying uveitis
    b. intravenous methylprednisolone 1 g daily for 3 days
    c. periocular sub-Tenon injection of triamcinolone
    d. pars plana vitrectomy

14. What is the pathogen associated with the development of Kaposi sarcoma?
    a. human herpes virus 4
    b. human herpes virus 8
    c. herpes simplex virus type 1
    d. cytomegalovirus

15. A patient with AIDS developed unilateral cytomegalovirus (CMV) retinitis. He was treated with oral valganciclovir and 3 intraocular injections of foscarnet, which halted the retinitis. At that time, his $CD4^+$ T-lymphocyte count was 49 cells/μL. He has since started antiretroviral treatment, with an improvement in $CD4^+$ T-lymphocyte count to 103 cells/μL. He presents with complaints of floaters in the eye with prior CMV and now exhibits a robust vitritis, although the prior area of CMV retinitis looks stable. What is the best initial therapy for this patient?
    a. pars plana vitrectomy with intravitreal injection of foscarnet
    b. continuation of oral valganciclovir and starting systemic corticosteroids
    c. discontinuation of oral valganciclovir and injection of intraocular triamcinolone 4 mg
    d. discontinuation of antiretroviral treatment and starting systemic corticosteroids

16. What condition produces a Th2-mediated response?
    a. acute anterior uveitis
    b. giant papillary conjunctivitis
    c. parasitic infection
    d. Vogt-Koyanagi-Harada syndrome

17. What is the term for antigenic sites on antibodies?
    a. isotopes
    b. epitopes
    c. allotopes
    d. idiotopes

18. What immune response is part of the innate immune response?
    a. antigen presentation
    b. B-cell induction
    c. induction of natural killer cells
    d. T-cell induction

19. The conjunctiva contains mucosa-associated lymphoid tissue (MALT). Aside from providing regional immunity in the setting of direct inoculation, what feature allows this system to mount a predominantly antibody-mediated effector response in the absence of direct prior exposure?
    a. an abundance of antigen-presenting cells
    b. a predominance of immunoglobulin A
    c. prior exposure at any MALT site
    d. any form of prior exposure

20. Corneal transplantation has success rates of over 90%, without the need for systemic immunosuppression. What is the reason for this, and what immunoregulatory processes are responsible?
    a. immune privilege site, intact limbal physiology, and anterior chamber–associated immune deviation
    b. effector blockade, attenuated antigen presentation
    c. immune privilege site, mucosa-associated lymphoid tissue, and blood–aqueous barrier
    d. effector blockade, attenuated natural killer cells, and lymphocyte activity

21. A 23-year-old patient presents with 2 days of discharge, itching, and redness of the right eye. The patient states that she was just getting over a cold, and has noticed waking up with her eyelids stuck together for the past 2 mornings. On examination, in addition to conjunctival follicles, what else is the ophthalmologist likely to find?
    a. inflamed adenoids
    b. swollen submandibular nodes
    c. dense pseudomembranes
    d. similar findings in the other eye

22. Given that the immunoregulatory processes of the retina and choroid are not well understood, what tissue currently seems to provide immunoregulatory properties in this area?
    a. retina
    b. retinal pigment epithelium
    c. choroid
    d. choriocapillaris

23. Aside from effector blockade and anterior chamber–associated immune deviation, what is the major mechanism that affords immune privilege to the cornea?
    a. cytokines (eg, IL-1)
    b. mucosa-associated lymphoid tissue
    c. limbal physiology
    d. complement

24. A 23-year-old male medical student is very anxious about some test results and seeks further information from an ophthalmologist. He reports that during a class about human leukocyte antigen (HLA) haplotypes, his medical school performed HLA screening on all of the students, and he learned that he is positive for HLA-B27. He is now exceedingly worried about developing acute anterior uveitis (AAU). What counseling should the ophthalmologist provide to this patient after a normal eye examination?
    a. Almost 10% of individuals who are HLA-B27 positive manifest AAU, but it typically affects females, so he does not need to worry.
    b. Approximately 8% of the population is positive for HLA-B27, while only 0.012% of the population will develop AAU, so it is much more likely that he will never manifest AAU.
    c. Almost two-thirds of individuals who are HLA-B27 positive manifest AAU, so there is real risk of his developing the disease, and he should be monitored closely.
    d. There is no need to worry, because HLA-B27 is not associated with AAU. It is recommended that he see a rheumatologist, because HLA-B27 is associated with the seronegative spondyloarthropathies.

25. HLA-DR4 is weakly associated with what diseases?
    a. acute anterior uveitis
    b. Behçet disease
    c. birdshot chorioretinopathy
    d. sympathetic ophthalmia

26. A 12-year-old patient with juvenile idiopathic arthritis (JIA)–associated chronic anterior uveitis (CAU) presents for her regular follow-up appointment. She has been a patient at this clinic for 7 years. Her CAU has been very well controlled on a daily topical steroid, and she remains asymptomatic. What finding can be expected on examination?
    a. band keratopathy
    b. fibrinous anterior chamber reaction
    c. hypopyon
    d. vitritis

27. How has the Standardization of Uveitis Nomenclature (SUN) Working Group classified recurrent uveitis?
    a. episodes of uveitis that recur less than 3 months after treatment has been discontinued
    b. episodes of uveitis that recur more than 3 months after treatment has been discontinued
    c. episodes of uveitis that recur irrespective of when treatment has been discontinued
    d. episodes of uveitis that resolve in fewer than 3 months

28. What medication can be used in the treatment of intermediate uveitis associated with multiple sclerosis?
    a. subcutaneous adalimumab
    b. intravenous infliximab
    c. intravenous methylprednisolone
    d. subcutaneous etanercept

29. What agent used in the therapy of uveitis may induce antichimeric antibodies?
    a. abatacept
    b. infliximab
    c. interferon alfa-2a/2b
    d. tacrolimus

30. What treatment can be used for recurrent, noninfectious, refractory anterior scleritis?
    a. topical corticosteroid drops
    b. topical nonsteroidal anti inflammatory drops
    c. systemic steroids
    d. systemic nonsteroidal anti-inflammatory drugs

31. What type of scleritis prompts more evaluation for possible infection before initiation of immunosuppression?
    a. nodular scleritis
    b. diffuse scleritis
    c. posterior scleritis
    d. scleromalacia perforans

32. Abnormal urinalysis findings, with increased β_2-microglobulin level, in a patient with uveitis should prompt initiation of what systemic treatment?
    a. anticoagulation
    b. steroids
    c. xanthine oxidase inhibitor
    d. antibiotics

33. What further testing may be required in a patient with nongranulomatous anterior uveitis with hypopyon and HLA-B27-positive ankylosing spondylitis?
    a. urinalysis
    b. pathergy test
    c. aqueous tap for polymerase chain reaction testing
    d. chest x-ray and cardiac echogram

34. A 50-year-old woman presents with chronic scleritis, headaches, a history of branch retinal artery occlusion, and tracheomalacia. What test may further assist in the diagnosis and treatment?
    a. quantitative and qualitative antinuclear antibody testing
    b. lumbar puncture and spinal fluid analysis
    c. urinalysis
    d. anti–cyclic citrullinated antibody test

35. Central nervous system involvement is unlikely in what condition?
    a. sarcoidosis
    b. multifocal choroiditis and panuveitis
    c. Vogt-Koyanagi-Harada syndrome
    d. Behçet disease

36. What chorioretinopathy or white dot syndrome may be associated with infectious etiology?
    a. acute posterior multifocal placoid pigment epitheliopathy
    b. birdshot chorioretinopathy or vitiliginous chorioretinitis
    c. punctate inner choroiditis
    d. serpiginous choroiditis or geographic/helicoid choroidopathy

Answer Sheet for Section 9 Study Questions

Question	Answer	Question	Answer
1	a b c d	19	a b c d
2	a b c d	20	a b c d
3	a b c d	21	a b c d
4	a b c d	22	a b c d
5	a b c d	23	a b c d
6	a b c d	24	a b c d
7	a b c d	25	a b c d
8	a b c d	26	a b c d
9	a b c d	27	a b c d
10	a b c d	28	a b c d
11	a b c d	29	a b c d
12	a b c d	30	a b c d
13	a b c d	31	a b c d
14	a b c d	32	a b c d
15	a b c d	33	a b c d
16	a b c d	34	a b c d
17	a b c d	35	a b c d
18	a b c d	36	a b c d

Answers

1. **a.** The innate immune response is fast acting, nonspecific, and the same for all pathogen exposures. Of the reactions listed, only the production of reactive oxygen species is part of the innate immune response. Plasma cell induction, the formation of antibodies, and establishing memory B cells are all part of the more pathogen-specific, targeted, and slower adaptive immune response.
2. **a.** Basophils are the blood-borne equivalent of the tissue-bound mast cell. Once basophils leave the bloodstream and take residence in tissue, they become mast cells. The other answer choices are incorrect pairings of blood- and tissue-equivalent cells.
3. **c.** Given the lack of symptoms and this being the patient's first presentation at 78 years of age, the diagnosis is unlikely to be uveitic in nature. While his age places him in the right demographic for lymphoma, his vitreous cavity was clear and the diagnosis of primary intraocular lymphoma is unlikely (although this should certainly be considered, as it is one of the masquerade syndromes for uveitis). While extensive intraocular surgery can result in breakdown of the blood–aqueous barrier, it does not typically result after cataract surgery (nor would it explain his hypotony and absence of cells in the left eye). The most likely diagnosis is ocular ischemia, a masquerade syndrome for uveitis, and carotid Doppler images should be ordered to assess for right-sided stenosis of the carotid artery.
4. **a.** Whipple disease is a rare multisystem disease caused by the *Tropheryma whipplei* bacterium. It is most common in middle-aged White men. Migratory arthritis occurs in 80% of cases, and diarrhea, steatorrhea, and malabsorption occur in 75%. Central nervous system involvement occurs in 10% of cases and results in seizures, dementia, and coma. Neuro-ophthalmic signs can include cranial nerve palsies, nystagmus, and ophthalmoplegia. Intraocular involvement occurs in less than 5% of cases. Patients can present with bilateral panuveitis, retinal vasculitis, and multifocal chorioretinitis. The gold standard for diagnosis of Whipple disease is a duodenal biopsy that demonstrates a periodic acid–Schiff–positive bacillus in macrophages within intestinal villi.
5. **c.** Syphilis should be considered in the differential diagnosis of every individual with uveitis. It is caused by the spirochete *Treponema pallidum* and is associated with numerous ocular manifestations. Posterior segment findings of acquired syphilis include vitritis, chorioretinitis, focal/multifocal retinitis, necrotizing retinochoroiditis, retinal vasculitis, exudative retinal detachment, isolated papillitis, and neuroretinitis. Syphilis may present as a focal retinitis or as a peripheral necrotizing retinochoroiditis that may resemble acute retinal necrosis or progressive outer retinal necrosis.
6. **d.** Diabetes mellitus and advanced age in someone with West Nile virus (WNV)-associated uveitis are associated with the development of severe neurologic disease (meningitis or encephalitis). In addition, diabetes mellitus has been implicated as a risk factor for WNV-related death. Systemically, a patient may present with fever, myalgias, headache, conjunctivitis, and a maculopapular rash. Cardiomyopathy has not been associated with an increased risk of WNV-associated mortality.
7. **a.** Stellate keratic precipitates (KPs) are very suggestive of a viral intraocular infection and are frequently seen. However, in herpetic intraocular infections, particularly with herpes simplex viruses 1 and 2 as well as varicella-zoster virus, there may be nongranulomatous or granulomatous KPs as well. In this question, stellate KPs are identified and, when pre-

sent, often are found diffusely. The KPs localizing only to the Arlt triangle are classically found in noninfectious etiologies of intraocular inflammation and may be either granulomatous or nongranulomatous. Coin-shaped lesions are found in cytomegalovirus anterior uveitis.

8. **b.** While intravenous acyclovir 10 mg/kg every 8 hours for 10–14 days may be used for induction treatment in acute retinal necrosis, oral valacyclovir 2 g 3 times/day may be used; it is twice the dose used for active herpetic keratitis. Oral valganciclovir is reserved for cytomegalovirus-associated intraocular infections.
9. **b.** When hematogenous dissemination of *Candida* involves only the choroid, systemic antifungals may be used. However, when there is vitreal involvement as well, pars plana vitrectomy in conjunction with systemic antifungals should be considered. In addition, at the time of surgery, intraocular injection of antifungals may be considered. Oral voriconazole for this particular case is the best option, given that it will have excellent intraocular penetration and there is not vitreal involvement at this time, so vitrectomy is not required. Periocular or intraocular depot corticosteroid injection should be avoided, because this can make the endophthalmitis worse. Intravitreal injection of an antifungal alone is unlikely to result in adequate treatment of the current chorioretinal lesions, and systemic therapy is warranted.
10. **a.** The most common ocular manifestation of coccidioidomycosis (caused by *Coccidioides immitis*) is a phlyctenular and granulomatous conjunctivitis. The granulomas may resemble follicles, but histopathologically are granulomas. Uveal/intraocular involvement is less common than conjunctival involvement. The anterior segment features may include granulomatous keratic precipitates (ocular hypertension is not a classic feature), as well as iris nodules, which are granulomas on histopathology. Choroidal involvement presents as multifocal choroidal granulomas with a preferential location for the postequatorial region of the fundus.
11. **d.** The case described clinically is consistent with primary vitreoretinal lymphoma (PVRL). The cytopathology secures the diagnosis. In more than two-thirds of cases of PVRL, patients will have or will go on to develop intracranial disease. In fact, PVRL is a subset of primary central nervous system lymphoma (PCNSL). Approximately 20% of patients with PCNSL (who do not yet have intraocular involvement) will go on to develop PVRL.
12. **d.** Band keratopathy results from the deposition of calcium hydroxyapatite at the level of the Bowman membrane. Aside from chronic inflammation associated with uveitis, other causes of calcific band keratopathy include systemic disorders that cause hypercalcemia or elevated serum phosphorus, as well as silicone oil (particularly in an aphakic eye), exposure to mercurial vapors or preservative, and primary hereditary band keratopathy.
13. **c.** Uveitic macular edema is a frequent complication of uveitis and may occur even when inflammation is otherwise controlled. Optical coherence tomography of the macula can help identify contributing factors to the macular edema, such as vitreomacular traction. If there is prominent vitreomacular traction, a pars plana vitrectomy may be considered. In this case, however, while there is uveitic macular edema, the imaging is otherwise unremarkable. If there was persistently active intraocular inflammation that may be driving the uveitic macular edema, advancing a patient's systemic therapy may be beneficial. However, this patient's intraocular inflammation is inactive. In addition, advancing therapy from an antimetabolite (mycophenolate mofetil) to an alkylating agent (cyclophosphamide) is not indicated, because

alkylating agents are reserved for aggressive, sight-threatening causes of ocular inflammation due to their significant side effects. Similarly, intravenous methylprednisolone would not be indicated as the first step in managing this patient's macular edema, although such therapy can be used initially for robust intraocular inflammation that needs to be managed quickly and requires doses higher than what may be needed with oral corticosteroids. The use of periocular sub-Tenon triamcinolone, then, is the best initial choice in managing this patient's uveitic macular edema.

14. **b.** The pathogen involved with the development of Kaposi sarcoma is human herpes virus (HHV)-8. HHV-4 is also known as *Epstein-Barr virus* and is associated with the development of primary central nervous system lymphomas and primary vitreoretinal lymphomas in HIV-infected individuals. Herpes simplex virus type 1 and cytomegalovirus (HHV-5) are not associated with any specific neoplasias in HIV.

15. **b.** This patient is likely exhibiting immune recovery uveitis associated with improvement of his $CD4^+$ T-lymphocyte count and ability to mount an inflammatory response to retinal cytomegalovirus (CMV) antigens. Such inflammation can be managed with systemic corticosteroids. The best answer choice listed is to continue oral valganciclovir and start systemic corticosteroids. Use of periocular steroids should proceed with caution, because there is a chance that there may be a recurrence of the CMV retinitis. Intraocular steroids should be avoided as a first-line therapy for managing immune recovery uveitis. Certainly, if periocular steroids were to be considered, antivirals should be continued. There is no role for pars plana vitrectomy as a first-line therapy for this patient. While there may be a significant amount of vitreous debris associated with inflammation, a trial of systemic corticosteroids may preclude the development of significant debris. Discontinuing antiretroviral therapy is not advisable, as the goal of therapy is to improve the $CD4^+$ T-lymphocyte count and decrease the patient's overall risk for the development of opportunistic infections.

16. **c.** Acute anterior uveitis, giant papillary conjunctivitis, and Vogt-Koyanagi-Harada syndrome are all Th1-mediated responses. The response to parasitic infections is thought to be a Th2-mediated response.

17. **d.** Because they are proteins, antibodies themselves can be antigenic. Their antigenic sites are called *idiotopes*, as distinguished from *epitopes*, which are the antigenic sites on foreign molecules. An allotope is a site on the constant or nonvarying portion of an antibody molecule that can be recognized by a combining site of other antibodies. An isotope is 1 of 2 or more atoms whose nuclei have the same number of protons but different numbers of neutrons.

18. **c.** Antigen presentation, T-cell induction, and B-cell induction are all parts of the adaptive immune response. Activation of natural killer cells is a rapid, nonspecific, "generic" response to any pathogen and is part of the innate immune response (although natural killer cells can also take part in the adaptive immune response; on the other hand, antigen presentation, B cells, and T cells do not also take part in the innate immune response).

19. **c.** There is an abundance of antigen-presenting cells (macrophages, dendritic cells) in mucosa-associated lymphoid tissue (MALT). However, their role is to convey antigen to local lymph nodes for processing; they do not create a population of memory B cells. While immunoglobulin A (IgA) is present abundantly in tears, IgA does not provide for a secondary adaptive immune response. One defining feature of the MALT system is that it is an interconnected system of lymphatic function, such that prior exposure at any MALT site will allow for a secondary adaptive immune response (eg, via a population of memory

B cells) at every MALT site. However, prior exposure anywhere in the body (eg, a skin abrasion) does not sensitize and prime the MALT system for future exposure.

20. **a.** The high success rates of corneal transplantation are due to effective corneal immunoregulation that renders the cornea immune privileged. The 2 major mechanisms that establish this are intact limbal physiology (which prevents blood vessels from crossing over onto the corneal surface) and anterior chamber–associated immune deviation, which attenuates inflammatory reactions in the anterior chamber and on the endothelial surface. The answer choices "effector blockade, attenuated antigen presentation" (b) and "immune privilege site, mucosa-associated lymphatic tissue, and blood–aqueous barrier" (c) are not paired with the proper effector mechanisms. The answer choice "effector blockade, attenuated natural killer cells and lymphocyte activity" (d), while paired with the appropriate effectors, does not modulate corneal immune responses, but rather anterior uveal immune responses.
21. **b.** Although the patient is just getting over a cold and may have had swollen adenoids at its onset, it is unlikely that her adenoids are still swollen, given that she is getting over the cold. Dense pseudomembranes can certainly form in the setting of viral conjunctivitis secondary to aggressive strains of adenovirus; however, these are not present at the onset of symptoms and tend to appear after days of prolonged inflammation. Also, while viral conjunctivitis commonly spreads to the other eye, not only does it typically take a few days to occur, but the patient would not be asymptomatic in the fellow eye, and she did not report any symptoms in her left eye. The most likely finding in this setting is the presence of swollen submandibular glands, given that the preauricular and submandibular lymphatics drain the conjunctival surface.
22. **b.** The retinal pigment epithelium (RPE) is currently thought to modulate T-cell activity and convert effector cells into regulatory cells. Although a process similar to anterior chamber–associated immune deviation has been observed after subretinal injections of antigen, it is not clear if this is a retinal or RPE process. The immunoregulatory functions of the choroid and choriocapillaris are poorly understood.
23. **c.** Cytokines and complement help recruit immune mediators to the central cornea, which is otherwise relatively devoid of immune effectors. Mucosa-associated lymphoid tissue is responsible for conjunctival antigenic processing, but the effector limb of this system can spill over onto the corneal surface and recruit immune effectors to the cornea. Limbal physiology is the only answer choice that keeps immune effectors from reaching the central cornea (ie, makes the cornea immune privileged), mainly by serving as a barrier to vascularization of the cornea, which would provide great immune access to the central cornea, but at the cost of severe reduction in vision.
24. **b.** In the population as a whole, 8% will be positive for HLA-B27, while only 0.012% will develop acute anterior uveitis (AAU); that is, of all the individuals who are HLA-B27 positive, only 1 in approximately 667 will manifest AAU.
25. **d.** HLA-DR4 has been weakly associated with both Vogt-Koyanagi-Harada syndrome and sympathetic ophthalmia.
26. **a.** Chronic anterior uveitis (CAU) associated with juvenile idiopathic arthritis is an indolent, relatively asymptomatic, yet destructive anterior uveitis in children. Typically, these patients have had years of low-grade inflammation in their eyes and manifest signs of chronic inflammation, which includes band keratopathy, cataracts, and/or synechiae. Fibrinous anterior chamber reactions and hypopyons typically present in the setting of brisk

anterior chamber inflammatory reactions that are typically quite symptomatic (eg, acute anterior uveitis). Vitritis is a feature of intermediate and posterior uveitis, but is typically not seen in the setting of CAU (patients can manifest anterior vitreous cell in the setting of CAU, but this is not the same as vitritis).

27. **b.** Episodes of uveitis that recur less than 3 months after treatment has been discontinued are classified as chronic uveitis. Acute uveitis is defined as resolving in fewer than 3 months. The answer choice "episodes of uveitis that recur irrespective of when treatment has been discontinued" (c) is not a currently accepted classification of uveitis. Recurrent uveitis is classified as disease in which patients exhibit periods of quiescence that last longer than 3 months, off of therapy.

28. **c.** Tumor necrosis factor α (TNF-α) is believed to play a major role in the pathogenesis of juvenile idiopathic arthritis, ankylosing spondylitis, and other spondyloarthropathies. Adalimumab, infliximab, certolizumab, golimumab, and etanercept are TNF-α inhibitors. TNF inhibitors have been associated with central nervous system demyelination (promoting or unmasking multiple sclerosis), increased risk of malignancy such as lymphoma, hepatitis B reactivation, and deep fungal and other serious atypical infections. Their use is not recommended in patients with demyelinating disease, such as multiple sclerosis. Latent tuberculosis must be ruled out or completely treated, with the oversight of an infectious disease specialist, prior to their use.

    A number of immunomodulatory agents, including interferon β preparations, alemtuzumab, dimethyl fumarate, natalizumab, ocrelizumab, and teriflunomide, have important beneficial effects for patients with multiple sclerosis. Acute attacks of multiple sclerosis are typically treated with glucocorticoids. Intravenous steroids can safely be used in intermediate uveitis associated with multiple sclerosis.

29. **b.** Infliximab is a mouse/human-chimeric, immunoglobulin G1 kappa (IgG1κ) monoclonal antibody directed against tumor necrosis factor α. As many as 75% of patients receiving more than 3 infusions developed antinuclear antibodies, thus causing drug-induced lupus syndrome and the formation of human antichimeric antibodies, which can lead to reduced efficacy of infliximab. Abatacept is a T-cell costimulation inhibitor given as an intravenous infusion. Interferon alfa-2a/2b (IFN-α2a/2b), administered subcutaneously, has been reported to be beneficial in some patients with uveitis. IFN-α2a has antiviral, immunomodulatory, and antiangiogenic effects. Tacrolimus, a product of *Streptomyces tsukubaensis,* is a calcineurin inhibitor that eliminates T-cell receptor signal transduction and downregulates interleukin-2 gene transcription and receptor expression of $CD4^+$ T lymphocytes. Abatacept, IFN-α2a/2b, and tacrolimus are not associated with formation of antibodies.

30. **c.** Topical treatment is usually insufficient to treat scleritis; therefore, systemic treatment is indicated. This may range from oral nonsteroidal anti-inflammatory drops to systemic immunomodulatory agents. In individuals with no specific contraindications, mild to moderate noninfectious anterior scleritis, either diffuse or nodular, may be primarily managed with oral nonsteroidal anti-inflammatory drugs (NSAIDs) for a few weeks. More severe noninfectious cases, refractory to NSAIDs, or with posterior or necrotizing disease, are managed with systemic corticosteroids, typically with an initial dose of prednisone 1 mg/kg/day or equivalent, followed by a slow tapering regimen.

31. **a.** Infectious etiology should be ruled out in all cases of scleritis or ocular inflammation. Infectious etiologies should be ruled out especially in cases of nodular anterior scleritis,

particularly in the presence of necrosis. Anterior diffuse scleritis is mainly associated with rheumatoid arthritis, systemic lupus erythematosus, and relapsing polychondritis. Posterior scleritis can be associated with inflammatory conditions at rates similar to anterior uveitis. Necrotizing scleritis without (overt) inflammation, is called *scleromalacia perforans*. Patients with scleromalacia perforans are often elderly women with long-standing rheumatoid arthritis.

32. **b.** Tubulointerstitial nephritis and uveitis (TINU) syndrome occurs in adolescent girls and women. The mean age of onset is 21 years. Uveitis is typically a bilateral, nongranulomatous, anterior uveitis. Posterior segment involvement is rare but may include vitritis, multifocal chorioretinal lesions, and retinal vascular leakage, as well as optic nerve and macular edema. More commonly, patients may present with systemic symptoms before the development of uveitis. These patients may have abnormal serum creatinine level or decreased creatinine clearance; abnormal urinalysis findings, with increased β_2-microglobulin level, proteinuria, presence of eosinophils, pyuria or hematuria, urinary white cell casts, and normoglycemic glycosuria. TINU syndrome is responsive to high-dose oral corticosteroids. A small proportion of patients with a prolonged course may require immunomodulatory therapy.
33. **d.** Ankylosing spondylitis (AS) may range in severity from asymptomatic to severe, crippling disease. Up to 90% of patients with AS test positive for HLA-B27. About 25% of HLA-B27-positive patients will develop spondyloarthritis or eye disease. Sacroiliac imaging studies should be obtained when indicated by a suggestive history. Patients should be informed of the risk of deformity and referred to a rheumatologist. Pulmonary apical fibrosis and cardiovascular disease (aortic valvular insufficiency) may also develop, so if the patient is symptomatic, it may be worthwhile to do chest imaging or cardiac echogram to rule these out. Although these patients may present with hypopyon, this is usually sterile, so aqueous tap is not indicated unless for research purposes. Pathergy is a skin condition in which a minor trauma such as a bump or bruise leads to the development of skin lesions or ulcers that may be resistant to healing. Pathergy is seen with both Behçet disease and pyoderma gangrenosum. Urinalysis is usually not indicated in patients with ankylosing spondylitis.
34. **c.** Granulomatosis with polyangiitis (GPA; formerly known as *Wegener granulomatosis*), is a multisystem autoimmune disorder characterized by the classic triad of necrotizing granulomatous vasculitis of the upper and lower respiratory tract causing, in some cases, tracheomalacia, focal segmental glomerulonephritis, and necrotizing vasculitis of small arteries and veins, leading to branch or central retinal artery or vein occlusion. It may present only with scleritis, initially. In addition to testing for antineutrophil cytoplasmic antibodies, early detection of renal involvement with urinalysis is important, as glomerulonephritis develops in up to 85% of patients during the course of the disease and carries significant mortality if left untreated. Antinuclear antibodies are autoantibodies that bind to contents of the cell nucleus. They are found in systemic lupus erythematosus, Sjögren syndrome, scleroderma, mixed connective tissue disease, polymyositis, dermatomyositis, autoimmune hepatitis, and drug-induced lupus. Anti–cyclic citrullinated peptide (anti-CCP) antibody testing is particularly useful in the diagnosis of rheumatoid arthritis, with high specificity.
35. **b.** Central nervous system (CNS) involvement has been described in sarcoidosis, Behçet disease, and Vogt-Koyanagi-Harada syndrome. There is no report of CNS involvement with multifocal choroiditis and panuveitis.

36. **d.** It is important to distinguish presumed immune-mediated serpiginous choroiditis from infectious entities that can simulate the disease. Although herpetic and syphilitic choroiditis can occasionally mimic serpiginous choroiditis, much more commonly, *Mycobacterium tuberculosis* can cause inflammation in a similar pattern. Results of tuberculin skin testing and the interferon-gamma release assay are usually positive for tuberculosis, although the chest x-ray often appears normal. The disease usually responds to anti-tuberculosis treatment, and corticosteroids may also be needed to control inflammation. An infectious etiology has not been suggested for acute posterior multifocal placoid pigment epitheliopathy (although it may be preceded by viral prodrome), birdshot chorioretinopathy, or punctate inner choroiditis.

Index

(*f* = figure; *t* = table)